Advances in Neonatology

Guest Editors

LUCKY JAIN, MD, MBA
DAVID P. CARLTON, MD

PEDIATRIC CLINICS
OF NORTH AMERICA

www.pediatric.theclinics.com

June 2009 • Volume 56 • Number 3

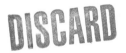

SAUNDERS an imprint of ELSEVIER, Inc.

W.B. SAUNDERS COMPANY
A Division of Elsevier Inc.

1600 John F. Kennedy Boulevard • Suite 1800 • Philadelphia, Pennsylvania 19103-2899

http://www.theclinics.com

THE PEDIATRIC CLINICS OF NORTH AMERICA Volume 56, Number 3
June 2009 ISSN 0031-3955, ISBN-13: 978-1-4377-0520-1, ISBN-10: 1-4377-0520-0

Editor: Carla Holloway
Developmental Editor: Theresa Collier

The Pediatric Clinics of North America (ISSN 0031-3955) is published bimonthly by Elsevier Inc., 360 Park Avenue South, New York, NY 10010-1710. Months of publication are February, April, June, August, October, and December. Business and Editorial Offices: 1600 John F. Kennedy Blvd., Suite 1800, Philadelphia, PA 19103-2899. Customer Service Office: 11830 Westline Industrial Drive, St. Louis, MO 63146. Periodicals postage paid at New York, NY and additional mailing offices. Subscription prices are $162.00 per year (US individuals), $350.00 per year (US institutions), $220.00 per year (Canadian individuals), $466.00 per year (Canadian institutions), $262.00 per year (international individuals), $466.00 per year (international institutions), $81.00 per year (US students and residents), and $138.00 per year (international and Canadian residents and students). To receive students/resident rare, orders must be accompanied by name of affiliated institution, date of term, and the signature of program/residency coordinator on institution letterhead. Orders will be billed at individual rate until proof of status is received. Foreign air speed delivery is included in all *Clinics* subscription prices. All prices are subject to change without notice. **POSTMASTER:** Send address changes to *The Pediatric Clinics of North America*, Elsevier Journals Customer Service, 11830 Westline Industrial Drive, St. Louis, MO 63146. **Customer Service: 1-800-654-2452 (US and Canada). From outside of the US and Canada: 1-314-453-7041. Fax: 1-314-453-5170. For print support, e-mail: JournalsCustomerService-usa@elsevier.com. For online support, e-mail: JournalsOnlineSupport-usa@elsevier.com.**

Reprints. For copies of 100 or more, of articles in this publication, please contact the Commercial Reprints Department, Elsevier Inc., 360 Park Avenue South, New York, NY 10010-1710. Tel.: 212-633-3812; Fax: 212-462-1935; E-mail: reprints@elsevier.com.

The Pediatric Clinics of North America is also published in Spanish by McGraw-Hill Inter-americana Editores S.A., Mexico City, Mexico; in Portuguese by Riechmann and Affonso Editores, Rua Comandante Coelho 1085, CEP 21250, Rio de Janeiro, Brazil; and in Greek by Althayia SA, Athens, Greece.

The Pediatric Clinics of North America is covered in *MEDLINE/PubMed (Index Medicus), Excerpta Medica, Current Contents, Current Contents/Clinical Medicine, Science Citation Index, ASCA, ISI/BIOMED,* and *BIOSIS.*

Printed in the United States of America.

GOAL STATEMENT

The goal of the *Pediatric Clinics of North America* is to keep practicing physicians and residents up to date with current clinical practice in pediatrics by providing timely articles reviewing the state-of-the-art in patient care.

ACCREDITATION

The *Pediatric Clinics of North America* is planned and implemented in accordance with the Essential Areas and Policies of the Accreditation Council for Continuing Medical Education (ACCME) through the joint sponsorship of the University of Virginia School of Medicine and Elsevier. The University of Virginia School of Medicine is accredited by the ACCME to provide continuing medical education for physicians.

The University of Virginia School of Medicine designates this educational activity for a maximum of 15 *AMA PRA Category 1 Credits*™. Physicians should only claim credit commensurate with the extent of their participation in the activity.

The American Medical Association has determined that physicians not licensed in the US who participate in this CME activity are eligible for 15 *AMA PRA Category 1 Credits*™.

Credit can be earned by reading the text material, taking the CME examination online at http://www.theclinics.com/home/cme, and completing the evaluation. After taking the test, you will be required to review any and all incorrect answers. Following completion of the test and evaluation, your credit will be awarded and you may print your certificate.

FACULTY DISCLOSURE/CONFLICT OF INTEREST

The University of Virginia School of Medicine, as an ACCME accredited provider, endorses and strives to comply with the Accreditation Council for Continuing Medical Education (ACCME) Standards of Commercial Support, Commonwealth of Virginia statutes, University of Virginia policies and procedures, and associated federal and private regulations and guidelines on the need for disclosure and monitoring of proprietary and financial interests that may affect the scientific integrity and balance of content delivered in continuing medical education activities under our auspices.

The University of Virginia School of Medicine requires that all CME activities accredited through this institution be developed independently and be scientifically rigorous, balanced and objective in the presentation/discussion of its content, theories and practices.

All authors/editors participating in an accredited CME activity are expected to disclose to the readers relevant financial relationships with commercial entities occurring within the past 12 months (such as grants or research support, employee, consultant, stock holder, member of speakers bureau, etc.). The University of Virginia School of Medicine will employ appropriate mechanisms to resolve potential conflicts of interest to maintain the standards of fair and balanced education to the reader. Questions about specific strategies can be directed to the Office of Continuing Medical Education, University of Virginia School of Medicine, Charlottesville, Virginia.

The faculty and staff of the University of Virginia Office of Continuing Medical Education have no financial affiliations to disclose.

The authors/editors listed below have identified no financial or professional relationships for themselves or their spouse/partner:
Sarah L. Berga, MD; David P. Carlton, MD (Guest Editor); Ritu Chitkara, MD; Donald J. Dudley, MD; Emily F. Durkin, MD; Darren Farley, MD; Paul M. Fernhoff, MD, FAAP, FACMG; Carla Holloway (Acquisitions Editor); Scott T. Holmstrom, BA; Jay D. Iams, MD; Lucky Jain, MD, MBA (Guest Editor); Pei-Ni Jone, MD; William J. Keenan, MD; Una Olivia Kim, MD; Joyce M. Koenig, MD; Girija Ganesh Konduri, MD; Christopher T. Lang, MD; Abbot R. Laptook, MD; Samuel A. Pauli, MD; Ciaran S. Phibbs, PhD; Anand K. Rajani, MD; Ashwin Ramachandrappa, MD, MPH; Karen Rheuban, MD (Test Author); Kenneth O. Schowengerdt, Jr., MD; Donna R. Session, MD; Aimen F. Shaaban, MD; Weirong Shang, PhD; Rebecca A. Simmons, MD; Bonnie E. Stephens, MD; Betty R. Vohr, MD; and Jon F. Watchko, MD.

The authors/editors listed below identified the following professional or financial affiliations for themselves or their spouse/partner:
Louis P. Halamek, MD is a consultant for Laerdal Medical and Advanced Medical Stimulation and has received a grant from Laerdal Foundation.

Disclosure of Discussion of Non-FDA Approved Uses for Pharmaceutical and/or Medical Devices:
The University of Virginia School of Medicine, as an ACCME provider, requires that all authors identify and disclose any "off label" uses for pharmaceutical and medical device products. The University of Virginia School of Medicine recommends that each physician fully review all the available data on new products or procedures prior to clinical use.

TO ENROLL

To enroll in the *Pediatric Clinics of North America* Continuing Medical Education program, call customer service at 1-800-654-2452 or visit us online at www.theclinics.com/home/cme. The CME program is available to subscribers for an additional fee of $195.00.

Contributors

GUEST EDITORS

LUCKY JAIN, MD, MBA
Richard Bloomberg Professor of Pediatrics and Executive Vice Chairman, Department of Pediatrics, Emory University School of Medicine, Atlanta, Georgia

DAVID P. CARLTON, MD
Marcus Professor of Pediatrics and Chief, Division of Neonatal-Perinatal Medicine, Emory University School of Medicine, Atlanta, Georgia

AUTHORS

SARAH L. BERGA, MD
James Robert McCord Professor and Chairman, Department of Gynecology and Obstetrics, Emory University School of Medicine, Atlanta, Georgia

RITU CHITKARA, MD
Fellow, Division of Neonatal and Developmental Medicine, Department of Pediatrics, Stanford University School of Medicine, Palo Alto, California

DONALD J. DUDLEY, MD
Professor, Division of Maternal-Fetal Medicine, Department of Obstetrics and Gynecology, University of Texas Health Science Center at San Antonio, San Antonio, Texas

EMILY F. DURKIN, MD
General Surgery Resident, Department of Surgery, University of Wisconsin, School of Medicine and Public Health, Madison, Wisconsin

DARREN FARLEY, MD
Instructor/MFM Fellow, Division of Maternal-Fetal Medicine, Department of Obstetrics and Gynecology, University of Texas Health Science Center at San Antonio, San Antonio, Texas

PAUL M. FERNHOFF, MD, FAAP, FACMG
Division of Medical Genetics, Department of Human Genetics; and Department of Pediatrics, Emory University School of Medicine, Atlanta, Georgia

LOUIS P. HALAMEK, MD
Associate Professor, Division of Neonatal and Developmental Medicine, Department of Pediatrics, Stanford University School of Medicine, Palo Alto, California

SCOTT T. HOLMSTROM, BA
Health Economics Resource Center; and Center for Health Care Evaluation, Veterans Affairs Palo Alto Health Care System, Menlo Park, California

JAY D. IAMS, MD
Frederick P. Zuspan Professor and Endowed Chair, Division of Maternal-Fetal Medicine, Department of Obstetrics and Gynecology, The Ohio State University College of Medicine, Columbus, Ohio

LUCKY JAIN, MD, MBA
Richard Bloomberg Professor of Pediatrics and Executive Vice Chairman, Department of Pediatrics, Emory University School of Medicine, Atlanta, Georgia

PEI-NI JONE, MD
Clinical Instructor, Division of Pediatric Cardiology, University of Colorado, Denver, Colorado

WILLIAM J. KEENAN, MD
Professor of Pediatrics and Director, Division of Neonatal-Perinatal Medicine, Department of Pediatrics, Saint Louis University, Saint Louis, Missouri

U. OLIVIA KIM, MD
Assistant Professor of Pediatrics, Division of Neonatology, Department of Pediatrics, Children's Research Institute and Medical College of Wisconsin, Milwaukee, Wisconsin

JOYCE M. KOENIG, MD
Professor of Pediatrics, Molecular Immunology and Microbiology, Division of Neonatal-Perinatal Medicine; and Associate Chair for Research, Department of Pediatrics, Saint Louis University, Saint Louis, Missouri

G. GANESH KONDURI, MD
Professor of Pediatrics, Division of Neonatology, Department of Pediatrics, Children's Research Institute and Medical College of Wisconsin, Milwaukee, Wisconsin

CHRISTOPHER T. LANG, MD
Senior Fellow, Division of Maternal-Fetal Medicine, Department of Obstetrics and Gynecology, The Ohio State University College of Medicine, Columbus; and Mount Carmel St. Ann's Hospital, Westerville, Ohio

ABBOT R. LAPTOOK, MD
Medical Director Neonatal Intensive Care Unit, Women and Infants' Hospital of Rhode Island; and Department of Pediatrics, Warren Alpert Medical School of Brown University, Providence, Rhode Island

SAMUEL A. PAULI, MD
Fellow, Division of Reproductive Endocrinology and Fertility, Department of Gynecology and Obstetrics, Emory University School of Medicine, Atlanta, Georgia

CIARAN S. PHIBBS, PhD
Department of Pediatrics, Department of Health Research and Policy; and Center for Primary Care Outcomes Research, Stanford University School of Medicine, Stanford, California; Health Economics Resource Center; and Center for Health Care Evaluation, Veterans Affairs Palo Alto Health Care System, Menlo Park, California

ANAND K. RAJANI, MD
Fellow, Division of Neonatal and Developmental Medicine, Department of Pediatrics, Stanford University School of Medicine, Palo Alto, California

ASHWIN RAMACHANDRAPPA, MD, MPH
Division of Neonatology, Department of Pediatrics, Emory University School of Medicine, Atlanta, Georgia

KENNETH O. SCHOWENGERDT, Jr., MD
Wieck-Sullivan Professor of Pediatrics and Director of Pediatric Cardiology, Cardinal Glennon Children's Medical Center, Saint Louis University School of Medicine, Saint Louis, Missouri

DONNA R. SESSION, MD
Associate Professor and Chief, Division of Reproductive Endocrinology and Fertility, Department of Gynecology and Obstetrics, Emory University School of Medicine, Atlanta, Georgia

AIMEN SHAABAN, MD
Associate Professor, Department of Surgery, University of Iowa, Carver College of Medicine, Iowa City, Iowa

WEIRONG SHANG, PhD
Assistant Professor and Director, Andrology and Embryology Laboratory, Division of Reproductive Endocrinology and Fertility, Department of Gynecology and Obstetrics, Emory University School of Medicine, Atlanta, Georgia

REBECCA A. SIMMONS, MD
Associate Professor of Pediatrics, Department of Pediatrics, Children's Hospital; and University of Pennsylvania School of Medicine, Philadelphia, Pennsylvania

BONNIE E. STEPHENS, MD
Assistant Professor of Pediatrics, Women and Infants Hospital, The Warren Alpert School of Brown University; and Neonatal Follow-up Program, Women and Infants Hospital, Providence, Rhode Island

BETTY R. VOHR, MD
Professor of Pediatrics, Women and Infants Hospital, The Warren Alpert School of Brown University; and Director, Neonatal Follow-up Program, Women and Infants Hospital, Providence, Rhode Island

JON F. WATCHKO, MD
Professor of Pediatrics, Obstetrics, Gynecology, and Reproductive Sciences, Division of Newborn Medicine, Department of Pediatrics, University of Pittsburgh; and Senior Scientist, Magee-Womens Research Institute, Magee-Womens Hospital, Pittsburgh, Pennsylvania

Advances in Neonatology

JUHAHī

FORSYTH TECHNICAL COMMUNITY COLLEGE
2100 SILAS CREEK PARKWAY
WINSTON-SALEM, NC 27103-5197

Contents

Intrauterine growth retardation (IUGR) has been linked to development of type 2 diabetes in adulthood. Using a rat model, we tested the hypothesis that uteroplacental insufficiency disrupts the function of the electron transport chain in the fetal β-cell and leads to a debilitating cascade of events. The net result is progressive loss of β-cell function and eventual development of type 2 diabetes in the adult. Studies in the IUGR rat demonstrate that an abnormal intrauterine environment induces epigenetic modifications of key genes regulating β-cell development; experiments directly link chromatin remodeling with suppression of transcription. Future research will be directed at elucidating the mechanisms underlying epigenetic modifications in offspring.

Assisted reproductive technologies are important tools in the clinical armamentarium used to treat both female and male infertility disorders. Pre-implantation genetic diagnosis offers couples at risk of having children with inheritable disorders the ability to analyze the genetic make-up of embryos before transfer. For patients undergoing treatment of cancer with chemotherapy or radiation therapy, these technologies offer the potential for the preservation of future fertility. As technology evolves, it is likely the clinical applications of assisted reproduction will continue to develop and expand in the future to enhance fertility.

Fetal monitoring during pregnancy is used to prevent fetal death. This article addresses the goals of fetal monitoring during pregnancy. Methods of fetal surveillance are reviewed, as well as the meaning of abnormal fetal testing and how these results relate to fetal and neonatal outcome. Overall, pediatricians who understand the goals, methods, and interpretation of fetal testing can communicate more effectively with the delivering obstetric team in anticipation of optimizing obstetric and pediatric outcomes.

Newborn screening has become an integral part of the evaluation of more than 4 million newborns a year in the United States and of most newborns in industrialized countries and many in developing countries. Because the term "newborn screening" refers to many procedures performed in a nursery such as screening for hearing loss or congenital heart disease, this discussion is limited to screening for genetic or congenital disorders with blood spotted on filter paper cards. This discussion reflects primarily the experiences and current status of NBS programs in the United States.

Neonatal resuscitation is an attempt to facilitate the dynamic transition from fetal to neonatal physiology. This article outlines the current practices in delivery room management of the neonate. Developments in cardiopulmonary resuscitation techniques for term and preterm infants and advances in the areas of cerebral resuscitation and thermoregulation are reviewed. Resuscitation in special circumstances (such as the presence of congenital anomalies) are also covered. The importance of communication with other members of the health care team and the family is discussed. Finally, future trends in neonatal resuscitation are explored.

Complications of prematurity surpass congenital malformations as the leading cause of infant mortality in the United States. Since 1990, there has been a steady rise in preterm birth, alarming health professionals from all disciplines. This review from a prenatal perspective confirms those concerns and describes the risks and opportunities that may attend efforts to improve the health of fetuses, newborns, and infants. Fetal and live-born outcomes are included.

"Late preterm" birth is not such an unusual occurrence; in fact these infants were the first group of premature infants who pediatricians learned to treat, and did so with such remarkable success that physicians no longer consider them to be of high risk. So, why the sudden interest in this group? There is now enough evidence that this population is not as benign as previously thought. They have increased mortality when compared to term infants and are at increased risk for complications including transient tachypnea of newborn (TTN), respiratory distress syndrome (RDS), persistent pulmonary hypertension (PPHN), respiratory failure, temperature instability, jaundice, feeding difficulties and prolonged neonatal intensive care unit (NICU) stay. Evidence is currently emerging that late preterm infants make up a majority of preterm births, take up significant resources, have increased mortality/morbidity, and may even have long-term neurodevelopmental consequences secondary to their late prematurity.

Rapid evaluation of a neonate who is cyanotic and in respiratory distress is essential for achieving a good outcome. Persistent pulmonary hypertension of the newborn (PPHN) can be a primary cause or a contributing factor to respiratory failure, particularly in neonates born at 34 weeks or more of gestation. PPHN represents a failure of normal postnatal adaptation that occurs at birth in the pulmonary circulation. Rapid advances in therapy in recent years have led to a remarkable decrease in mortality for the affected infants. Infants who survive PPHN are at significant risk for long-term hearing and neurodevelopmental impairments, however. This review focuses on the diagnosis, recent advances in management, and recommendations for the long-term follow-up of infants who have PPHN.

Newborn encephalopathy represents a clinical syndrome with diverse causes, many of which may result in brain injury. Hypoxic-ischemic encephalopathy represents a subset of newborns with encephalopathy and, in contrast to other causes, may have a modifiable outcome. Laboratory research has demonstrated robust neuroprotection associated with reductions of brain temperature following hypoxia-ischemia in animals. The neuroprotective effects of hypothermia reflect antagonism of multiple cascades of events that contribute to brain injury. Clinical trials have translated laboratory observations into successful interventions. Hypoxici-schemic encephalopathy is often unanticipated, unavoidable, and may occur in any obstetric setting. Pediatricians and other providers based in community hospitals play a critical role in the initial assessment, recognition, and stabilization of infants who may be candidates for therapeutic hypothermia.

This article examines the outcome data for very low birth weight infants in low-volume, mid-volume, and high-volume neonatal ICUs (NICUs) and argues for regionalization of NICU services on the basis of both medical outcomes and economic rationality. It recognizes some of the obstacles to regionalization of these services and presents ways to surmount them.

Advances in antenatal medicine and neonatal intensive care have successfully resulted in improved survival rates of preterm infants. These improvements have been most dramatic in infants born extremely low birth weight (ELBW, $\leq$ 1000 g) and at the limits of viability (22 to 25 weeks). But improvements in survival have not been accompanied by proportional reductions in the incidence of disability in this population. Thus, survival is not an adequate measure of success in these infants who remain at high risk for neurodevelopmental and behavioral morbidities. There is now increasing evidence of sustained adverse outcomes into school age and adolescence, not only for ELBW infants but for infants born late preterm.

Neonatal surgical care requires a current understanding of pre- and postnatal intervention for a myriad of congenital anomalies. This article includes an update of the recent information on commonly encountered fetal and neonatal surgical problems, highlighting specific areas of controversy and challenges in diagnosis. The authors hope that this article is useful for trainees and practitioners involved in any aspect of fetal and neonatal care.

Hyperbilirubinemia is the most common condition requiring evaluation and treatment in neonates. Identifying among all newborns those few at risk to develop marked hyperbilirubinemia is a clinical challenge. Clinical, epidemiologic, and genetic risk factors associated with severe hyperbilirubinemia include late preterm gestational age, exclusive breastfeeding, glucose-6-phosphate dehydrogenase deficiency, ABO hemolytic disease, East Asian ethnicity, jaundice observed in the first 24 hours of life, cephalohematoma or significant bruising, and history of a previous sibling treated with phototherapy. It is increasingly apparent that the etiopathogenesis of severe hyperbilirubinemia is often multifactorial, and emerging evidence suggests that combining risk factor assessment with measurement of predischarge total serum or transcutaneous bilirubin levels will improve hyperbilirubinemia risk prediction.

Despite an era of marked success with universal screening, Group B *Streptococcus* (GBS) continues to be an important cause of early-onset sepsis, and thus remains a significant public health issue. Improved eradication of GBS colonization and disease may involve universal screening in conjunction with rapid diagnostic technologies or other novel approaches. Given the complications and potential limitations associated with maternal intrapartum prophylaxis, however, vaccines may be the most effective means of preventing neonatal GBS disease. The global utility of conjugated GBS vaccines may be hampered by the variability of serotypes in diverse populations and geographic locations. Modern technologies, such as those involving proteomics and genomic sequencing, are likely to hasten the development of a universal vaccine against GBS.

This article presents advancements in the field of fetal echocardiography and the significant impact of these within the fields of pediatric cardiology, perinatology, and neonatology. A prenatal diagnosis of congenital heart disease allows for improved counseling of the parents, guides the timing and optimal location of delivery, and allows appropriate planning and consultation between the cardiologist and neonatologist. It also facilitates accurate diagnosis and management of fetal arrhythmias, identifies potential candidates for in utero cardiac intervention, and serves as the imaging guidance technique for these procedures. The goals, indications, advantages, limitations, and spectrum of congenital heart disease that can be diagnosed are reviewed.

RELATED INTEREST

Advances in Pediatrics (Volume 55)
Michael S. Kappy, *Editor-in-Chief*

Clinics in Perinatology
Volume 36, Issue 1 (March 2009)
Current Controversies in Perinatology
Michael R. Uhing and Robert Kliegman, *Guest Editors*
www.perinatology.theclinics.com

Clinics in Perinatology
Volume 33, Issue 4 (December 2006)
Late Preterm Pregnancy and the Newborn
Lucky Jain and Tonse N.K. Raju, *Guest Editors*
www.perinatology.theclinics.com

THE CLINICS ARE NOW AVAILABLE ONLINE!

Access your subscription at:
www.theclinics.com

Preface

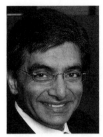 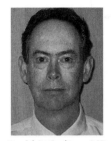

Lucky Jain, MD, MBA   David P. Carlton, MD
Guest Editors

Had he been alive today, Patrick Bouvier Kennedy would have been hailed as a triumph of neonatal care—after all, he was the son of the former United States President, John F. Kennedy and former First Lady Jacqueline B. Kennedy. Born prematurely at 34-weeks gestation, he would have been aptly labeled as a late preterm neonate; however, based on his birth weight (2.1 kg) and gestational age, few would have predicted the outcome he had then, were he to be born in 2009. But then, in 1963, little was available to the clinician for the management of hyaline membrane disease— no routine use of neonatal ventilators, no device to provide airway positive pressure, no surfactant, and no antenatal steroids. He died two days after his birth; the New York Times obituary said that "the battle for the Kennedy baby was lost because medical science has not advanced far enough."

In the last few decades, since the death of Patrick Kennedy, we have witnessed unprecedented progress in the field of neonatology. Neonatal mortality has seen a four-fold decline since 1960, and there has been a remarkable increase in neonatal intensive care units and neonatologists throughout the world. Birth weight and gestational age-specific mortality has decreased significantly, although the progress has been slower as we approach gestation <23 weeks, where we may have reached the limits of viability. Other problems remain—our efforts to decrease prematurity have been poorly rewarded, and, while outcomes of infants with congenital anomalies have improved, the overall frequency of such occurrences has not decreased; together, neonates who have complex anomalies and those with extreme prematurity continue to be a substantial drain on healthcare resources.

In this issue of *Pediatric Clinics of North America*, we have attempted to cover a broad array of topics in neonatology that are relevant to the practicing pediatrician. We are grateful to Carla Holloway at Elsevier for her support of this issue and to all of our colleagues who have contributed thoughtfully written articles for this undertaking.

Pediatr Clin N Am 56 (2009) xv–xvi
doi:10.1016/j.pcl.2009.04.007
0031-3955/09/$ – see front matter © 2009 Elsevier Inc. All rights reserved.

pediatric.theclinics.com

We hope that this update on neonatology will serve as a useful source of current information for the busy pediatrician. Although gaps in our knowledge remain, we should all be proud of the progress and advances that have been made!

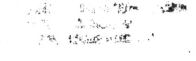

Lucky Jain, MD, MBA
Emory University School of Medicine
2015 Uppergate Dr. NE
Atlanta, GA 30322

David P. Carlton, MD
Emory University School of Medicine
2015 Uppergate Drive NE
Atlanta, GA 30322

E-mail addresses:
ljain@emory.edu (L. Jain)
dpcarlt@emory.edu (D.P. Carlton)

Developmental Origins of Adult Disease

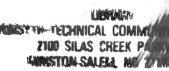

Rebecca A. Simmons, MD[a,b,*]

KEYWORDS

- Intrauterine growth retardation • Type 2 diabetes
- Fetal origins of adult disease • Epigenetics
- Mitochondria • Oxidative stress

The period from conception to birth is a time of rapid growth, cellular replication and differentiation, and functional maturation of organ systems. These processes are very sensitive to alterations in the intrauterine milieu. Programming describes the mechanisms whereby a stimulus or insult at a critical period of development has lasting or lifelong effects. This review discusses the human and animal data supporting the Developmental Origin's of Adult Disease hypothesis and some of the underlying cellular and molecular mechanisms responsible for the observed defects in β-cell function and development.

LOW BIRTH WEIGHT

It is becoming increasingly apparent that the in utero environment in which a fetus develops may have long-term effects on subsequent health and survival.[1,2] The landmark cohort study of 300,000 men by Ravelli and colleagues[3] showed that exposure to the Dutch famine of 1944 to 1945 during the first one half of pregnancy resulted in significantly higher obesity rates at age 19 years. Subsequent studies of English men demonstrated a relationship between low birth weight and the later development of cardiovascular disease[4] and impaired glucose tolerance.[5–8] Other studies of populations in the United States,[9–11] Sweden,[12] France,[13,14] Norway,[15] and Finland[16] have demonstrated a significant correlation between low birth weight and the later development of adult diseases. The associations with low birth weight and increased risk of coronary heart disease, stroke, and type 2 diabetes remain strong, even after adjusting for lifestyle factors (eg, smoking, physical activity, occupation, income, dietary habits, childhood socioeconomic status) and occur independent of the current level of obesity or exercise.[17]

Grant Support: Dr. Rebecca Simmons is supported by the National Institutes of Health grants #DK55704 and AG20898.
[a] Department of Pediatrics, Children's Hospital, Philadelphia, PA, USA
[b] University of Pennsylvania School of Medicine, BRB II/III, Room 1308, 421 Curie Boulevard, Philadelphia, PA 19104, USA
* University of Pennsylvania School of Medicine, BRB II/III, Room 1308, 421 Curie Boulevard, Philadelphia, PA 19104.
E-mail address: rsimmons@mail.med.upenn.edu

Pediatr Clin N Am 56 (2009) 449–466
doi:10.1016/j.pcl.2009.03.004
0031-3955/09/$ – see front matter © 2009 Elsevier Inc. All rights reserved.

pediatric.theclinics.com

HIGH BIRTH WEIGHT

An increased birth weight is associated with an enhanced body mass index (BMI) and an elevated prevalence of adulthood obesity.[18] Those individuals who are obese as adults tend to have been heavier at birth and to have had an accelerated gain in body mass through childhood and adolescence. Factors in early childhood may lead to obesity through metabolic programming (discussed later in this article) or establishment of lifestyle behaviors. During infancy, breastfeeding may protect against the development of excess weight during childhood. Most, but not all, epidemiologic studies demonstrate this protective effect, which could be mediated by behavioral and/or physiologic mechanisms. Confounding cultural factors associated with both the decision to breastfeed and later obesity, however, are possible. Recent data also suggest that rapid weight gain during infancy is associated with obesity later in childhood, perhaps reflecting a combination of genetically determined catch-up growth and postnatal environmental factors.[18]

LOW BIRTH WEIGHT AND INSULIN SECRETION

It remains controversial as to whether the adverse effects of intrauterine growth retardation on glucose homeostasis are mediated through programming of the fetal endocrine pancreas.[1] Growth-retarded fetuses and newborns have been reported to have both a reduced population of pancreatic β-cells[19] or a normal percentage of pancreatic area occupied by β-cells.[20] Both of these studies were observational, morphometric analyses were not optimal, and only a small number of fetuses/newborns were examined. It is likely that a significant proportion, but not all growth-retarded fetuses will have reduced β-cell numbers. A more clinically relevant consideration is the impact of fetal growth retardation upon β-cell function.

Intrauterine growth retarded (IUGR) fetuses have been found to exhibit lower insulin and glucose levels and higher glucose/insulin ratio in the third trimester as measured by cordocentesis.[21] Two recent studies showed that IUGR infants display decreased pancreatic β-cell function, but increased insulin sensitivity at birth.[22,23] Low birth weight has been associated with reduced insulin response after glucose ingestion in young nondiabetic men, whereas other studies have found no impact of low birth weight on insulin secretion.[17,18] However, none of these earlier studies adjusted for the corresponding insulin sensitivity, which has a profound impact on insulin secretion. Therefore, Jensen and colleagues[24] measured insulin secretion and insulin sensitivity in a well-matched white population of 19-year-old glucose tolerant men with birth weights of either below the 10th percentile (small for gestational age [SGA]) or between the 50th and 75th percentile (controls). To eliminate the major confounders such as "diabetes genes," none of the participants had a family history of diabetes, hypertension, or ischemic heart disease. There was no difference between the groups with regard to current weight, body mass index (BMI), body composition, and lipid profile. When controlled for insulin sensitivity, insulin secretion was reduced by 30%. Insulin sensitivity, however, was normal in the SGA subjects. The investigators hypothesized that defects in insulin secretion may precede defects in insulin action and that once SGA individuals accumulate body fat, they will develop insulin resistance.[24]

INSULIN SECRETION IN OFFSPRING OF DIABETIC MOTHERS

Several epidemiologic studies show that the risk for diabetes is significantly higher in the offspring of mothers who have type 2 diabetes.[25–28] It is likely that impaired β-cell function contributes to this increased risk. Islet hypertrophy and β-cell hyperplasia are typical features of fetuses and newborns of diabetic mothers.[29] Most studies have focused on altered glucose homeostasis during the newborn period; two clinical investigations done at older ages, however, demonstrate altered insulin secretion.[28,30] Thus, both a deficiency and a surfeit of nutrient availability to the fetus during development have profound lasting effects on β-cell function.

GENETICS VERSUS ENVIRONMENT

Several epidemiologic and metabolic studies of twins and first-degree relatives of patients with type 2 diabetes have demonstrated an important genetic component of diabetes.[31–34] The association between low birth weight and risk of type 2 diabetes in some studies could theoretically be explained by a genetically determined reduced fetal growth rate. In other words, the genotype responsible for type 2 diabetes may itself cause retarded fetal growth in utero. This forms the basis for the fetal insulin hypothesis, which suggests that genetically determined insulin resistance could result in low insulin-mediated fetal growth in utero as well as insulin resistance in childhood and adulthood.[35] Insulin is one of the major growth factors in fetal life and monogenic disorders that affect fetal insulin secretion or fetal insulin resistance also affect fetal growth. Mutations in the gene encoding glucokinase have been identified that result in low birth weight and maturity onset diabetes of the young.[36,37]

The recently described type 2 diabetes susceptibility gene Transcription Factor7-like 2 (TCF7L2) confers a risk-allele frequency of approximately 30%.[38] Studies of nondiabetic subjects show that TCF7L2 diabetes-risk genotypes alter insulin secretion.[39–41] A large study of 24,053 subjects from six studies demonstrated that TCF7L2 is the first type 2 diabetes gene to be reproducibly associated with altered birth weight. Each maternal copy of the T allele at re7903146 increased offspring birth weight by 30 g, and the investigators suggest that the most likely mechanism is through reduced maternal-insulin secretion resulting in maternal hyperglycemia and increased insulin-mediated fetal growth.[42]

Recent genetic studies suggest that the increased susceptibility to type 2 diabetes of subjects who are born SGA also results from the combination of both genetic factors and an unfavorable fetal environment. Polymorphisms of Peroxisome Proliferator-Activated Receptor-gamma 2 (PPARg2), a gene involved in the development and in the metabolic function of adipose tissue, have been shown to modulate the susceptibility of subjects who are born SGA to develop insulin resistance later in life.[43,44] The polymorphism is associated with a higher risk of type 2 diabetes only if birth weight is reduced.[43,44] There is obviously a close relationship between genes and the environment. Not only can maternal gene expression alter the fetal environment, the maternal intrauterine environment also affects fetal gene expression, and both influence birth weight.

WHAT ANIMAL MODELS CAN TELL US

Animal models have a normal genetic background upon which environmental effects during gestation or early postnatal life can be tested for their role in inducing diabetes. Ontogeny of β-cell development in the rodent approximates what has been observed in the human.[45,46] The most commonly used animal models for IUGR are caloric or protein restriction, glucocorticoid administration, or induction of uteroplacental insufficiency in the pregnant rodent. In the rat, maternal dietary protein restriction (approximately 40% to 50% of normal intake, termed LP) throughout gestation and lactation has been reported to alter insulin secretory capacity and reduce β-cell mass through a reduction in β-cell proliferation rate and an increase in apoptosis.[47–55] Expression of Pdx-1 (pancreatic duodenal homeobox-1), a homeodomain-containing transcription factor that regulates early development of both endocrine and exocrine pancreas, and later differentiation and function of β cells,[56] is also reduced in islets from pups of LP mothers.[57] In adulthood, rats born from LP mothers still have reductions in β-cell mass and insulin secretion and show glucose intolerance, but usually not overt diabetes.[47,48,55] In old age, LP offspring develop fasting hyperglycemia associated with insulin resistance.[58–62]

Total caloric restriction during the last week of pregnancy and throughout lactation also reduces β-cell mass and impairs insulin secretion in the offspring.[63,64] When maternal undernutrition is prolonged until weaning and normal nutrition is given to the offspring from weaning onwards, growth retardation and beta-cell mass reduction persists into adulthood.[64]

Treatment of pregnant rats with dexamethasone during the last week of gestation retards fetal growth.[65] Insulin content of fetal beta-cells is reduced and is associated with a reduction in Pdx-1.[65]

An ovine model of IUGR induced by placental insufficiency (heat-induced) results in a significant reduction in β-cell mass in fetuses near term (0.9 of gestation) from decreased rates of β-cell proliferation and neogenesis.[66] Plasma insulin concentrations in the IUGR fetuses are lower at baseline and glucose-stimulated insulin secretion is impaired. Similar deficits occur with arginine-stimulated insulin secretion. A deficiency in islet glucose metabolism also occurs in the rate of islet glucose oxidation at maximal stimulatory glucose concentrations. Thus, pancreatic islets from nutritionally deprived IUGR fetuses caused by chronic placental insufficiency have impaired insulin secretion caused by reduced glucose–stimulated glucose oxidation rates, insulin biosynthesis, and insulin content. This impaired glucose-stimulated insulin secretion (GSIS) occurs despite an increased fractional rate of insulin release from a greater proportion of releasable insulin as a result of diminished insulin stores.[67]

To extend these experimental studies of growth retardation, we developed a model of IUGR in the rat that restricts fetal growth.[68–70] Growth-retarded fetal rats have critical features of a metabolic profile characteristic of growth-retarded human fetuses: decreased levels of glucose, insulin, insulin-like growth factor I, amino acids, and oxygen.[68–72] Birth weights of IUGR animals are significantly lower than those of controls until approximately 7 weeks of age, when IUGR rats catch up to controls. Between 7 and 10 weeks of age, the growth of IUGR rats accelerates and surpasses that of controls, and by 26 weeks of age, IUGR rats are obese.[69] No significant differences are observed in blood glucose and plasma insulin levels at 1 week of age. Between 7 and 10 weeks of age, however, IUGR rats develop mild fasting hyperglycemia and hyperinsulinemia. IUGR animals are glucose-intolerant and insulin-resistant at an early age. First-phase insulin secretion in response to glucose is also impaired early in life in IUGR rats, before the onset of hyperglycemia. There are no significant differences in beta-cell mass, islet size, or pancreatic weight between IUGR and control animals at 1 and 7 weeks of age. In 15-week-old IUGR rats, however, the relative beta-cell mass is 50% that of controls, and by 26 weeks of age, beta-cell mass is less than one third that of controls. This loss of β-cell mass is accompanied by a reduction in Pdx-1 expression that is greater than that in β-cell mass.[73] By 6 months of age, IUGR rats develop diabetes with a phenotype remarkably similar to that observed in the human with type 2 diabetes: progressive dysfunction in insulin secretion and insulin action.[69] Thus, despite different animal models of IUGR, these studies support the hypothesis that an abnormal intrauterine milieu can induce permanent changes in β-cell function after birth and lead to type 2 diabetes in adulthood.

CELLULAR MECHANISMS: MITOCHONDRIAL DYSFUNCTION AND OXIDATIVE STRESS

Uteroplacental insufficiency, caused by such disorders as preeclampsia, maternal smoking, and abnormalities of uteroplacental development, is one of the most common causes of fetal growth retardation. The resultant abnormal intrauterine milieu restricts the supply of crucial nutrients to the fetus, thereby limiting fetal growth. Multiple studies have shown that intrauterine growth retardation is associated with increased oxidative stress in the human fetus.[73–80] A major consequence of limited nutrient availability is an alteration in the redox state in susceptible fetal tissues leading to oxidative stress. In particular, low levels of oxygen, evident in growth-retarded fetuses, will decrease the activity of complexes of the electron transport chain, which will generate increased levels of reactive oxygen species (ROS). Overproduction of ROS initiates many oxidative reactions that lead to oxidative damage not only in the mitochondria but also in cellular proteins, lipids, and nucleic acids. Increased ROS levels inactivate the iron-sulfur centers of the electron transport chain complexes, and tricarboxylic acid cycle aconitase, resulting in shutdown of mitochondrial energy production.

A key adaptation enabling the fetus to survive in a limited energy environment may be the reprogramming of mitochondrial function. However, these alterations in mitochondrial function can have deleterious effects, especially in cells that have a high-energy requirement, such as the β-cell. The β-cell depends on the normal production of ATP for nutrient-induced insulin secretion[81–88] and proliferation.[89] Thus, an interruption of mitochondrial function can have profound consequences for the β-cell.

Mitochondrial dysfunction can also lead to increased production of ROS, which causes oxidative stress if the defense mechanisms of the cell are overwhelmed. β-cells are especially vulnerable to ROS because expression of antioxidant enzymes in pancreatic islets is very low,[90,91] and β-cells have a high oxidative energy requirement. Increased ROS impair glucose-stimulated insulin secretion,[92,93] decrease gene expression of key β-cell genes,[94–98] and induce cell death.[98–103]

We have examined the causal role of mitochondrial dysfunction in the impairment of β-cell function and development in IUGR offspring.[104] ROS production and oxidative stress gradually increase in IUGR islets. ATP production is impaired and continues to deteriorate with age. The activities of complex I and III of the electron transport chain progressively decline in IUGR islets. Mitochondrial DNA point mutations accumulate with age and are associated with decreased mitochondrial DNA content and reduced expression of mitochondria-encoded genes in IUGR islets. Mitochondrial dysfunction results in impaired insulin secretion. These results demonstrate that IUGR induces mitochondrial dysfunction in the fetal β-cell, leading to increased production of ROS, which in turn damage mitochondrial DNA. A self-reinforcing cycle of progressive deterioration in mitochondrial function leads to a corresponding decline in β-cell function. Finally, a threshold in mitochondrial dysfunction and ROS production is reached, and diabetes ensues.[104]

MOLECULAR MECHANISMS: EPIGENETIC REGULATION

An adverse intrauterine milieu impacts the development of the fetus by modifying gene expression in both pluripotential cells and terminally differentiated, poorly replicating cells such as the β-cell. The long-range effects on the offspring (into adulthood) depend on the cells undergoing differentiation, proliferation, and/or functional maturation at the time of the disturbance in maternal fuel economy. Permanent alterations to the phenotype of the offspring suggest that fetal growth retardation is associated with stable changes in gene expression.

Epigenetic modifications of the genome provide a mechanism that allows the stable propagation of gene activity states from one generation of cells to the next. Excellent reviews on this topic appear frequently, reflecting the rapid advances of knowledge in the field.[105–108] Epigenetic states can be modified by environmental factors, which may contribute to the development of abnormal phenotypes. There are at least two distinct classes of epigenetic information that can be inherited with chromosomes. One class of epigenetic control of gene expression involves changes in chromatin proteins, usually involving modifications of histone tails. The amino termini of histones can be modified by acetylation, methylation, sumoylation, phosphorylation, glycosylation, and ADP ribosylation. The most common modifications involve acetylation and methylation of lysine residues in the amino termini of H3 and H4. Increased acetylation induces transcription activation, whereas decreased acetylation usually induces transcription repression. Methylation of histones is associated with both transcription repression and activation.

The second class of epigenetic regulation is DNA methylation, in which a cytosine base is modified by a DNA methyltransferase at the C5 position of cytosine, a reaction that is performed by various members of a single family of enzymes. Approximately 70% of CpG (cytosine-guanine) dinucleotides in human DNA are constitutively methylated, whereas most of the unmethylated CpGs are located in CpG islands. CpG islands are cytosine guanine-rich sequences located near coding sequences, and serve as promoters for the associated genes. Approximately half of mammalian genes have CpG islands. Methylation of CpG sites is also maintained by DNA methyltransferases. DNA methylation is commonly associated with gene silencing and contributes to X-chromosomal inactivation, genomic imprinting, and transcriptional regulation of tissue-specific genes during cellular differentiation.[108]

Most CpG islands remain unmethylated in normal cells; however, under some circumstances such as cancer[109–114] and oxidative stress (see later in this article), they can become methylated de novo. This aberrant methylation is accompanied by local changes in histone modification and chromatin structure, such that the CpG island and its embedded promoter acquire a repressed conformation that is incompatible with gene transcription. It is not known why particular CpG islands are susceptible to aberrant methylation. A study by Feltus and colleagues[115] suggests that there is a "sequence signature associated with aberrant methylation." Of major significance to type 2 diabetes is their finding that Pdx-1 is one of only 15 CpG genes (a total of 1749 genes with CpG islands were examined) that is susceptible to increased methylation from overexpression of a DNA methyltransferase.

Hypermethylation of specific genes has also been observed in tissues of aging individuals.[113] As an age-related disease, type 2 diabetes increases in prevalence in older populations as the metabolic profile of individuals deteriorates with time. DNA methylation errors that accumulate with increasing age could explain this phenomenon, perhaps through induction of oxidative stress.

ROS can also lead to alterations in DNA methylation, without changing the DNA base sequence.[116] Such changes in DNA methylation patterns have been shown to affect the expression of multiple genes.[116] Replacement of guanine with the oxygen radical adduct 8-hydroxyguanine profoundly alters methylation of adjacent cytosines.[116] Histones, because of their abundant lysine residues, are also very susceptible to oxidative stress.[117–119]

EPIGENETIC REGULATION OF GENE EXPRESSION IN FETAL GROWTH RETARDATION

A number of studies have suggested that uteroplacental insufficiency induces epigenetic modifications in the offspring.[120–124] Genome-wide DNA hypomethylation has been found in postnatal IUGR liver and is associated with an increase in total H3 acetylation.[120] Acetylation of histone H3 and acetylation of H3 lysine-9 (H3/K9), lysine-14 (H3/K14), and lysine-18 (H3/K18) is increased at the promoters of PPAR-coactivator-1 (PGC-1) and carnitine palmitoyltransferase 1 (CPT1), respectively, in IUGR liver.[122] At day 21 of life, the neonatal pattern of H3 hyperacetylation persists only in the IUGR males. Whether hyperacetylation at these sites actually causes increased transcription of PGC-1 or CPT1 and how these findings relate to a phenotype in the offspring remains to be determined.

CHROMATIN REMODELING IN THE β-CELL OF INTRAUTERINE GROWTH RETARDED RATS

Studies in the IUGR rat also demonstrate that fetal growth retardation induces epigenetic modifications of key genes regulating β-cell development.[125] Pdx-1 is a homeodomain-containing transcription factor that plays a critical role in the early development of both endocrine and exocrine pancreas, and then in the later differentiation and function of the β-cell. As early as 24 hours after the onset of growth retardation, Pdx-1 mRNA levels are reduced by more than 50% in IUGR fetal rats. Suppression of Pdx-1 expression persists after birth and progressively declines in the IUGR animal, implicating an epigenetic mechanism.

Chromatin modification mechanisms serve a critical function in affecting the transcriptional status of genes. Our data demonstrate that the open chromatin domain marked by histone H3 and H4 acetylation at the proximal promoter of Pdx1 is essential for transcription. Robust Pdx1 expression in islets from control animals is coincident with the presence of acetylated histones H3 and H4 as well as trimethylated H3K4. Loss of these marks results in Pdx1 silencing and reversal of IUGR-induced epigenetic modifications normalizes Pdx1 expression. These data suggest that histone modifications can be stably propagated throughout life.

The first epigenetic mark that is modified in β-cells of IUGR animals is histone acetylation (**Fig. 1**). Islets isolated from IUGR fetuses show a significant decrease in H3 and H4 acetylation at the proximal promoter of Pdx1. These changes in H3 and H4 acetylation are associated with a loss of binding of upstream stimulatory factor (USF)-1 to the proximal promoter of Pdx1. USF-1 is a critical activator of Pdx1 transcription and decreased binding markedly decreases Pdx1 transcription.[126,127] After birth, histone deacetylation progresses and is followed by a marked decrease in H3K4 trimethylation and a significant increase in dimethylation of H3K9 in IUGR islets (see **Fig. 1**). Progression of these histone modifications parallels the progressive decrease in Pdx1 expression as glucose homeostasis deteriorates and oxidative stress increases in IUGR animals. Nevertheless, in the IUGR pup (at 2 weeks of age) these silencing histone modifications alone suppress Pdx1 expression because there is no appreciable methylation in the CpG island and reversal of histone deacetylation in IUGR islets (in the presence of active β-cell replication) is sufficient to nearly normalize Pdx1 mRNA levels.

The initial mechanism by which IUGR silences Pdx1 is by recruitment of co-repressors, including HDAC1 and mSin3A, which catalyze histone deacetylation—the first repressive mark observed at Pdx1 in IUGR islets. Binding of these deacetylases in turn facilitates loss of trimethylation of H3K4 further repressing Pdx1 expression

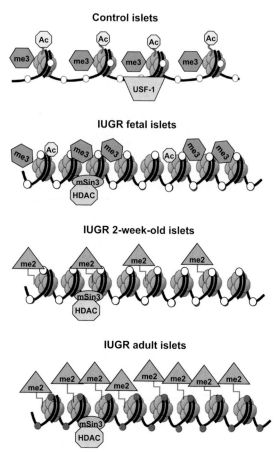

Fig.1. Summary of epigenetic changes at *Pdx1* in IUGR rats during the development of type 2 diabetes. In pancreatic β-cells (*top*), the *Pdx1* proximal promoter is normally found in an unmethylated (*white circles*) open chromatin state allowing access to transcription factors such as USF-1 and associated with nucleosomes characterized by acetylated (Ac, *blue octagons*) histones H3 and H4 and with trimethylated H3K4 (Me, *green hexagons*). In IUGR fetal and 2-week islets (*middle*) histone acetylation is progressively lost through association with a mSin3A-HDAC1-DNMT1 repressor complex, with trimethylated H3K4 disappearing and dimethylated H3K9 (Me, *red hexagons*) appearing after birth. IUGR adult islets are characterized by inactive chromatin with dimethylated H3K9 and extensive DNA methylation (*red circles*) locking in the transcriptionally silent state of *Pdx1*.

(see **Fig. 1**). Our observation that inhibition of HDAC activity by Trichostatin A treatment normalizes H3K4me3 levels at *Pdx1* in IUGR islets suggests that the association of HDAC1 at *Pdx1* in IUGR islets likely serves as a platform for the recruitment of a demethylase, which catalyzes demethylation of H3K4.

As described above, DNA methylation of a CpG island in the promoter is a key mechanism for silencing gene expression. Most CpG islands remain unmethylated in normal cells; however, under conditions of oxidative stress,[116,128–130] CpG islands can become methylated de novo. This is particularly relevant to type 2 diabetes, as there are now substantial data that show that oxidative stress plays a significant role in the progression of β-cell deterioration.[93,96,103,131,132] Further, IUGR induces mitochondrial dysfunction in the β-cell leading to increased production of ROS and oxidative stress.[104] It is not known why particular CpG islands are susceptible to aberrant methylation. A study by Feltus and colleagues[115] suggests that there is a "sequence signature associated with aberrant methylation." Of particular relevance to this study is their finding that *Pdx1* and a flanking gene, *Cdx*-2 (also encoding a homeobox protein), were 2 of only 15 genes (a total of 1749 genes with CpG islands were examined) that were methylation susceptible under conditions of increased methylation induced by overexpression of DNMT1.

The molecular mechanism responsible for DNA methylation in IUGR islets is likely to involve H3K9 methylation. A number of studies have shown that methylation of H3K9 precedes DNA methylation.[133,134] It has also been suggested that DNA methyltransferases may act only on chromatin that is methylated at lysine 9 on histone H3 (H3K9).[134] Histone methyltransferases bind to the DNA methylases DNMT3A and DNMT3B thereby initiating DNA methylation.[133]

These results demonstrate that IUGR induces a self-propagating epigenetic cycle in which the mSin3A/HDAC complex is first recruited to the *Pdx1* promoter, histone tails are subjected to deacetylation and *Pdx1* transcription is repressed. At the neonatal stage, this epigenetic process is reversible and may define an important developmental window for therapeutic approaches. However, as dimethylated H3K9 accumulates, DNMT3A is recruited to the promoter and initiates de novo DNA methylation, which locks in the silenced state in the IUGR adult pancreas resulting in diabetes. Our studies indicate novel mechanisms of epigenetic regulation of gene expression in vivo that link gene silencing in the β-cell to the development of type 2 diabetes and suggest novel therapeutic agents for the prevention of common diseases with late-onset phenotypes.

How do these events lead to diabetes? Targeted homozygous disruption of *Pdx 1* in mice results in pancreatic agenesis, and homozygous mutations yield a similar phenotype in humans.[135] Milder reductions in *Pdx 1* protein levels, as occurs in the *Pdx* ± mice, allow for the development of a normal mass of β cells,[135] but result in the impairment of several events in glucose-stimulated insulin secretion.[135] These results indicate that *Pdx 1* plays a critical role, distinct from its developmental role, in the normal function of β cells.[135] This may be the reason that humans with heterozygous missense mutations in *Pdx 1* exhibit early- and late-onset forms of type 2 diabetes.[135]

CHROMATIN REMODELING IN MUSCLE OF INTRAUTERINE GROWTH RETARDED RATS

A reduction in glucose transport in muscle has been shown to be a central basis for insulin resistance in the IUGR offspring.[60,136] Glucose transport, a rate-limiting step in glucose use under normal physiologic circumstances, occurs by facilitated diffusion.[137] This process is mediated by a family of structurally related membrane-spanning glycoproteins, termed the facilitative glucose transporters (GLUT; Slc2 family of transport proteins).[138] Of the isoforms cloned to date, GLUT4 is the major insulin-responsive isoform expressed in insulin-sensitive tissues such as skeletal muscle, adipose tissue, and cardiac muscle.[138] The promoter region of GLUT4 has been well characterized and disruption of the myocyte enhancer factor 2 (MEF2) binding site ablates tissue-specific glut4 expression in transgenic mice.[138] MyoD on the other hand is responsible for glut4 expression in vitro during myoblast to myocyte differentiation.[139] MyoD binding with that of MEF2 and TR 1 spans the 502- to 420-bp region of the *glut4* gene in skeletal muscle. These two proteins synergistically increase skeletal muscle *glut4* transcription and gene expression.[139] It has recently been shown by Devaskar and colleagues[140] that IUGR increases MEF2D (inhibitor) and decreases MEF2A (activator) and MyoD (co-activator) binding to the *glut4* promoter in skeletal muscle. Interestingly, no differential methylation of these three and other CpG clusters in the *glut4* promoter was found. They found that DNMT1 in postnatal, DNMT3a, and DNMT3b in adult were differentially recruited with increased MeCP2 (methyl CpG-binding protein) concentrations to bind the IUGR *glut4* gene. Covalent modifications of the histone (H) code consisted of H3 K14 de-acetylation mediated by recruitment of histone deacetylase (HDAC) 1 and enhanced association of HDAC4 enzymes. This set the stage for Suv39H1 methylase-mediated di-methylation of H3 K9 and increased recruitment of heterochromatin protein 1, which partially inactivates postnatal and adult IUGR *glut4* gene transcription. To date, it has not been demonstrated that these histone modifications are directly responsible for altered glut4 expression. Nonetheless, these studies show that histone modifications can be propagated.

SUMMARY

The human and animal studies described in this article clearly show that an adverse intrauterine environment associated with fetal growth retardation or fetal overgrowth results in impaired function and development of the β-cell, which in turn leads to the development of type 2 diabetes. Animal models demonstrate that the cellular and molecular mechanisms underlying altered β-cell development are related to abnormal mitochondrial function and epigenetic alterations of key β-cell genes.

Much of the recent progress in understanding epigenetic phenomena is directly attributable to technologies that allow researchers to pinpoint the genomic location of proteins that package and regulate access to the DNA. The advent of DNA microarrays and inexpensive DNA sequencing has allowed many of those technologies to be applied to the whole genome. It is possible that epigenetic profiling of CpG islands in the human genome can be used as a tool to identify genomic loci that are susceptible to DNA methylation or loss of DNA methylation.

The genome-wide mapping of histone modifications by ChIP-chip and DNA methylation has led to important insights regarding the mechanism of transcriptional and epigenetic memory, and how different chromatin states are propagated through the genome.[141–145] In the near future it is likely that technologies will be developed that will allow genome-wide epigenetics studies, especially applied to the limited number of cells that can be isolated to a high degree of purity by techniques such as laser capture microscopy. Epigenetic modifications can then be used as biomarkers for disease.

REFERENCES

1. Hales CN, Barker DJP. Type 2 diabetes mellitus: the thrifty phenotype hypothesis. Diabetologia 1992;35:595–601.
2. Kermack WO. Death rates in Great Britain and Sweden. Lancet 1934;1:698–703.
3. Ravelli GP, Stein ZA, Susser MW. Obesity in young men after famine exposure in utero and early infancy. N Engl J Med 1976;295:349–53.
4. Barker DJP. The developmental origins of adult disease. J Am Coll Nutr 2004;23:588S–95S.
5. Valdez R, Athens MA, Thompson GH, et al. Birthweight and adult health outcomes in a biethnic population in the USA. Diabetologia 1994;37:624–31.

6. Jaquet D, Gaboriau A, Czernichow P, et al. Insulin resistance early in adulthood in subjects born with intrauterine growth retardation. J Clin Endocrinol Metab 2000;85:1401–6.

7. Egeland GM, Skjaerven R, Irgrens LM. Birth characteristics of women who develop gestational diabetes: population based study. BMJ 2000;321:546–7.

8. Forsen T, Eriksson J, Tuomilehto J, et al. The fetal and childhood growth of persons who develop type 2 diabetes. Ann Intern Med 2000;133:176–82.

9. Rich-Edwards JW, Colditz GA, Stampfer MJ, et al. Birthweight and the risk for type 2 diabetes mellitus in adult women. Ann Intern Med 1999;130:278–84.

10. Eriksson J, Forsen T, Tuomilehto J, et al. Fetal and childhood growth and hypertension in adult life. Hypertension 2000;36:790–4.

11. Bhargava SK, Sachdev HS, Fall CH, et al. Relation of serial changes in childhood body-mass index to impaired glucose tolerance in young adulthood. N Engl J Med 2004;350:865–75.

12. Whincup PH, Cook DG, Adshead T, et al. Childhood size is more strongly related than size at birth to glucose and insulin levels in 10–11 year-old children. Diabetologia 1997;40:319–26.

13. Martin RM, McCarthy A, Smith GD, et al. Infant nutrition and blood pressure in early adulthood: the Barry Caerphilly Growth study. Am J Clin Nutr 2003;77:1489–97.

14. Law CM, Shiell AW, Newsome CA, et al. Fetal, infant, and childhood growth and adult blood pressure: a longitudinal study from birth to 22 years of age. Circulation 2002;105:1088–92.

15. Li C, Johnson MS, Goran MI. Effects of low birth weight on insulin resistance syndrome in Caucasian and African-American children. Diabetes Care 2001; 24:2035–42.

16. Boney CM, Verma A, Tucker R, et al. Metabolic syndrome in childhood: association with birth weight, maternal obesity, and gestational diabetes mellitus. Pediatrics 2005;115:290–6.

17. Clausen JO, Borch-Johnsen K, Pedersen O. Relation between birth weight and the insulin sensitivity index in a population sample of 331 young, healthy Caucasians. Am J Epidemiol 1997;146:23–31.

18. Flanagan DE, Moore VM, Godsland IF, et al. Fetal growth and the physiological control of glucose tolerance in adults: a minimal model analysis. Am J Physiol Endocrinol Metab 2000;278:E700–6.

19. Van Assche FA, De Prins F, Aerts L, et al. The endocrine pancreas in small-for dates infants. Br J Obstet Gynaecol 1977;84:751–3.

20. Beringue F, Blondeau B, Castellotti MC, et al. Endocrine pancreas development in growth-retarded human fetuses. Diabetes 2005;51:385–91.

21. Econimides DL, Proudler A, Nicolaides KH. Plasma insulin in appropriate and small for gestational age fetuses. Am J Obstet Gynecol 1989;160:1091–4.

22. Setia S, Sridhar MG, Bhat V, et al. Insulin sensitivity and insulin secretion at birth in intrauterine growth retarded infants. Pathology 2006;38:236–8.

23. Bazaes RA, Salazar TE, Pittaluga E. Glucose and lipid metabolism in small for gestational age infants at 48 hours of age. Pediatrics 2003;111:804–9.

24. Jensen CB, Storgaard H, Dela F, et al. Early differential defects of insulin secretion and action in 19-year-old Caucasian men who had low birth weight. Diabetes 2002;51:1271–80.

25. Pettitt DJ, Baird HR, Aleck KA, et al. Excessive obesity in offspring of Pima Indian women with diabetes during pregnancy. N Engl J Med 1983;308:242–5.

26. Pettitt DJ, Aleck KA, Baird HA, et al. Congenital susceptibility to NIDDM: role of the intrauterine environment. Diabetes 1988;37:622–8.

27. Martin AO, Simpson JL, Ober C, et al. Frequency of diabetes mellitus in mothers of probands with gestational diabetes: possible maternal influence on the predisposition to gestational diabetes. Am J Obstet Gynecol 1985;151:471–5.

28. Silverman B, Metzger BE, Cho NH, et al. Impaired glucose tolerance in adolescent offspring of diabetic mothers: relationship to fetal hyperinsulinism. Diabetes Care 1995;18:611–7.

29. Holemans K, Aerts L, Van Assche FA. Lifetime consequences of abnormal fetal pancreatic development. J Physiol 2003;547:11–20.

30. Plagemann A, Harder T, Kohlhoff R, et al. Glucose tolerance and insulin secretion in children of mothers with pregestational IDDM or gestational diabetes. Diabetologia 1997;40:1094–100.

31. Barnett AH, Eff C, Leslie RD, et al. Diabetes in identical twins. Diabetologia 1981; 20:87–93.

32. Newman B, Selby JV, King MC, et al. Concordance for type 2 diabetes mellitus in male twins. Diabetologia 1987;30:763–8.

33. Warram JH, Martin BC, Krolewski AS, et al. Slow glucose removal rate and hyperinsulinemia precede the development of type II diabetes in the offspring of diabetic parents. Ann Intern Med 1990;113:909–15.

34. Vaag A, Henricksen JE, Madsbad S, et al. Insulin secretion, insulin action, and hepatic glucose production in identical twins discordant for NIDDM. J Clin Invest 1995;95:690–8.

35. Hattersley AT, Tooke JE. The fetal insulin hypothesis: an alternative explanation of the association of low birthweight with diabetes and vascular disease. Lancet 1999;353:1789–92.

36. Froguel P, Zouali H, Vionnet N. Familial hyperglycemia due to mutations in glucokinase: definition of a subtype of diabetes mellitus. N Engl J Med 1993;328: 697–702.

37. Hattersley AT, Beards F, Ballantyne E, et al. Mutations in the glucokinase gene of the fetus result in reduced birth weight. Nat Genet 1998;19:268–70.

38. Grant SF, Thorleifsson G, Reynisdottir I, et al. Variant of transcription factor 7-like 2 (TCF7L2) gene confers risk of type 2 diabetes. Nat Genet 2006;38: 320–3.

39. Damcott CM, Pollin TI, Reinhart LJ, et al. Polymorphisms in the transcription factor 7-like 2 (TCF7L2) gene are associated with type 2 diabetes in the Amish: replication and evidence for a role in both insulin secretion and insulin resistance. Diabetes 2006;55:2654–9.

40. Saxena R, Gianniny L, Burtt NP, et al. Common single nucleotide polymorphisms in TCF7L2 are reproducibly associated with type 2 diabetes and reduce the insulin response to glucose in nondiabetic individuals. Diabetes 2006;55: 2890–5.

41. Munoz J, Lok KH, Gower BA, et al. Polymorphism in the transcription factor 7-like 2 (TCF7L2) gene is associated with reduced insulin secretion in nondiabetic women. Diabetes 2006;55:3630–4.

42. Freathy RM, Weedon MN, Bennett A, et al. Type 2 diabetes TCF7L2 risk genotypes alter birth weight: a study of 24,053 individuals. Am J Hum Genet 2007; 80:1150–61.

43. Kubaszek A, Markkanen A, Eriksson JG, et al. The association of the K121Q polymorphism of the plasma cell glycoprotein-1 gene with type 2 diabetes and hypertension depends on size at birth. J Clin Endocrinol Metab 2004;89: 2044–7.

44. Eriksson JG, Lindi V, Uusitupa M, et al. The effects of the Pro12Ala polymorphism of the peroxisome proliferator-activated receptor-gamma2 gene on insulin sensitivity and insulin metabolism interact with size at birth. Diabetes 2002;517: 2321–4.

45. Rahier J, Wallon J, Henquin JC. Cell populations in the endocrine pancreas of human neonates and infants. Diabetologia 1981;20:540–6.

46. Von Dorsche H, Reiher H, Hahn HJ. Phases in the early development of the human islet organ. Anat Anz 1988;166:69–76.

47. Dahri S, Reusens B, Remacle C, et al. Nutritional influences on pancreatic development and potential links with non-insulin-dependent diabetes. Proc Nutr Soc 1995;54:345–56.

48. Dahri S, Snoeck A, Reusens-Billen B, et al. Islet function in off-spring of mothers on low-protein diet during gestation. Diabetes 1991;40:115–20.

49. Snoeck A, Remacle C, Reusens B, et al. Effect of a low protein diet during pregnancy on the fetal rat endocrine pancreas. Biol Neonate 1990;57:107–18.

50. Berney DM, Desai M, Palmer DJ, et al. The effects of maternal protein deprivation on the fetal rat pancreas: major structural changes and their recuperation. J Pathol 1997;183:109–15.

51. Wilson MR, Hughes SJ. The effect of maternal protein deficiency during pregnancy and lactation on glucose tolerance and pancreatic islet function in adult rat offspring. J Endocrinol 1997;154:177–85.

52. Bertin E, Gangnerau MN, Bellon G, et al. Development of beta-cell mass in fetuses of rats deprived of protein and/or energy in last trimester of pregnancy. Am J Physiol Regul Integr Comp Physiol 2002;283:R623–30.

53. Boujendar S, Reusens B, Merezak S, et al. Taurine supplementation to a low protein diet during foetal and early postnatal life restores a normal proliferation and apoptosis of rat pancreatic islets. Diabetologia 2002;45:856–66.

54. Petrik J, Reusens B, Arany E, et al. A low protein diet alters the balance of islet cell replication and apoptosis in the fetal and neonatal rat, and is associated with a reduced pancreatic expression of insulin-like growth factor-II. Endocrinology 1999;140:4861–73.

55. Reusens B, Remacle C. Effects of maternal nutrition and metabolism on the developing endocrine pancreas. In: Barker DJP, editor. Fetal origins of cardiovascular and lung disease. New York: Marcel Dekker Inc.; 2000. p. 339–58.

56. Arantes VC, Teixeira VP, Reis MA, et al. Expression of PDX-1 is reduced in pancreatic islets from pups of rat dams fed a low protein diet during gestation and lactation. J Nutr 2002;132:3030–5.

57. Melloul D. Transcription factors in islet development and physiology: role of PDX-1 in beta-cell function. Ann N Y Acad Sci 2004;1014:28–37.

58. Petry CJ, Dorling MW, Pawlak DB, et al. Diabetes in old male offspring of rat dams fed a reduced protein diet. Int J Exp Diabetes Res 2001;2:139–43.

59. Ozanne SE, Wang CL, Coleman N, et al. Altered muscle insulin sensitivity in the male offspring of protein-malnourished rats. Am J Physiol 1996;271: E1128–34.

60. Ozanne SE, Jensen CB, Tingey KJ, et al. Low birthweight is associated with specific changes in muscle insulin-signalling protein expression. Diabetologia 2005;48:547–52.

61. Ozanne SE, Olsen GS, Hansen LL, et al. Early growth restriction leads to down regulation of protein kinase C zeta and insulin resistance in skeletal muscle. J Endocrinol 2003;177:235–41.

62. Fernandez-Twinn DS, Wayman A, Ekizoglou S, et al. Maternal protein restriction leads to hyperinsulinemia and reduced insulin-signaling protein expression in 21-mo-old female rat offspring. Am J Physiol Regul Integr Comp Physiol 2005; 288:R368–73.

63. Garofano A, Czernichow P, Bréant B. In utero undernutrition impairs rat beta-cell development. Diabetologia 1997;40:1231–4.

64. Garofano A, Czernichow P, Bréant B. Effect of ageing on beta-cell mass and function in rats malnourished during the perinatal period. Diabetologia 1999; 42:711–8.

65. Shen CN, Seckl JR, Slack JM, et al. Glucocorticoids suppress beta-cell development and induce hepatic metaplasia in embryonic pancreas. Biochem J 2003; 375(Pt 1):41–50.

66. Limesand SW, Jensen J, Hutton JC, et al. Diminished β-cell replication contributes to reduced ß-cell mass in fetal sheep with intrauterine growth restriction. Am J Physiol Regul Integr Comp Physiol 2005;288:R1297–305.

67. Limesand SW, Rozance PJ, Zerbe GO, et al. Attenuated insulin release and storage in fetal sheep pancreatic islets with intrauterine growth restriction. Endocrinology 2006;147:1488–97.

68. Ogata ES, Bussey M, Finley S. Altered gas exchange, limited glucose, branched chain amino acids, and hypoinsulinism retard fetal growth in the rat. Metabolism 1986;35:950–77.

69. Simmons RA, Templeton L, Gertz S, et al. Intrauterine growth retardation leads to type II diabetes in adulthood in the rat. Diabetes 2001;50:2279–86.

70. Boloker J, Gertz S, Simmons RA. Offspring of diabetic rats develop obesity and type II diabetes in adulthood. Diabetes 2002;51:1499–506.

71. Simmons RA, Gounis AS, Bangalore SA, et al. Intrauterine growth retardation: fetal glucose transport is diminished in lung but spared in brain. Pediatr Res 1991;31:59–63.

72. Unterman T, Lascon R, Gotway M, et al. Circulating levels of insulin-like growth factor binding protein-1 (IGFBP-1) and hepatic mRNA are increased in the small for gestational age fetal rat. Endocrinology 1990;127:2035–7.

73. Stoffers DA, Desai BM, DeLeon DD, et al. Neonatal exendin-4 prevents the development of diabetes in the intrauterine growth retarded rat. Diabetes 2003;52:734–40.

74. Myatt L, Eis AL, Brockman DE, et al. Differential localization of superoxide dismutase isoforms in placental villous tissue of normotensive, pre-eclamptic, and intrauterine growth-restricted pregnancies. J Histochem Cytochem 1997; 45:1433–8.

75. Karowicz-Billinska A, Suzin J, Sieroszewski P. Evaluation of oxidative stress indices during treatment in pregnant women with intrauterine growth retardation. Med Sci Monit 2002;8:CR211–6.

76. Ejima K, Nanri H, Toki N, et al. Localization of thioredoxin reductase and thioredoxin in normal human placenta and their protective effect against oxidative stress. Placenta 1999;20:95–101.

77. Kato H, Yoneyama Y, Araki T. Fetal plasma lipid peroxide levels in pregnancies complicated by preeclampsia. Gynecol Obstet Invest 1997;43:158–61.

78. Bowen RS, Moodley J, Dutton MF, et al. Oxidative stress in pre-eclampsia. Acta Obstet Gynecol Scand 2001;80:719–25.

79. Wang Y, Walsh SW. Increased superoxide generation is associated with decreased superoxide dismutase activity and mRNA expression in placental trophoblast cells in pre-eclampsia. Placenta 2001;22:206–12.

80. Wang Y, Walsh SW. Placental mitochondria as a source of oxidative stress in preeclampsia. Placenta 1998;19:581–6.
81. Panten U, Zielman S, Langer J, et al. Regulation of insulin secretion by energy metabolism in pancreatic ß-cell mitochondria. Biochem J 1984;219:189–96.
82. Newgard CB, McGarry JD. Metabolic coupling factors in pancreatic ß-cell signal transduction. Annu Rev Biochem 1995;64:689–719.
83. Schuit F. Metabolic fate of glucose in purified islet cells. Glucose regulated anaplerosis in ß-cells. J Biol Chem 1997;272:18572–9.
84. Mertz RJ, Worley JF III, Spencer B, et al. Activation of stimulus-secretion coupling in pancreatic ß-cells by specific products of glucose metabolism. J Biol Chem 1996;271:4838–45.
85. Ortsater H, Liss P, Akerman KE. Contribution of glycolytic and mitochondrial pathways in glucose-induced changes in islet respiration and insulin secretion. Pflugers Arch 2002;444:506–12.
86. Antinozzi PA, Ishihara H, Newgard CB, et al. Mitochondrial metabolism sets the maximal limit of fuel-stimulated insulin secretion in a model pancreatic beta cell. A survey of four fuel secretagogues. J Biol Chem 2002;277:11746–55.
87. Malaisse WJ, Hutton JC, Carpinelli AR, et al. The stimulus-secretion coupling of amino acid-induced insulin release. Metabolism and cationic effects of leucine. Diabetes 1980;29:431–7.
88. Lenzen S, Schmidt W, Rustenbeck I, et al. 2-Ketoglutarate generation in pancreatic ß-cell mitochondria regulates insulin secretory action of amino acids and 2-keto acids. Biosci Rep 1986;6:163–9.
89. Noda M, Yamashita S, Takahashi N, et al. Switch to anaerobic glucose metabolism with NADH accumulation in the beta-cell model of mitochondrial diabetes. Characteristics of beta HC9 cells deficient in mitochondrial DNA transcription. J Biol Chem 2002;277:41817–26.
90. Lenzen S, Drinkgern J, Tiedge M. Low antioxidant enzyme gene expression in pancreatic islets compared with various other mouse tissues. Free Radic Biol Med 1996;20:463–6.
91. Tiedge M, Lortz S, Drinkgern J, et al. Relationship between antioxidant enzyme gene expression and antioxidant defense status of insulin-producing cells. Diabetes 1997;46:1733–42.
92. Maechler P, Jornot L, Wollheim CB. Hydrogen peroxide alters mitochondrial activation and insulin secretion in pancreatic beta cells. J Biol Chem 1999;274:27905–13.
93. Sakai K, Matsumoto K, Nishikawa T, et al. Mitochondrial reactive oxygen species reduce insulin secretion by pancreatic ß-cells. Biochem Biophys Res Commun 2003;300:216–22.
94. Kaneto H, Xu G, Fujii N, et al. Involvement of c-Jun N-terminal kinase in oxidative stress-mediated suppression of insulin gene expression. J Biol Chem 2002;277:30010–8.
95. Kaneto HH, Xu G, Fujii N, et al. Involvement of protein kinase C beta 2 in c-myc induction by high glucose in pancreatic beta-cells. J Biol Chem 2002;277:3680–5.
96. Kaneto H, Xu G, Song KH, et al. Activation of the hexosamine pathway leads to deterioration of pancreatic beta-cell function through the induction of oxidative stress. J Biol Chem 2001;276:31099–104.
97. Kaneto H, Kajimoto Y, Fujitani Y, et al. Oxidative stress induces p21 expression in pancreatic islet cells: possible implication in beta-cell dysfunction. Diabetologia 1999;42:1093–7.

98. Jonas JC, Laybutt DR, Steil GM, et al. High glucose stimulates early response gene c-Myc expression in rat pancreatic beta cells. J Biol Chem 2001;276: 35375–81.

99. Jonas JC, Sharma A, Hasenkamp W, et al. Chronic hyperglycemia triggers loss of pancreatic beta cell differentiation in an animal model of diabetes. J Biol Chem 1999;274:14112–21.

100. Efanova IB, Zaitsev SV, Zhivotovsky B, et al. Glucose and tolbutamide induce apopotosis in pancreatic ß-cells. J Biol Chem 1998;273:22501–7.

101. Moran A, Zhang HJ, Olsonm LK, et al. Differentiation of glucose toxicity from ß-cell exhaustion during the evolution of defective insulin gene expression in the pancreatic islet cell line, HIT-T15. J Clin Invest 2000;99:534–9.

102. Donath MY, Gross DJ, Cerasi E, et al. Hyperglycemia-induced ß-cell apoptosis in pancreatic islets of *Psammomys obesus* during development of diabetes. Diabetes 1999;48:738–44.

103. Silva JP, Kohler M, Graff C, et al. Impaired insulin secretion and ß-cell loss in tissue specific knockout mice with mitochondrial diabetes. Nat Genet 2000; 26:336–40.

104. Simmons RA, Suponitsky-Kroyter I, Selak M. Progressive accumulation of mito-chondrial DNA mutations and decline in mitochondrial function lead to beta-cell failure. J Biol Chem 2005;280:28785–91.

105. Bannister AJ, Kouzarides T. Reversing histone methylation. Nature 2005;436: 1103–6.

106. Bernstein E, Allis CD. RNA meets chromatin. Genes Dev 2005;19:1635–55.

107. Sproul D, Gilbert N, Bickmore WA. The role of chromatin structure in regulating the expression of clustered genes. Nat Rev Genet 2005;6:775–81.

108. Schubeler D, Lorincz MC, Cimbora DM, et al. Genomic targeting of methylated DNA: influence of methylation on transcription, replication, chromatin structure, and histone acetylation. Mol Cell Biol 2000;20:9103–12.

109. Galm O, Yoshikawa H, Esteller M, et al. SOCS-1, a negative regulator of cytokine signaling, is frequently silenced by methylation in multiple myeloma. Blood 2003;101:2784–8.

110. Yoshikawa H, Matsubara K, Qian GS, et al. SOCS-1, a negative regulator of the JAK/STAT pathway, is silenced by methylation in human hepatocellular carci-noma and shows growth-suppression activity. Nat Genet 2001;28:29–35.

111. He B, You L, Uematsu K, et al. SOCS-3 is frequently silenced by hypermethyla-tion and suppresses cell growth in human lung cancer. Proc Natl Acad Sci U S A 2003;100:14133–8.

112. Shiraishi M, Sekiguchi A, Oates AJ, et al. HOX gene clusters are hotspots of de novo methylation in CpG islands of human lung adenocarcinomas. Oncogene 2002;21:3659–63.

113. So K, Tamura G, Honda T, et al. Multiple tumor suppressor genes are increas-ingly methylated with age in non-neoplastic gastric epithelia. Cancer Sci 2006;97:1155–8.

114. Takahashi T, Shigematsu H, Shivapurkar N, et al. Aberrant promoter methylation of multiple genes during multistep pathogenesis of colorectal cancers. Int J Cancer 2006;118:924–31.

115. Feltus FA, Lee EK, Costello JF, et al. Predicting aberrant CpG island methylation. Proc Natl Acad Sci U S A 2003;100:12253–8.

116. Cerda S, Weitzman SA. Influence of oxygen radical injury on DNA methylation. Mutat Res 1997;386:141–52.

117. Drake J, Petroze R, Castegna A, et al. 4-Hydroxynonenal oxidatively modifies histones: implications for Alzheimer's disease. Neurosci Lett 2004;356:155–8.

118. Gilmour PS, Rahman I, Donaldson K, et al. Histone acetylation regulates epithelial IL-8 release mediated by oxidative stress from environmental particles. Am J Physiol Lung Cell Mol Physiol 2003;284:L533–40.

119. Rahman I, Gilmour PS, Jimenez LA, et al. Oxidative stress and TNF-alpha induce histone acetylation and NF-kappaB/AP-1 activation in alveolar epithelial cells: potential mechanism in gene transcription in lung inflammation. Mol Cell Biochem 2002;234–5:239–48.

120. MacLennan NK, James SJ, Melnyk S, et al. Uteroplacental insufficiency alters DNA methylation, one-carbon metabolism, and histone acetylation in IUGR rats. Physiol Genomics 2004;18:43–50.

121. Pham TD, MacLennan NK, Chiu CT, et al. Uteroplacental insufficiency increases apoptosis and alters p53 gene methylation in the full-term IUGR rat kidney. Am J Physiol Regul Integr Comp Physiol 2003;285:R962–70.

122. Fu Q, McKnight RA, Yu X, et al. Uteroplacental insufficiency induces site-specific changes in histone H3 covalent modifications and affects DNA-histone H3 positioning in day 0 IUGR rat liver. Physiol Genomics 2004;20:108–16.

123. Ke X, Lei Q, James SJ, et al. Uteroplacental insufficiency affects epigenetic determinants of chromatin structure in brains of neonatal and juvenile IUGR rats. Physiol Genomics 2006;25:16–28.

124. Fu Q, McKnight RA, Yu X, et al. Growth retardation alters the epigenetic characteristics of hepatic dual specificity phosphatase 5. FASEB J 2006;20: 2127–9.

125. Park JH, Stoffers DA, Nicholls RD, et al. Development of type 2 diabetes following intrauterine growth retardation in rats is associated with progressive epigenetic silencing of Pdx1. J Clin Invest 2008;118:2316–24.

126. Qian J, Kaytor EN, Towle HC, et al. Upstream stimulatory factor regulates Pdx-1 gene expression in differentiated pancreatic ß-cells. Biochem J 1999;341: 315–22.

127. Sharma S, Leonard J, Lee S, et al. Pancreatic islet expression of the homeobox factor STF-1 (Pdx-1) relies on an E-box motif that binds USF. J Biol Chem 1996; 271:2294–9.

128. Franco R, Schoneveld O, Georgakilas AG, et al. Oxidative stress, DNA methylation and carcinogenesis. Cancer Lett 2008;266:6–11.

129. Yauk C, Polyzos A, Rowan-Carroll A, et al. Germ-line mutations, DNA damage, and global hypermethylation in mice exposed to particulate air pollution in an urban/industrial location. Proc Natl Acad Sci U S A 2008;105:605–10.

130. Hitchler MJ, Domann FE. An epigenetic perspective on the free radical theory of development. Free Radic Biol Med 2007;43:1023–36.

131. Ihara Y, Toyokuni S, Uchida K, et al. Hyperglycemia causes oxidative stress in pancreatic beta-cells of GK rats, a model of type 2 diabetes. Diabetes 1999; 48:927–32.

132. Sakuraba H, Mizukami H, Yagihashi N, et al. Reduced beta-cell mass and expression of oxidative stress-related DNA damage in the islet of Japanese type II diabetic patients. Diabetologia 2002;45:85–96.

133. Bachman KE, Park BH, Rhee I, et al. Histone modifications and silencing prior to DNA methylation of a tumor suppressor gene. Cancer Cell 2003;3:89–95.

134. Kouzarides T. Histone methylation in transcriptional control. Curr Opin Genet Dev 2002;12:198–209.

135. Bernardo AS, Hay CW, Docherty K. Pancreatic transcription factors and their role in the birth, life and survival of the pancreatic beta cell. Mol Cell Endocrinol 2008;294:1–9.
136. Thamotharan M, Shin BC, Suddirikku DT, et al. GLUT4 expression and subcellular localization in the intrauterine growth-restricted adult rat female offspring. Am J Physiol 2005;288:E935–47.
137. Fueger PT, Shearer J, Bracy DP, et al. Control of muscle glucose uptake: test of the rate-limiting step paradigm in conscious, unrestrained mice. J Physiol 2005; 562:925–35.
138. Karnieli E, Armoni M. Transcriptional regulation of the insulin-responsive glucose transporter GLUT4 gene: from physiology to pathology. Am J Physiol Endocrinol Metab 2008;295:E38–45.
139. Moreno H, Serrano AL, Santalucía T, et al. Differential regulation of the muscle-specific GLUT4 enhancer in regenerating and adult skeletal muscle. J Biol Chem 2003;278:40557–64.
140. Raychaudhuri N, Raychaudhuri S, Thamotharan M, et al. Histone code modifications repress glucose transporter 4 expression in the intrauterine growth-restricted offspring. J Biol Chem 2008;283:13611–26.
141. Gebhard C, Schwarzfischer L, Pham TH, et al. Genome-wide profiling of CpG methylation identifies novel targets of aberrant hypermethylation in myeloid leukemia. Cancer Res 2006;66:6118–28.
142. Korshunova Y, Maloney RK, Lakey N, et al. Massively parallel bisulphite pyrosequencing reveals the molecular complexity of breast cancer-associated cytosine-methylation patterns obtained from tissue and serum DNA. Genome Res 2008;18:19–29.
143. Mori Y, Cai K, Cheng Y, et al. A genome-wide search identifies epigenetic silencing of somatostatin, tachykinin-1, and 5 other genes in colon cancer. Gastroenterology 2006;131:797–808.
144. Lieb JD, Beck S, Bulyk ML, et al. Applying whole-genome studies of epigenetic regulation to study human disease. Cytogenet Genome Res 2006;114:1–15.
145. Kim TH, Barrera LO, Zheng M, et al. A high-resolution map of active promoters in the human genome. Nature 2005;436:876–80.

Current Status of the Approach to Assisted Reproduction

Samuel A. Pauli, MD[a],*, Sarah L. Berga, MD[b],
Weirong Shang, PhD[c], Donna R. Session, MD[a]

KEYWORDS

- ART • IVF • Infertility • Pediatric • Oncofertility
- Fertility preservation

Since the advent of in vitro fertilization (IVF) and the successful birth of Louise Brown on July 25, 1978, more than 3 million children have been born worldwide through assistive reproductive technologies (ART).[1] In 2005, the 422 fertility clinics in the United States reported performing 134,260 ART cycles resulting in 38,910 live births of 52,041 children.[2] Approximately 1% of all births and 18% of all multiple births in the United States are the result of assisted reproductive technologies.[2,3]

Assisted reproductive technology includes all treatments that involve manipulation of both eggs and sperm outside of the body. Most commonly, it refers to in vitro fertilization, although other forms of ART used include gamete intrafallopian transfer (GIFT), zygote intrafallopian transfer (ZIFT), tubal embryo transfer (TET), donor oocyte, and gestational carriers. Other commonly used strategies to treat infertility, including ovulation induction and intrauterine inseminations, are not considered forms of ART. Ovulation induction stimulates multifollicular development with the use of oral or injectable medication without retrieving oocytes. Intrauterine insemination involves the handling of only the male gametes outside of the body.

The purpose of this chapter is to describe the workup of infertility, provide an overview of the indications for ART, and explain the process of ovarian stimulation, sperm recovery, fertilization, and embryo transfer. Complications related to the use of ART

[a] Division of Reproductive Endocrinology and Infertility, Department of Gynecology and Obstetrics, Emory University School of Medicine, Emory Reproductive Center, Medical Office Tower, 550 Peachtree Street, Suite 1800, Atlanta, GA 30308, USA
[b] Department of Gynecology and Obstetrics, Emory University School of Medicine, 1639 Pierce Drive, Room 4208-WMB, Atlanta, Georgia 30322, USA
[c] Andrology and Embryology Laboratory, Division of Reproductive Endocrinology and Infertility, Department of Gynecology and Obstetrics, Emory University School of Medicine, Emory Reproductive Center, Medical Office Tower, 550 Peachtree Street, Suite 1800, Atlanta, GA 30308, USA
* Corresponding author.
E-mail address: spauli@emory.edu (S.A. Pauli).

Pediatr Clin N Am 56 (2009) 467–488
doi:10.1016/j.pcl.2009.04.001
0031-3955/09/$ – see front matter © 2009 Elsevier Inc. All rights reserved.

will be discussed with an emphasis on topics related to the care of the pediatric population. In addition, the use of ART in the preservation of fertility in pediatric and adolescent population undergoing chemotherapy or radiation therapy will be explored.

INDICATIONS AND EVALUATION BEFORE IN VITRO FERTILIZATION

Infertility has been defined as the inability of a couple to conceive after 12 months of unprotected and frequent intercourse. Women who have never conceived a child are classified as having primary infertility, whereas women who have had a prior child and are unable to subsequently conceive are classified as having secondary infertility. According to the 2002 National Survey of Family Growth published by the Center for Disease Control and Prevention, 7.4% of married women not using contraception, ages 15 through 44, were unable to become pregnant in the previous 12 months and thus classified as infertile.[4] They also noted that 7.1% of childless women and 11.9% of all women between the ages of 15 and 44 had received infertility treatment. In practice, patients may present with the inability to achieve pregnancy before 12 months and desire treatment options. Earlier evaluation and treatment may be warranted in women older than 35, because fecundity decreases with increasing maternal age. In addition, earlier evaluation is indicated in patients with suspected reproductive disorders, such as amenorrhea or oligomenorrhea, tubal disease, endometriosis, prior history of chemotherapy, or impending treatment with chemotherapy or radiation to the pelvis.

Although IVF was first developed for the treatment of tubal disease, today IVF is commonly used to treat a variety of causes of infertility (**Box 1**). With the birth of the first child from a cryopreserved embryo in 1983, the use of IVF was expanded to include patients facing chemotherapy or radiation therapy to preserve fertility.[5] The development of intracytoplasmic sperm injection (ICSI) allowed for the treatment of severe male-factor infertility.[6] Advances in molecular genetics and embryo biopsy have permitted IVF to be used to screen for single gene defects and aneuploidy, with the first two reported clinical pregnancies after preimplantation genetic diagnosis reported in 1990.[7] Alternatively, patients who carry a genetic disorder may opt for donor oocytes. Current work in cryobiology in the areas of ovarian tissue freezing and oocyte cryopreservation may further expand the role of ART in fertility preservation in women wishing to delay childbearing and women undergoing chemotherapy or radiation therapy.

The basic evaluation of the female partner includes an assessment of ovarian reserve, uterine abnormalities, and tubal patency. A day three follicle-stimulating hormone, estradiol level, or antral follicle count by ultrasound scan have all been shown to correlate with ovarian responsiveness to gonadotropins in patients undergoing assisted reproductive technologies.[8–14] Recently, serum anti-Mullerian hormone has also been associated with ovarian response.[15] The uterus should also be evaluated for the presence of polyps, submucosal fibroids, and adhesions. This may be performed via a sonohysterogram (saline infusion sonogram), hysterosalpingogram, or hysteroscopy. A hysterosalpingogram has the benefit of evaluating for the presence of hydrosalpinges (abnormally distended fluid filled fallopian tubes), which are most often the result of a prior inflammatory process. If structural abnormalities are found they should be addressed before starting an ART cycle, because structural irregularities of the uterus may interfere with implantation or be responsible for miscarriages. A mock or trial embryo transfer has been advocated to reduce the number of difficult embryo transfers and has been shown to improve IVF outcomes.[16] Male factor infertility can be evaluated through performing a routine semen analysis.

Box 1
Indications for ART
Tubal factor
Male factor
Endometriosis
Diminished ovarian reserve
Before radiation or chemotherapy treatment
Genetically transmitted disease
Fertility preservation
Donor egg
Uterine factor/gestational carrier
Uterine anomaly
Prior hysterectomy
Extensive fibroid disease
Asherman's syndrome–intrauterine adhesions
Maternal medical condition precluding pregnancy
Poor obstetric history
Ovulatory dysfunction
Polycystic ovarian syndrome
Hypogonadotropic hypogonadism
Unexplained infertility

OVARIAN STIMULATION

Assisted reproductive technologies refer to a large number of techniques by which a third party handles oocytes and sperm outside the body to create an embryo that is transferred to an intended recipient. IVF is a method of assisted reproduction whereby a woman's ovaries are stimulated with fertility medications; oocytes are aspirated from ovarian follicles, fertilized in the laboratory, and transferred to the uterus to implant and develop into a pregnancy.

The first IVF birth resulted from the retrieval of a single oocyte from a natural menstrual cycle.[1] To increase the number of embryos available for embryo transfer and cryopreservation, fertility medications often are given to enhance the number of oocytes. The goal of ovarian stimulation is to produce a cohort of uniform follicles that develop and mature in a controlled fashion to allow for retrieval of multiple mature oocytes.

There are various treatment regimens used for superovulation to stimulate multifollicular development in the ovaries. The use of clomiphene citrate and the combination of clomiphene citrate and exogenous gonadotropins have been used for ovarian stimulation; however, the most commonly used approach is exogenous gonadotropins alone. Clomiphene citrate is an oral medication that binds to nuclear estrogen receptors producing estrogen agonist and antagonist effects.[17] It interferes with estrogen negative feedback resulting in an augmentation of gonadotropin-releasing hormone (GnRH) secretion leading to increased pituitary release of gonadotropins, which stimulate ovarian follicular development. In addition to augmenting endogenous GnRH production, exogenous gonadotropins can be given to promote follicular growth. Typically, exogenous gonadotropins are given in combination with GnRH analogs, either agonist or antagonists in various stimulation protocols. The "long" protocol involves the administration of a GnRH agonist during the luteal phase of the preceding menstrual cycle before IVF to down-regulate pituitary production of endogenous gonadotropins, preventing a premature luteinizing hormone (LH) surge during stimulation. Alternatively, the "short" or "flare" protocol involves starting the GnRH agonists at the beginning of the menstrual cycle to take advantage of the initial surge of endogenous gonadotropins released before down-regulation. Unlike GnRH agonists that down-regulate GnRH receptors, thereby inhibiting endogenous pituitary gonadotropin secretion, GnRH antagonist competitively bind to GnRH receptors suppressing endogenous gonadotropin production and preventing a premature LH surge.[18] Because GnRH antagonists are fast acting, they may be given later in the cycle, therefore, decreasing the number of injections, length of the cycle, and potentially cost.

The stimulation protocol selected for a patient should take into account the patient's age, cause of infertility, ovarian reserve, and prior treatment history. It should also seek to minimize cost and risk while maximizing chance of pregnancy. A Cochrane meta-analysis of 22 trials comparing long and short GnRH agonist protocols found slight superiority in the number of clinical pregnancies using the long protocol; odds ratio (OR) 1.27 (95% confidence interval [CI], 1.04–1.56).[19] Both the short or flare protocol and GnRH antagonist protocols are used for patients with diminished ovarian reserve. A recent randomized study of 90 patients comparing microdose flare and GnRH antagonist protocols found a significantly higher number of oocytes retrieved and implantation rates, as well as a nonstatistically significant trend toward higher clinical pregnancy rates in the flare group.[20] However, GnRH antagonist protocols help suppress premature LH surges, preventing premature ovulation in poor responders, and can be used to decrease the incidence of ovarian hyperstimulation.[21,22]

Ovarian stimulation usually occurs for 8 to 12 days. Response to stimulation can be monitored by measuring serum estradiol levels and serial ultrasound measurements of follicular growth and endometrial thickness. The dose of gonadotropins given can be titrated up or down based on these findings to promote the desired follicular response. When the cohort of developing preovulatory follicles reaches an optimal size, human chorionic gonadotropin (hCG) is given to induce follicular maturation and the ovulatory cascade. Various criteria are used to judge when a cycle has reached the target threshold for hCG administration. Ideally, at least two follicles present measuring 17 to 18 mm in diameter with multiple other follicles 14 to 16 mm in diameter and serum estradiol concentrations consistent with the number of follicles in the cohort (approximately 200 pg/mL per follicle measuring greater than 14 mm) are optimal for hCG administration.[23]

OOCYTE RETRIEVAL

Oocyte retrieval occurs 34 to 36 hours after hCG administration. Oocyte retrievals were initially performed laparoscopically; however, this technique has been largely replaced by transvaginal ultrasound–guided oocyte aspiration, because of safety as well as increased number of oocytes retrieved. After analgesia, an ultrasound probe is inserted into the vagina and used to identify the follicles. A needle is then inserted though a needle guide, and the follicles are sequentially vacuum aspirated. Complications after oocyte retrieval are rare. Despite not being able to use antiseptics, which can be toxic to embryos, the risk of infection after retrieval is low, regardless of whether prophylactic antibiotics are administered.[24] Hemorrhage from the needle puncture site is uncommon.

FERTILIZATION AND EMBRYO CULTURE

Once oocytes are identified, they are placed in culture medium in an incubator. Oocytes that have extruded the first polar body identify mature metaphase II oocytes from immature oocytes. Oocytes are inseminated 2 to 8 hours after retrieval depending on the method of insemination. Fertilization may be achieved by conventional means whereby each oocyte is incubated with 50,000 to 100,000 motile sperm for 12 to 18 hours. Alternatively, individually selected sperm may be injected into the ooplasm of the oocyte in a process called *intracytoplasmic sperm injection* (ICSI) (**Fig. 1**). Unlike conventional fertilization in which the sperm must penetrate the zona pellucida of the oocyte, undergo the acrosome reaction, and fuse with the oocyte membrane to activate the oocyte, ICSI directly activates the oocyte. ICSI is performed primarily for severe male factor infertility, couples who have previously failed conventional fertilization, to limit contamination with extraneous DNA when performing preimplantation genetic diagnosis, and when small quantities of sperm remain. Fertilization rates of approximately 70% are observed for both conventional fertilization and ICSI. Sperm is most commonly obtained from a partner by masturbation, but ICSI can achieve fertilization with sperm retrieved by other methods. Retrograde ejaculation can be treated with sympathomimetics, or sperm can be recovered from a postejaculatory void after alkalinization of the urine. Men with spinal cord injuries below T6 or psychogenic ejaculatory failure may produce ejaculate with the aid of vibratory stimulation or electroejaculation. In patients with congenital bilateral absence of the vas deferens or uncorrectable duct obstructions, epididymal sperm aspiration can be performed. Testicular sperm extraction and aspiration can be used to retrieve sperm in men with nonobstructive azoospermia.

Fertilization can be confirmed by visualization of two pronuclei and two polar bodies the day after fertilization. The first cleavage division occurs within 24 hours after fertilization. Two days after retrieval, the embryo consists of two to four cells and reaches

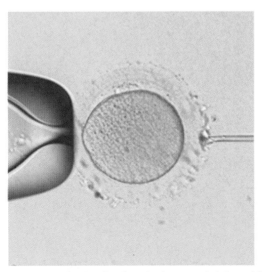

Fig. 1. Intracytoplasmic Sperm Injection (ICSI): a single sperm is injected into an oocyte.

eight cells by day 3.[25] DNA transcription begins between days 3 and 4 when compaction occurs at the 8 to 16 cells stage in which the previously visualized individual cells become an indistinguishable solid mass called a *morula*. By day 5, the embryo is called a blastocyst, which contains a fluid-filled cavity, an inner cell mass, and a trophoblast, which later develops into the placenta (**Fig. 2**).

Before implantation, the blastocyst hatches from the zona pellucida. A variety of embryo micromanipulation techniques called *assisted hatching* have been developed to artificially thin the zona to improve the interaction of the embryo and the endometrium. While multiple studies have failed to show that assisted hatching improves pregnancy rates in all patients, the procedure may be of value in selected populations.[26,27] Current guidelines support assisted hatching in patients with more than two failed IVF cycles, poor embryo quality, or women older than 37 years.[28]

EMBRYO TRANSFER

Embryo transfer typically is performed 3 days after oocyte retrieval at the cleavage stage or 5 days after retrieval at the blastocyst stage. The most common embryo transfer involves placing a catheter via the cervix into the uterus; however, embryos can also be placed in the fallopian tubes laparoscopically. The number of embryos transferred is based on the age of the patient, embryo quality and stage, and other patient characteristics that may influence success. A Cochrane meta-analysis of 16 trials comparing cleavage stage versus blastocyst embryo transfer showed no difference in live birth rates, clinical pregnancy rates, multiple gestations, higher-order multiple pregnancies, or miscarriages.[29] Blastocyst transfer was associated with a higher failure to transfer embryos and lower rates of embryo freezing. Blastocyst transfers have also been associated with a higher rate of monozygotic twins and may be associated with imprinting disorders caused by epigenetic alterations.[30–34] As technology has improved, the rates of success for patients undergoing ART has improved steadily throughout the years. In 2005, 34% of ART cycles resulted in a clinical pregnancy, and 28% of cycles resulted in

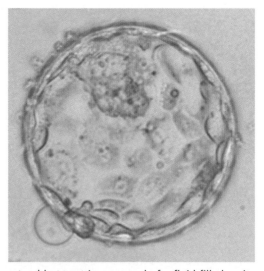

Fig. 2. Day 5 blastocyst: a blastocyst is composed of a fluid filled cavity, an inner cell mass, and an outer ring of trophoblastic cells.

a live birth.[2] Success rates correlate with the age of the patient, with the highest pregnancy rates observed in patients under the age of 35 (**Table 1**).

The ability to cryopreserve embryos has increased the success rate of ART. In patients with a high yield of good-quality embryos, freezing increases the cumulative pregnancy rate per retrieval and decreases the risk of higher-order multiples. Cryopreservation has also been used to decrease the risk of ovarian hyperstimulation syndrome, as the syndrome is worsened and prolonged in conception cycles.[35,36] Success rates of a frozen embryo transfer cycle are approximately one half to two thirds that observed for fresh cycles.[23] The lower pregnancy rate observed in frozen embryo transfers is likely secondary to cell damage from the freezing and thawing process as well as the best quality embryos most likely to result in pregnancy were transferred during the fresh cycle.

PREIMPLANTATION GENETIC DIAGNOSIS

The ability to biopsy embryos and advances in the field of molecular genetics have allowed for pretransfer analysis of the genetic make-up of embryos created through in vitro fertilization in a process called preimplantation genetic diagnosis (PGD). This technique can reduce the risk of conceiving a child with a genetic abnormality as long as the genetic abnormality has been identified and can be tested for in a single cell. Although PGD involves evaluating embryos for a specific known mutation or chromosomal rearrangement carried by one or both of the parents, preimplantation genetic screening (PGS) is a similar technology that screens embryos of presumed chromosomally normal parents for aneuploidy. One of the key advantages of preimplantation genetic testing over conventional prenatal diagnosis is that it allows for early detection of affected embryos before embryo transfer. This reduces the risk of having to decide to terminate an affected pregnancy before it has been established.

Although various methods of biopsying the embryo for PGD or PGS exist, the most commonly used process involves removing one or two cells from an eight-cell cleavage-stage embryo for genetic analysis. Gene analysis typically is performed using either fluorescence in situ hybridization (FISH) or polymerase chain reaction (PCR) for PGD. FISH and comparative genomic hybridization (CGH) are used for PGS. Although PGD has been a major advance for couples at risk of conceiving a child with an inheritable disease, the technology is limited by several factors, including the short amount of time available for analysis before the embryos must be transferred, limited genetic material available for amplification, and false-positive and false-negative results secondary to genetic mosaicism.[37] To limit the risk of misdiagnosis,

Table 1		
2005 Centers for Disease Control Assistive Reproductive Technology national success rates		
Age	**% Pregnancy**	**% Live Birth**
<35	43	37
35–37	36	29
38–40	27	20
41–42	18	11
>42	8	4
All cycles[a]	34	28
Donor egg[a]	55	47

[a] Regardless of age.

chorionic villus sampling (CVS) or amniocentesis is recommended during the pregnancy to confirm PGD results.

PGD was first used for sex selection to prevent the transmission of X-linked diseases to male offspring.[7] PGD has evolved and is now able to detect a variety of chromosomal abnormalities and gene mutations encompassing more than 100 inheritable genetic conditions (**Box 2**). PGS was proposed initially to increase the effectiveness of IVF in women of advanced maternal age by screening for aneuploidies. However, it is not routinely recommended because a recent randomized, controlled study found PGS reduced pregnancy rates and live births.[38] PGD has been used in IVF cycles of couples with known autosomal recessive single gene disorders, such as cystic fibrosis, beta-thalassemia, and sickle cell anemia, as well as autosomal dominant conditions such as hemophilia and myotonic dystrophy.[39–43] This technology has also recently been used to screen for mutations with high penetrance that predispose to cancer. PGD has been used to identify mutations in the APC gene that cause familial adenomatous polyposis coli, the BRCA1 gene that predisposes to breast and ovarian cancer, the NF2 mutation that causes neurofibromatosis 2, and mutations in the tumor suppressor gene p53.[44–48] PGD has detected early adult-onset syndromes associated with gene mutations such Huntington's disease and Alzheimer disease caused by a mutation in valine to leucine at codon 717.[49,50] Rhesus (Rh) D–negative embryos identified by PGD were transferred to an RhD alloimmunized mother with a heterozygous RhD-positive father to prevent hemolytic disease of a newborn.[51] PGD combined with human leukocyte antigen (HLA) typing has been used to establish unaffected donor progeny for cord blood cell transplantation for a sibling affected with Fanconi anemia.[52]

Couples at risk of having a child with a genetic disorder or parents with a child with an affected disorder should be made aware of the possibility of preimplantation genetic diagnosis before attempting to become pregnant. The advantage of PGD over prenatal diagnosis (amniocentesis or chorionic villus sampling) is that the

---

Box 2
Potential indications for preimplantation genetic diagnosis

X-linked disorders

Single gene disorders

  Autosomal recessive

  Autosomal dominant

Structural chromosome abnormalities

  Translocations

  Inversions

  Deletions

Detection of genetic susceptibility and late-onset disease

  Huntington's

  BRCA1/BRCA2

Human leukocyte antigen (HLA) typing to establish potential donor progeny

  Fanconi anemia

  Leukemia

detection of the condition is possible before the pregnancy is established. Unaffected embryos can be transferred, eliminating the need to make the difficult decision whether to terminate the pregnancy in the event of an affected fetus. For parents faced with a child needing a bone marrow transplant who desire further children, PGD offers a unique opportunity to preselect unaffected embryos that can be HLA-compatible with the sibling. Although currently not performed, preimplantation gene therapy may be possible as technology advances.

RISK OF ART

Risks of IVF can be divided into risks associated with the procedure and risks to the pregnancy. Relatively minor bruising at the site of injections and abdominal discomfort as the ovaries enlarge are common. Multiple studies have been performed to evaluate the effect of fertility medication on the risk of ovarian cancer. Although some of the early studies suggested a possible link of fertility medications to ovarian cancer, the most recent studies have failed to establish an association.[53,54] A poor response to medication can result in cycle cancellation of some women, whereas an exaggerated ovarian response is seen in some patients resulting in ovarian hyperstimulation syndrome (OHSS). Bleeding, anesthesia complications, or injury to bowel, bladder, or blood vessels at the time or retrieval are uncommon. Infection related to oocyte retrieval or embryo transfers is uncommon, and prophylactic antibiotics can be given to further minimize risks.

OHSS is one of the more serious complications of IVF with the potential for critical morbidity and death. OHSS is more common in younger patients and correlates with the number of developing follicles, high or rapidly rising serum estradiol levels, and number of retrieved oocytes.[55–57] The degree of ovarian hyperstimulation can be classified into three levels and five grades based on signs, symptoms, ultrasound, and laboratory findings.[58] The use of hCG for inducing oocyte maturation or for luteal support, as well as pregnancy, increases the risk of OHSS.[56,59] Mild hyperstimulation is common and occurs in approximately 30% of IVF cycles. Moderate OHSS is seen in 3% to 6% of cycles, and severe OHSS is observed in 0.25% to 1.8% of IVF cycles. Symptoms may include abdominal distention and discomfort with accompanying nausea, vomiting, and diarrhea. Moderate to severe OHSS can be associated with significant weight gain, ascites, pleural or pericardial effusions, hemoconcentration, electrolyte imbalance, hypovolemia, and thrombosis. If severe enough, this can place a patient at risk for respiratory distress, renal failure, stroke, and death. Hospitalization often is required for intravenous fluid replacement, correction of electrolyte disturbances, initiation of thrombosis prophylaxis, and drainage of third-spaced fluid if symptomatic. Ovarian enlargement seen in OHSS may place the patient at increased risk of ovarian torsion, necessitating urgent surgical correction. OHSS is self-limiting and typically resolves within 14 days.[60] Cryopreservation of all embryos, coined a "freeze all" cycle, with delayed interval transfer decreases the risk of ovarian hyperstimulation yet maintains pregnancy and live birth rates.[36,61]

First trimester bleeding before 13 weeks' gestation may occur in patients that conceive via ART. Bleeding can be clinically insignificant or may signal an impending miscarriage or ectopic pregnancy. First trimester bleeding requires medical evaluation to determine the cause. Very early spotting within a week after transfer may be associated with implantation bleeding. First trimester bleeding is associated with a twofold relative risk of a spontaneous miscarriage.[62] Bleeding may be associated with a subchorionic hemorrhage in which bleeding occurs between the uterine wall and the chorionic membranes that may leak through the cervical canal resulting in vaginal bleeding. Subchorionic hemorrhage is associated not only with an increased risk of miscarriage, but also stillbirth, placental abruption, and preterm labor.[63] Vaginal spotting, with or without unilateral pain, may be a harbinger of an ectopic pregnancy. In 2005, 0.6% of all ART cycles corresponding to 1.7% of all resulting pregnancies ended in an ectopic pregnancy.[2] Rates of ectopic pregnancy are increased in women electing for ZIFT in lieu of IVF and those with tubal factor infertility or endometriosis and are related to location of embryo transfer.[64,65] Studies have also found that rates are lower in women who have had a prior live birth, when embryos with a high implantation potential are transferred, in donor egg cycles, and when a gestational carrier or surrogate is used.[64] Although the rate of a spontaneous heterotopic pregnancy, where there is both an intrauterine and extrauterine pregnancy, is a rare event, occurring in 1 in 10,000 pregnancies, this condition can be observed in approximately 1 in 100 ART pregnancies.[66,67]

It has been estimated that 12% to 15% of clinically recognized pregnancies result in miscarriage.[23] This number is an underestimate of the miscarriage rate given the number of early pregnancies that end before they are detected clinically.[68] The risk of miscarriage for pregnancies conceived by ART is comparable with that observed in spontaneous pregnancies, with data from the Centers for Disease Control (CDC) 2005 Assisted Reproductive Technology Success Rate report indicating 15.8% of all pregnancies resulting from ART ended in miscarriage.[2] The risk of miscarriage increases as the age of the mother increases. Although miscarriage rates in 2005 were less than 13% for women under the age of 33 undergoing ART, the miscarriage rate reached 27% by age 40 and was 64% for women over the age of 43.[2] Pregnancies resulting from frozen embryo transfers have a higher rate of miscarriage when compared with pregnancies conceived with freshly fertilized embryos.[69]

ART increases the risk of multiple gestations. Although ART is responsible for approximately 1% of all births in the United States, it accounts for almost 18% of multiple births. In 2005, fresh nondonor ART cycles produced 33,101 pregnancies resulting in 60.4% singleton pregnancies, 28.5% twin pregnancies, and 4.4% triplet and higher-order multiple pregnancies; 6.7% of pregnancies were unknown secondary to early miscarriage.[2] Of the resulting 27,047 births, 68.0% were singletons, 29.6% twins, and 2.4% triplets and higher order multiples. Although most twins are dizygotic, ART increases the risk of monozygotic twinning. This may be related to ovulation induction, assisted hatching, and blastocyst transfer.[31–33,70,71] Multiple-order births pose significant risks to both the mothers and resulting infants of these pregnancies.[72] Mothers are more prone to pregnancy complications including hyperemesis, gestational diabetes, preeclampsia, preterm labor, cesarean delivery, and postpartum hemorrhage. Pregnancies are at a higher risk for intrauterine growth restriction and preterm delivery with increased rates of perinatal and infant morbidity and mortality. Monozygotic twins also have higher rates of congenital anomalies.[73]

The goal of IVF is to maximize chances of pregnancy while minimizing the risk of higher-order multiple gestations. The live birth rate increases as the number of embryos transferred increases to a threshold, after which, only the multiple pregnancy rate increases.[74] The most important factor in predicting success is the age of a women or oocyte donor undergoing IVF retrieval and embryo quality.[75] Other patient characteristics including prior IVF cycle response are also important in guiding the decision of how many embryos to transfer. Therefore, the American Society of Reproductive Medicine (ASRM) has established guidelines that delineate the ideal number of embryos to transfer based on age and prognosis (**Table 2**).[76] The current recommendation for women less than 35 years with a favorable prognosis is to transfer no more than two embryos. Women with a favorable prognosis and a high risk of multiple

	Cleavage-Stage Embryos		Blastocysts	
Age[a]	Favorable Prognosis[b]	Others	Favorable Prognosis	Others
<35	1–2	2	1	2
35–37	2	3	2	2
38–40	3	4	2	3
>40	5	5	3	3

Table 2
2006 American Society of Reproductive Medicine embryo transfer guidelines

In patients with two or more failed cycles or other unfavorable circumstances, additional embryos may be transferred with informed consent.
[a] In donor egg cycles use age of donor.
[b] First IVF cycle, good quality embryos, excess embryos for cryopreservation.

pregnancy may elect for single embryo transfer.[77,78] In the event of a multifetal pregnancy, selective reduction can be performed to reduce fetal number. The decision to perform the procedure is not a suitable option for some couples. Although reduction is associated with higher birth weights and lower rates of preterm delivery, this must be balanced against an approximately 5% risk of loss of the entire pregnancy.[79]

ART is associated with an increased risk of preterm delivery and low birth weight. It has been estimated that the cost to society per preterm birth is $51,600, with the medical cost in the first year being ten times greater for children born preterm compared with full-term babies.[80] Multiple studies and systematic reviews have found an increase in preterm delivery and low birth weight independent of the increase seen in multiple gestations.[81–86] A comparison of the 42,463 infants conceived with assisted reproductive technologies between 1996 and 1997 with the almost 3.4 million infants born in 1997 in the United States showed a 2.6 times (95% CI 2.3–2.6) increase in the risk of a low birth weight term (>37 weeks) infants for ART babies when compared with the general population.[81] This trend was also observed in preterm (<37 weeks) infants with a risk ratio of 1.4 (95% CI 1.3–1.5) but was not observed in twin ART pregnancies with a risk ratio of 1.0 (95% CI 1.0–1.1).[81] This observation has been supported by a recent meta-analysis that compared perinatal outcomes of in vitro fertilization twins with spontaneously conceived twins.[87] It showed that although IVF was associated with a very mild, if any, increase in preterm birth, it was not associated with an increase in low birth weight IVF twins.[87] Although the association between preterm birth and low birth weight infants has been established, the etiology remains unclear. The elevated risk ratio for preterm labor and low birth weight infants for singleton ART pregnancies in 2002 persisted when compared with the general population when analyzed by the cause for infertility, number of embryos cryopreserved, days of embryo culture, or the use of IVF, ICSI, or assisted hatching.[88] Proposed explanation for the difference in outcomes of ART pregnancies when compared with spontaneous pregnancies include the subset of infertility, maternal-fetal exposures to medications and ART procedures, treatment biases and obstetric practices of ART pregnancies, differences in the socioeconomic forces of the two populations, and altered circulating ovarian or uterine protein levels unique to ART pregnancies.

Although early studies failed to show an increased risk of congenital malformations among patients undergoing IVF and ICSI, more recent studies show a modest increase.[89,90] An Australian study found 26 of 301 infants conceived with ICSI (8.6%), 75 of 837 infants conceived with IVF (9.0%), and 168 of 4000 naturally conceived infants (4.2%) had a major birth defect identified before 1 year of age.[91]

This study highlighted that infants conceived with ICSI or IVF were twice as likely to have a major birth defect when compared with spontaneously conceived infants. This increase in congenital birth defects was confirmed by a recent meta-analysis of 25 studies that suggested a 30% to 40% increased risk of birth defects associated with ART.[90] A Swedish study that compared congenital malformations in 9175 infants born via IVF from 1982 to 1997 to the population base control group of 1,690,577 infants born in Sweden over the same period showed IVF was related with an almost threefold increase in neural tube defects, esophageal atresia, small gut atresia, anal atresia, omphalocele, and hypospadias.[92] The excess risk of hypospadias was seen only in infants that resulted from ISCI and was thought to be secondary to paternal subfertility. However, limitations of these studies, as well as other studies that have looked at the risk of congenital malformations in children born as a result of ART, include the relatively small number of defects detected and the possible increased diagnostic vigilance in ART-conceived pregnancies compared with spontaneously pregnancies. Furthermore, the increased risk of birth defects observed may be because of the underlying cause of infertility. Although most studies have used spontaneously conceived pregnancies from women without infertility as controls, a more appropriate control group would be spontaneously conceived pregnancies from women who sought infertility treatment or pregnancies resulting from couples undergoing ART after failed reversal of a tubal ligation or vasectomy.

Men with extreme oligozoospermia or azoospermia have an approximately 25% increased risk of genetic abnormalities.[93] ICSI in this population can result in an increased risk of unbalanced translocations, subsequent infertility of male offspring from inheritance of Y-chromosomal microdeletions, and cystic fibrosis if both parents are carriers of the CFTR gene mutation. A daughter conceived via ICSI from a father with an androgen-receptor gene defect caused by expansion of CAG trinucleotide repeats on the gene located on the X chromosome could have a son in the following generation affected by infertility and Kennedy's disease (spinal and bulbar atrophy).[94,95]

Many studies have looked at both short- and long-term neurologic sequelae in children born after IVF. IVF babies are at an increased risk of developing neurologic problems, especially cerebral palsy. However, this increase is likely secondary to the high frequency of twin pregnancies with associated increased risk of low birth weights and prematurity and not related to IVF directly.[96] A recent meta-analysis of nine studies reported that IVF had an increased risk of cerebral palsy associated with preterm delivery with an odds ratio of 2.18 (95% CI, 1.71–2.77), whereas eight studies looking at autism spectrum disorders, and 30 studies examining developmental delay failed to show any difference.[97] A Danish nationwide cohort study found similar rates of neurologic sequelae and cerebral palsy when twins conceived by assisted reproductive technologies were compared with spontaneously conceived twins or singleton pregnancies conceived by ART.[98] This same study also found similar rates of neurologic sequelae and cerebral palsy in children conceived with ICSI compared with children conceived by IVF with an odds ratios of 1.1 (95% CI, 0.7–1.7) and 0.9 (95% CI, 0.5–1.7), respectively. Multiple studies comparing children born with ICSI to spontaneously conceived children or children conceived by IVF have shown no difference in cognitive, psychomotor, and neurodevelopmental outcomes when examined 2, 5, and 10 years after birth.[99–103]

Assisted reproductive technologies may also influence imprinting disorders through epigenetic modifications. Rather than altering the DNA sequence, epigenetic changes involve modifications in DNA methylation of either maternal or paternal alleles, resulting in altered gene expression. Although nine human imprinting disorders exist, only 3 have been potentially linked to assisted reproductive technologies.[104] Angelman syndrome, a neurogenetic disorder characterized by mental retardation, developmental delays, seizures, jerky movements, hand-flapping, absence of speech, and a happy disposition, is caused by a loss of function of a gene on maternal chromosome 15.[105] A study of two children with Angelman syndrome conceived with ICSI found hypomethylation of the maternal chromosome 15, suggesting ICSI may increase the risk of imprinting disorders in children conceived by ART.[106] Epigenetic alterations LIT1 and H19 on chromosome 11 have also been seen in children with Beckwith-Wiedemann syndrome who were conceived by ART.[107] This syndrome is characterized by macroglossia, macrosomia, midline abdominal wall defects, ear creases/ear pits, and neonatal hypoglycemia.[108] It has been suggested that maternal hypomethylation syndrome may be associated with abnormal imprinting in patients conceived by ART.[104] Animal data in mice has suggested that the length of time in culture and certain culture conditions may predispose to imprinting disorders; however, it is still uncertain whether there is an association in humans.[109–112] Additionally, while the possible association between ART and imprinting disorders has been raised by the above studies, the infrequency of imprinting disorders makes them difficult to study and prone to selection bias. Further research on the effect of embryo culture conditions in humans, as well as large-scale epidemiologic studies with appropriate control groups are needed to clarify the relationship of imprinting disorders with impaired fertility and ART.

FERTILITY PRESERVATION AND ASSISTIVE REPRODUCTIVE TECHNOLOGIES

ARTs offer a unique opportunity to preserve fertility in pediatric and adolescent populations with cancer. Fortunately, survival and cure rates for childhood cancers have increased dramatically. However, both systemic chemotherapy and radiation therapy directed to areas that contain the gonads may result in premature gonadal failure, subfertility, or infertility. Various treatment strategies exist to minimize risk to the gonads and preserve fertility either before or during treatment. Discussions regarding fertility preservation and the available modalities should involve the patient and family and take into account the child's age and cancer type.

Various treatment strategies exist to preserve male fertility both during and before treatment. Although findings from studies in rats suggested gonadotropin-releasing agonist could protect the male gonads from cytotoxic chemotherapy, no benefit has been observed in humans.[113–117] For male patients undergoing radiation therapy, gonads can be shielded or relocated outside the radiation field to the thigh or anterior abdominal wall. The most common technique to preserve male fertility is cryopreservation of sperm obtained from masturbation. Cryopreserved sperm can be used later for intrauterine insemination or intracytoplasmic sperm injection in combination with in vitro fertilization. In boys not psychologically ready to produce a specimen for cryopreservation, penile vibratory stimulation and electroejaculation can be performed under general anesthesia.[118] Sperm production occurs around age 13, with one study showing the rate of spermaturia, a marker for spermarche, occurs in almost 69% of adolescent boys by age 13 compared with less than 1% of boys at age 11.[119] Discussions of masturbation and future fertility should be approached with sensitivity, as this can be a source of embarrassment for adolescent boys. The use of testicular cryopreservation, spermatogonial stem cell transplantation, and in vitro maturation of sperm are experimental. These are areas of ongoing research and may be available in the future when these techniques are developed further.

Similarly, there are a variety of approaches to preserving female fertility during chemotherapy, radiation treatment, and surgery for early-stage tumors. The use of gonadotropin-releasing hormone agonists to reduce chemotherapy-induced ovarian damage may be of benefit. A recent prospective, randomized study in young adult women undergoing combination chemotherapy for breast cancer found women that received gonadotropin-releasing agonists were more likely to have resumption of menses (90% versus 33%), return to spontaneous ovulation (69% versus 26%), and decreased risk of premature ovarian failure (11% versus 67%) compared with controls.[120] Ovarian shielding or ovarian transposition can be performed to minimize radiation exposure for those receiving pelvic radiation.[121–123] Children and women who have not completed childbearing undergoing surgery for ovarian stromal tumors, germ cell tumors, and borderline and stage Ia epithelial ovarian cancers should be offered conservative fertility-sparing surgery.[124–127] This includes exploratory laparotomy with unilateral salingo-oophorectomy and surgical staging, with preservation of the contralateral ovary and uterus.

Before treatment, cryopreservation of embryos, oocytes, and ovarian tissue may be performed.[128] Cryopreservation of embryos and mature oocytes requires postponement of treatment as well as hormonal stimulation. These methods are not recommended for individuals with advanced stage or aggressive cancers or in cases of estrogen receptor sensitive tumors. Although cryopreservation of embryos is a well-established technique commonly used to store surplus embryos from in vitro fertilization cycles, it requires an immediately available partner or the use of donor sperm. Oocyte cryopreservation circumvents the need for a current partner. This procedure is investigational with limited long-term follow-up studies. Although pregnancies have been reported from cryopreserved oocytes, pregnancy rates are lower than those observed using cryopreserved embryos.[129,130] Ovarian tissue cryopreservation is also an investigational technique for fertility preservation with limited safety and efficacy data. The advantage of this method over embryo and oocyte cryopreservation is that ovarian tissue can be obtained quickly without delaying treatment and does not require ovarian stimulation. Similar to oocyte cryopreservation, ovarian cryopreservation does not require a current partner. Immature oocytes from ovarian tissue can be harvested and matured in vitro either before freezing or after thawing. Alternatively, ovarian tissue can be reimplanted after treatment is complete. In addition to possible fertility preservation, autotransplantation also preserves the endocrine function of the ovary.[131–133] Although the use of both oocyte and ovarian tissue cryopreservation holds promise in preserving fertility, their use is investigational. These procedures should only be performed in a research setting with informed consent and institutional review board approval until optimal protocols have been developed and the safety of these methods has been validated.[134,135]

The approach to fertility preservation in children with cancer is a complex issue and requires a comprehensive approach from an interdisciplinary team. It is imperative that the child and family be explained the potential impact of treatment on future fertility potential and made aware of available fertility preservation options. Both informed assent by the child and informed consent of the parents are paramount in establishing a plan for cancer treatment and fertility preservation.[136,137] This requires close communication between the family and the medical team, which may involve pediatricians, medical oncologists, radiation oncologists, oncologic surgeons, reproductive endocrinologists, reproductive biologists, geneticists, embryologists, psychiatrists, and medical ethicists.

SUMMARY

Assisted reproductive technologies are important tools in the clinical armamentarium used to treat both female and male infertility disorders. Preimplantation genetic diagnosis offers couples at risk of having children with inheritable disorders the ability to analyze the genetic make-up of embryos before transfer. For patients undergoing treatment of cancer with chemotherapy or radiation therapy, these technologies offer the potential for the preservation of future fertility. Assisted reproductive technologies are not without risks, and it is imperative to continue to perfect treatment strategies to increase success rates, while at the same time reducing the risk of treatment complications, higher-order multiple pregnancies, and preterm birth. Concerns regarding the possible association of assisted reproductive technologies with congenital malformations and epigenetic modifications have been proposed in the literature. Further research with large-scale, carefully controlled studies is necessary to analyze the outcomes of these pregnancies. As technology evolves, it is likely the clinical applications of assisted reproduction will continue to develop and expand in the future to enhance fertility.

REFERENCES

1. Steptoe PC, Edwards RG. Birth after the reimplantation of a human embryo. Lancet 1978;2(8085):366.
2. Available at: www.cdc.gov/art/art2005/. Accessed Jan 19, 2009.
3. Hamilton BE, Martin JA, Ventura SJ. Births: preliminary data for 2005. Natl Vital Stat Rep 2006;55(11):1–18.
4. Chandra A, Martinez GM, Mosher WD, et al. Fertility, family planning, and reproductive health of U.S. women: data from the 2002 National Survey of Family Growth. Vital Health Stat 2005;23(25):1–160.
5. Trounson A, Mohr L. Human pregnancy following cryopreservation, thawing and transfer of an eight-cell embryo. Nature 1983;305(5936):707–9.
6. Palermo G, Joris H, Devroey P, et al. Pregnancies after intracytoplasmic injection of single spermatozoon into an oocyte. Lancet 1992;340(8810):17–8.
7. Handyside AH, Kontogianni EH, Hardy K, et al. Pregnancies from biopsied human preimplantation embryos sexed by Y-specific DNA amplification. Nature 1990;344(6268):768–70.
8. Muasher SJ, Oehninger S, Simonetti S, et al. The value of basal and/or stimulated serum gonadotropin levels in prediction of stimulation response and in vitro fertilization outcome. Fertil Steril 1988;50(2):298–307.
9. Scott RT, Toner JP, Muasher SJ, et al. Follicle-stimulating hormone levels on cycle day 3 are predictive of in vitro fertilization outcome. Fertil Steril 1989;51(4):651–4.
10. Toner JP, Philput CB, Jones GS, et al. Basal follicle-stimulating hormone level is a better predictor of in vitro fertilization performance than age. Fertil Steril 1991;55(4):784–91.
11. Licciardi FL, Liu HC, Rosenwaks Z. Day 3 estradiol serum concentrations as prognosticators of ovarian stimulation response and pregnancy outcome in patients undergoing in vitro fertilization. Fertil Steril 1995;64(5):991–4.
12. Smotrich DB, Widra EA, Gindoff PR, et al. Prognostic value of day 3 estradiol on in vitro fertilization outcome. Fertil Steril 1995;64(6):1136–40.
13. Tomas C, Nuojua-Huttunen S, Martikainen H. Pretreatment transvaginal ultrasound examination predicts ovarian responsiveness to gonadotrophins in in-vitro fertilization. Hum Reprod 1997;12(2):220–3.

14. Chang MY, Chiang CH, Hsieh TT, et al. Use of the antral follicle count to predict the outcome of assisted reproductive technologies. Fertil Steril 1998;69(3):505–10.
15. Seifer DB, MacLaughlin DT, Christian BP, et al. Early follicular serum mullerian-inhibiting substance levels are associated with ovarian response during assisted reproductive technology cycles. Fertil Steril 2002;77(3):468–71.
16. Mansour R, Aboulghar M, Serour G. Dummy embryo transfer: a technique that minimizes the problems of embryo transfer and improves the pregnancy rate in human in vitro fertilization. Fertil Steril 1990;54(4):678–81.
17. Clark JH, Markaverich BM. The agonistic-antagonistic properties of clomiphene: a review. Pharmacol Ther 1981;15(3):467–519.
18. Matikainen T, Ding YQ, Vergara M, et al. Differing responses of plasma bioactive and immunoreactive follicle-stimulating hormone and luteinizing hormone to gonadotropin-releasing hormone antagonist and agonist treatments in postmenopausal women. J Clin Endocrinol Metab 1992;75(3):820–5.
19. Daya S. Gonadotropin releasing hormone agonist protocols for pituitary desensitization in in vitro fertilization and gamete intrafallopian transfer cycles. Cochrane Database Syst Rev 2000;(2):CD001299.
20. Demirol A, Gurgan T. Comparison of microdose flare-up and antagonist multiple-dose protocols for poor-responder patients: a randomized study. Fertil Steril 2008; [epub ahead of print].
21. Leroy I, d'Acremont M, Brailly-Tabard S, et al. A single injection of a gonadotropin-releasing hormone (GnRH) antagonist (Cetrorelix) postpones the luteinizing hormone (LH) surge: further evidence for the role of GnRH during the LH surge. Fertil Steril 1994;62(3):461–7.
22. Ludwig M, Felberbaum RE, Devroey P, et al. Significant reduction of the incidence of ovarian hyperstimulation syndrome (OHSS) by using the LHRH antagonist Cetrorelix (Cetrotide) in controlled ovarian stimulation for assisted reproduction. Arch Gynecol Obstet 2000;264(1):29–32.
23. Speroff L, Fritz MA. Clinical gynecologic endocrinology and infertility. 7th edition. Philadelphia: Lippincott Williams & Wilkins; 2005.
24. Bennett SJ, Waterstone JJ, Cheng WC, et al. Complications of transvaginal ultrasound-directed follicle aspiration: a review of 2670 consecutive procedures. J Assist Reprod Genet 1993;10(1):72–7.
25. Veeck LL. An atlas of human gametes and conceptuses: an illustrated reference for assisted reproductive technology. New York: Parthenon Pub. Group; 1999.
26. Edi-Osagie E, Hooper L, Seif MW. The impact of assisted hatching on live birth rates and outcomes of assisted conception: a systematic review. Hum Reprod 2003;18(9):1828–35.
27. Seif MM, Edi-Osagie EC, Farquhar C, et al. Assisted hatching on assisted conception (IVF & ICSI). Cochrane Database Syst Rev 2006;(1):CD001894.
28. The role of assisted hatching in in vitro fertilization: a review of the literature. A Committee opinion. Fertil Steril 2008;90(Suppl 5):S196–8.
29. Blake D, Proctor M, Johnson N, et al. Cleavage stage versus blastocyst stage embryo transfer in assisted conception. Cochrane Database Syst Rev 2005;(4):CD002118.
30. Sheiner E, Har-Vardi I, Potashnik G. The potential association between blastocyst transfer and monozygotic twinning. Fertil Steril 2001;75(1):217–8.
31. Milki AA, Jun SH, Hinckley MD, et al. Incidence of monozygotic twinning with blastocyst transfer compared to cleavage-stage transfer. Fertil Steril 2003; 79(3):503–6.

32. Jain JK, Boostanfar R, Slater CC, et al. Monozygotic twins and triplets in association with blastocyst transfer. J Assist Reprod Genet 2004;21(4):103–7.
33. Wright V, Schieve LA, Vahratian A, et al. Monozygotic twinning associated with day 5 embryo transfer in pregnancies conceived after IVF. Hum Reprod 2004; 19(8):1831–6.
34. Blastocyst culture and transfer in clinical-assisted reproduction. Fertil Steril 2008;90(Suppl 5):S174–7.
35. Amso NN, Ahuja KK, Morris N, et al. The management of predicted ovarian hyperstimulation involving gonadotropin-releasing hormone analog with elective cryopreservation of all pre-embryos. Fertil Steril 1990;53(6):1087–90.
36. Ferraretti AP, Gianaroli L, Magli C, et al. Elective cryopreservation of all pronucleate embryos in women at risk of ovarian hyperstimulation syndrome: efficiency and safety. Hum Reprod 1999;14(6):1457–60.
37. Preimplantation genetic testing: a Practice Committee opinion. Fertil Steril 2008; 90(Suppl 5):S136–43.
38. Mastenbroek S, Twisk M, van Echten-Arends J, et al. In vitro fertilization with preimplantation genetic screening. N Engl J Med 2007;357(1):9–17.
39. Handyside AH, Lesko JG, Tarin JJ, et al. Birth of a normal girl after in vitro fertilization and preimplantation diagnostic testing for cystic fibrosis. N Engl J Med 1992;327(13):905–9.
40. Ray PF, Kaeda JS, Bingham J, et al. Preimplantation genetic diagnosis of beta-thalassaemia major. Lancet 1996;347(9016):1696.
41. Xu K, Shi ZM, Veeck LL, et al. First unaffected pregnancy using preimplantation genetic diagnosis for sickle cell anemia. JAMA 1999;281(18):1701–6.
42. Grifo JA, Tang YX, Cohen J, et al. Pregnancy after embryo biopsy and coamplification of DNA from X and Y chromosomes. JAMA 1992;268(6):727–9.
43. Sermon K, Lissens W, Joris H, et al. Clinical application of preimplantation diagnosis for myotonic dystrophy. Prenat Diagn 1997;17(10):925–32.
44. Ao A, Wells D, Handyside AH, et al. Preimplantation genetic diagnosis of inherited cancer: familial adenomatous polyposis coli. J Assist Reprod Genet 1998;15(3):140–4.
45. Spits C, De Rycke M, Van Ranst N, et al. Preimplantation genetic diagnosis for cancer predisposition syndromes. Prenat Diagn 2007;27(5):447–56.
46. Abou-Sleiman PM, Apessos A, Harper JC, et al. First application of preimplantation genetic diagnosis to neurofibromatosis type 2 (NF2). Prenat Diagn 2002;22(6):519–24.
47. Verlinsky Y, Rechitsky S, Verlinsky O, et al. Preimplantation diagnosis for neurofibromatosis. Reprod Biomed Online 2002;4(3):218–22.
48. Verlinsky Y, Rechitsky S, Verlinsky O, et al. Preimplantation diagnosis for p53 tumour suppressor gene mutations. Reprod Biomed Online 2001;2(2):102–5.
49. Schulman JD, Black SH, Handyside A, et al. Preimplantation genetic testing for Huntington disease and certain other dominantly inherited disorders. Clin Genet 1996;49(2):57–8.
50. Verlinsky Y, Rechitsky S, Verlinsky O, et al. Preimplantation diagnosis for early-onset Alzheimer disease caused by V717L mutation. JAMA 2002;287(8): 1018–21.
51. Seeho SK, Burton G, Leigh D, et al. The role of preimplantation genetic diagnosis in the management of severe rhesus alloimmunization: first unaffected pregnancy: case report. Hum Reprod 2005;20(3):697–701.
52. Verlinsky Y, Rechitsky S, Schoolcraft W, et al. Preimplantation diagnosis for Fanconi anemia combined with HLA matching. JAMA 2001;285(24):3130–3.

53. Klip H, Burger CW, Kenemans P, et al. Cancer risk associated with subfertility and ovulation induction: a review. Cancer Causes Control 2000;11(4): 319–44.

54. Venn A, Watson L, Lumley J, et al. Breast and ovarian cancer incidence after infertility and in vitro fertilisation. Lancet 1995;346(8981):995–1000.

55. Navot D, Relou A, Birkenfeld A, et al. Risk factors and prognostic variables in the ovarian hyperstimulation syndrome. Am J Obstet Gynecol 1988;159(1):210–5.

56. Enskog A, Henriksson M, Unander M, et al. Prospective study of the clinical and laboratory parameters of patients in whom ovarian hyperstimulation syndrome developed during controlled ovarian hyperstimulation for in vitro fertilization. Fertil Steril 1999;71(5):808–14.

57. Haning RV Jr, Austin CW, Carlson IH, et al. Plasma estradiol is superior to ultrasound and urinary estriol glucuronide as a predictor of ovarian hyperstimulation during induction of ovulation with menotropins. Fertil Steril 1983;40(1):31–6.

58. Golan A, Ron-el R, Herman A, et al. Ovarian hyperstimulation syndrome: an update review. Obstet Gynecol Surv 1989;44(6):430–40.

59. Herman A, Ron-El R, Golan A, et al. Pregnancy rate and ovarian hyperstimulation after luteal human chorionic gonadotropin in in vitro fertilization stimulated with gonadotropin-releasing hormone analog and menotropins. Fertil Steril 1990;53(1):92–6.

60. Whelan JG III, Vlahos NF. The ovarian hyperstimulation syndrome. Fertil Steril 2000;73(5):883–96.

61. Pattinson HA, Hignett M, Dunphy BC, et al. Outcome of thaw embryo transfer after cryopreservation of all embryos in patients at risk of ovarian hyperstimulation syndrome. Fertil Steril 1994;62(6):1192–6.

62. Pezeshki K, Feldman J, Stein DE, et al. Bleeding and spontaneous abortion after therapy for infertility. Fertil Steril 2000;74(3):504–8.

63. Ball RH, Ade CM, Schoenborn JA, et al. The clinical significance of ultrasonographically detected subchorionic hemorrhages. Am J Obstet Gynecol 1996; 174(3):996–1002.

64. Clayton HB, Schieve LA, Peterson HB, et al. Ectopic pregnancy risk with assisted reproductive technology procedures. Obstet Gynecol 2006;107(3):595–604.

65. Nazari A, Askari HA, Check JH, et al. Embryo transfer technique as a cause of ectopic pregnancy in in vitro fertilization. Fertil Steril 1993;60(5):919–21.

66. Reece EA, Petrie RH, Sirmans MF, et al. Combined intrauterine and extrauterine gestations: a review. Am J Obstet Gynecol 1983;146(3):323–30.

67. Tal J, Haddad S, Gordon N, et al. Heterotopic pregnancy after ovulation induction and assisted reproductive technologies: a literature review from 1971 to 1993. Fertil Steril 1996;66(1):1–12.

68. Wilcox AJ, Weinberg CR, O'Connor JF, et al. Incidence of early loss of pregnancy. N Engl J Med 1988;319(4):189–94.

69. Schieve LA, Tatham L, Peterson HB, et al. Spontaneous abortion among pregnancies conceived using assisted reproductive technology in the United States. Obstet Gynecol 2003;101(5 Pt 1):959–67.

70. Derom C, Vlietinck R, Derom R, et al. Increased monozygotic twinning rate after ovulation induction. Lancet 1987;1(8544):1236–8.

71. Schieve LA, Meikle SF, Peterson HB, et al. Does assisted hatching pose a risk for monozygotic twinning in pregnancies conceived through in vitro fertilization? Fertil Steril 2000;74(2):288–94.

72. Schieve LA, Peterson HB, Meikle SF, et al. Live-birth rates and multiple-birth risk using in vitro fertilization. JAMA 1999;282(19):1832–8.

73. Schinzel AA, Smith DW, Miller JR. Monozygotic twinning and structural defects. J Pediatr 1979;95(6):921–30.
74. Templeton A, Morris JK. Reducing the risk of multiple births by transfer of two embryos after in vitro fertilization. N Engl J Med 1998;339(9):573–7.
75. Shulman A, Ben-Nun I, Ghetler Y, et al. Relationship between embryo morphology and implantation rate after in vitro fertilization treatment in conception cycles. Fertil Steril 1993;60(1):123–6.
76. Guidelines on number of embryos transferred. Fertil Steril 2006;86(Suppl 5): S51–2.
77. Strandell A, Bergh C, Lundin K. Selection of patients suitable for one-embryo transfer may reduce the rate of multiple births by half without impairment of overall birth rates. Hum Reprod 2000;15(12):2520–5.
78. Martikainen H, Tiitinen A, Tomas C, et al. One versus two embryo transfer after IVF and ICSI: a randomized study. Hum Reprod 2001;16(9):1900–3.
79. Stone J, Ferrara L, Kamrath J, et al. Contemporary outcomes with the latest 1000 cases of multifetal pregnancy reduction (MPR). Am J Obstet Gynecol 2008; 199(4):e401–4.
80. Behrman RE, Butler AS. Institute of medicine (US). Committee on understanding premature birth and assuring healthy outcomes. Preterm birth: causes, consequences, and prevention. Washington, DC: National Academies Press; 2007.
81. Schieve LA, Meikle SF, Ferre C, et al. Low and very low birth weight in infants conceived with use of assisted reproductive technology. N Engl J Med 2002; 346(10):731–7.
82. McGovern PG, Llorens AJ, Skurnick JH, et al. Increased risk of preterm birth in singleton pregnancies resulting from in vitro fertilization-embryo transfer or gamete intrafallopian transfer: a meta-analysis. Fertil Steril 2004;82(6):1514–20.
83. Jackson RA, Gibson KA, Wu YW, et al. Perinatal outcomes in singletons following in vitro fertilization: a meta-analysis. Obstet Gynecol 2004;103(3):551–63.
84. Helmerhorst FM, Perquin DA, Donker D, et al. Perinatal outcome of singletons and twins after assisted conception: a systematic review of controlled studies. BMJ 2004;328(7434):261.
85. Halliday J. Outcomes of IVF conceptions: are they different? Best Pract Res Clin Obstet Gynaecol 2007;21(1):67–81.
86. Wang YA, Sullivan EA, Black D, et al. Preterm birth and low birth weight after assisted reproductive technology-related pregnancy in Australia between 1996 and 2000. Fertil Steril 2005;83(6):1650–8.
87. McDonald S, Murphy K, Beyene J, et al. Perinatal outcomes of in vitro fertilization twins: a systematic review and meta-analyses. Am J Obstet Gynecol 2005; 193(1):141–52.
88. Schieve LA, Ferre C, Peterson HB, et al. Perinatal outcome among singleton infants conceived through assisted reproductive technology in the United States. Obstet Gynecol 2004;103(6):1144–53.
89. Van Steirteghem A. Outcome of assisted reproductive technology. N Engl J Med 1998;338(3):194–5.
90. Hansen M, Bower C, Milne E, et al. Assisted reproductive technologies and the risk of birth defects–a systematic review. Hum Reprod 2005;20(2):328–38.
91. Hansen M, Kurinczuk JJ, Bower C, et al. The risk of major birth defects after intracytoplasmic sperm injection and in vitro fertilization. N Engl J Med 2002; 346(10):725–30.
92. Ericson A, Kallen B. Congenital malformations in infants born after IVF: a population-based study. Hum Reprod 2001;16(3):504–9.

93. Dohle GR, Halley DJ, Van Hemel JO, et al. Genetic risk factors in infertile men with severe oligozoospermia and azoospermia. Hum Reprod 2002; 17(1):13–6.

94. Dowsing AT, Yong EL, Clark M, et al. Linkage between male infertility and trinucleotide repeat expansion in the androgen-receptor gene. Lancet 1999; 354(9179):640–3.

95. Patrizio P, Leonard DG, Chen KL, et al. Larger trinucleotide repeat size in the androgen receptor gene of infertile men with extremely severe oligozoospermia. J Androl 2001;22(3):444–8.

96. Stromberg B, Dahlquist G, Ericson A, et al. Neurological sequelae in children born after in-vitro fertilisation: a population-based study. Lancet 2002; 359(9305):461–5.

97. Hvidtjorn D, Schieve L, Schendel D, et al. Cerebral palsy, autism spectrum disorders, and developmental delay in children born after assisted conception: a systematic review and meta-analysis. Arch Pediatr Adolesc Med 2009; 163(1):72–83.

98. Pinborg A, Loft A, Schmidt L, et al. Neurological sequelae in twins born after assisted conception: controlled national cohort study. BMJ 2004;329(7461):311.

99. Agarwal P, Loh SK, Lim SB, et al. Two-year neurodevelopmental outcome in children conceived by intracytoplasmic sperm injection: prospective cohort study. BJOG 2005;112(10):1376–83.

100. Bonduelle M, Ponjaert I, Steirteghem AV, et al. Developmental outcome at 2 years of age for children born after ICSI compared with children born after IVF. Hum Reprod 2003;18(2):342–50.

101. Place I, Englert Y. A prospective longitudinal study of the physical, psychomotor, and intellectual development of singleton children up to 5 years who were conceived by intracytoplasmic sperm injection compared with children conceived spontaneously and by in vitro fertilization. Fertil Steril 2003;80(6):1388–97.

102. Ponjaert-Kristoffersen I, Bonduelle M, Barnes J, et al. International collaborative study of intracytoplasmic sperm injection-conceived, in vitro fertilization-conceived, and naturally conceived 5-year-old child outcomes: cognitive and motor assessments. Pediatrics 2005;115(3):e283–9.

103. Leunens L, Celestin-Westreich S, Bonduelle M, et al. Follow-up of cognitive and motor development of 10-year-old singleton children born after ICSI compared with spontaneously conceived children. Hum Reprod 2008;23(1):105–11.

104. Amor DJ, Halliday J. A review of known imprinting syndromes and their association with assisted reproduction technologies. Hum Reprod 2008;23(12):2826–34.

105. Knoll JH, Nicholls RD, Magenis RE, et al. Angelman and Prader-Willi syndromes share a common chromosome 15 deletion but differ in parental origin of the deletion. Am J Med Genet 1989;32(2):285–90.

106. Cox GF, Burger J, Lip V, et al. Intracytoplasmic sperm injection may increase the risk of imprinting defects. Am J Hum Genet 2002;71(1):162–4.

107. DeBaun MR, Niemitz EL, Feinberg AP. Association of in vitro fertilization with Beckwith-Wiedemann syndrome and epigenetic alterations of LIT1 and H19. Am J Hum Genet 2003;72(1):156–60.

108. DeBaun MR, Niemitz EL, McNeil DE, et al. Epigenetic alterations of H19 and LIT1 distinguish patients with Beckwith-Wiedemann syndrome with cancer and birth defects. Am J Hum Genet 2002;70(3):604–11.

109. Doherty AS, Mann MR, Tremblay KD, et al. Differential effects of culture on imprinted H19 expression in the preimplantation mouse embryo. Biol Reprod 2000;62(6):1526–35.

110. Khosla S, Dean W, Brown D, et al. Culture of preimplantation mouse embryos affects fetal development and the expression of imprinted genes. Biol Reprod 2001;64(3):918–26.

111. Ecker DJ, Stein P, Xu Z, et al. Long-term effects of culture of preimplantation mouse embryos on behavior. Proc Natl Acad Sci U S A 2004;101(6):1595–600.

112. Fernandez-Gonzalez R, Moreira P, Bilbao A, et al. Long-term effect of in vitro culture of mouse embryos with serum on mRNA expression of imprinting genes, development, and behavior. Proc Natl Acad Sci U S A 2004;101(16):5880–5.

113. Ward JA, Robinson J, Furr BJ, et al. Protection of spermatogenesis in rats from the cytotoxic procarbazine by the depot formulation of Zoladex, a gonadotropin-releasing hormone agonist. Cancer Res 1990;50(3):568–74.

114. Johnson DH, Linde R, Hainsworth JD, et al. Effect of a luteinizing hormone releasing hormone agonist given during combination chemotherapy on post-therapy fertility in male patients with lymphoma: preliminary observations. Blood 1985;65(4):832–6.

115. Waxman JH, Ahmed R, Smith D, et al. Failure to preserve fertility in patients with Hodgkin's disease. Cancer Chemother Pharmacol 1987;19(2):159–62.

116. Krause W, Pfluger KH. Treatment with the gonadotropin-releasing hormone agonist buserelin to protect spermatogenesis against cytotoxic treatment in young men. Andrologia 1989;21(3):265–70.

117. Kreuser ED, Hetzel WD, Hautmann R, et al. Reproductive toxicity with and without LHRHA administration during adjuvant chemotherapy in patients with germ cell tumors. Horm Metab Res 1990;22(9):494–8.

118. Schmiegelow ML, Sommer P, Carlsen E, et al. Penile vibratory stimulation and electroejaculation before anticancer therapy in two pubertal boys. J Pediatr Hematol Oncol 1998;20(5):429–30.

119. Hirsch M, Lunenfeld B, Modan M, et al. Spermarche–the age of onset of sperm emission. J Adolesc Health Care 1985;6(1):35–9.

120. Badawy A, Elnashar A, El-Ashry M, et al. Gonadotropin-releasing hormone agonists for prevention of chemotherapy-induced ovarian damage: prospective randomized study. Fertil Steril 2009;91(3):694–7.

121. Husseinzadeh N, Nahhas WA, Velkley DE, et al. The preservation of ovarian function in young women undergoing pelvic radiation therapy. Gynecol Oncol 1984;18(3):373–9.

122. Covens AL, van der Putten HW, Fyles AW, et al. Laparoscopic ovarian transposition. Eur J Gynaecol Oncol 1996;17(3):177–82.

123. Morice P, Castaigne D, Haie-Meder C, et al. Laparoscopic ovarian transposition for pelvic malignancies: indications and functional outcomes. Fertil Steril 1998; 70(5):956–60.

124. Perrin LC, Low J, Nicklin JL, et al. Fertility and ovarian function after conservative surgery for germ cell tumours of the ovary. Aust N Z J Obstet Gynaecol 1999; 39(2):243–5.

125. Zanetta G, Bonazzi C, Cantu M, et al. Survival and reproductive function after treatment of malignant germ cell ovarian tumors. J Clin Oncol 2001;19(4): 1015–20.

126. Morice P, Camatte S, El Hassan J, et al. Clinical outcomes and fertility after conservative treatment of ovarian borderline tumors. Fertil Steril 2001;75(1):92–6.

127. Morice P, Wicart-Poque F, Rey A, et al. Results of conservative treatment in epithelial ovarian carcinoma. Cancer 2001;92(9):2412–8.

128. Jeruss JS, Woodruff TK. Preservation of fertility in patients with cancer. N Engl J Med 2009;360(9):902–11.

129. Porcu E, Venturoli S. Progress with oocyte cryopreservation. Curr Opin Obstet Gynecol 2006;18(3):273–9.
130. Oktay K, Cil AP, Bang H. Efficiency of oocyte cryopreservation: a meta-analysis. Fertil Steril 2006;86(1):70–80.
131. Oktay K, Karlikaya G. Ovarian function after transplantation of frozen, banked autologous ovarian tissue. N Engl J Med 2000;342(25):1919.
132. Donnez J, Dolmans MM, Demylle D, et al. Live birth after orthotopic transplantation of cryopreserved ovarian tissue. Lancet 2004;364(9443):1405–10.
133. Meirow D, Levron J, Eldar-Geva T, et al. Pregnancy after transplantation of cryopreserved ovarian tissue in a patient with ovarian failure after chemotherapy. N Engl J Med 2005;353(3):318–21.
134. Ovarian tissue and oocyte cryopreservation. Fertil Steril 2008;90(Suppl 5): S241–6.
135. ACOG Committee Opinion No. 405: Ovarian tissue and oocyte cryopreservation. Obstet Gynecol 2008;111(5):1255–6.
136. Dudzinski DM. Ethical issues in fertility preservation for adolescent cancer survivors: oocyte and ovarian tissue cryopreservation. J Pediatr Adolesc Gynecol 2004;17(2):97–102.
137. Patrizio P, Butts S, Caplan A. Ovarian tissue preservation and future fertility: emerging technologies and ethical considerations. J Natl Cancer Inst Monogr 2005;34:107–10.

Fetal Assessment During Pregnancy

Darren Farley, MD, Donald J. Dudley, MD*

KEYWORDS
- Fetal monitoring • Pregnancy
- Antepartum • Intrapartum • Fetal heart rate

The use of fetal monitoring in pregnancy varies depending on the clinical scenario. The goal of fetal monitoring during pregnancy is to prevent fetal death.[1] In the first and early second trimesters, maternal symptoms may prompt further evaluation of the pregnancy to ensure there is not a problem with the pregnancy that puts the mother or fetus at risk. Throughout the rest of the pregnancy, the fetal heart rate is periodically auscultated with a handheld Doppler device, depending on the gestational age. Uterine fundal height is measured at each prenatal visit to assess for fetal growth, especially after 20 weeks, as the height in centimeters corresponds to the weeks of gestational age. Frequently, sonography is used to assess fetal anatomy in the second trimester. While sonography is a frequently ordered test, universal screening with ultrasound is controversial. If the pregnancy is progressing without complication, prenatal visits occur every 4 weeks through 28 weeks, every 2 weeks through 36 weeks, and then weekly for the remainder of the pregnancy. Should complications occur, fetal surveillance is initiated. Fetal surveillance may include nonstress testing, biophysical profiles, and Doppler velocimetry in a variety of possible combinations. Depending on the results of testing, gestational age, and overall clinical situation, delivery may be warranted if the risks of continuing the pregnancy outweigh the benefits.

BRIEF REVIEW OF PERTINENT FETAL PHYSIOLOGY

According to the American College of Obstetricians and Gynecologists (ACOG), the primary goal of antepartum fetal surveillance is the prevention of fetal death.[1] Most testing methods have high negative predictive values, meaning that the chance of fetal death within 1 week of a reassuring test is rare.[1] The various forms of fetal surveillance carry a wide range of positive predictive values, making interpretation somewhat difficult and often requiring the obstetrician to employ further testing. Studies have shown that fetal heart-rate (FHR) pattern, level of activity, and degree of fetal muscular tone are sensitive predictors of hypoxemia and acidemia.[2,3] Oligohydramnios, or

Division of Maternal-Fetal Medicine, Department of Obstetrics and Gynecology, University of Texas Health Science Center at San Antonio, 7703 Floyd Curl Drive, MSC 7836, San Antonio, TX 78229-3900, USA
* Corresponding author.
E-mail address: dudleyd@uthscsa.edu (D.J. Dudley).

Pediatr Clin N Am 56 (2009) 489–504
doi:10.1016/j.pcl.2009.03.001
0031-3955/09/$ – see front matter © 2009 Elsevier Inc. All rights reserved.

diminished amniotic fluid volume, may occur with redistribution of fetal blood flow in response to hypoxemia.[4]

These principles provide the basis for fetal surveillance, in that fetal oxygenation status as related to physiologic parameters can be indirectly tested. The ability of a fetus to have breathing and body movements, and accelerate its heart rate in response to these movements, is related to fetal oxygenation and metabolic state. Fetal movements begin early in pregnancy, as on average maternal perception of fetal movements occurs at about 20-week's gestation. As pregnancy advances, fetal movements become more synchronized and sophisticated. Nijhuis and colleagues[5] originally described several fetal behavioral states and categorized these as states 1F through 4F.[6] These states are present in most fetuses in the late third trimester. State 1F is quiescence, or quiet sleep, with low FHR variability. State 2F is an active sleep state, similar to rapid eye movement, and includes frequent gross body movements, continuous eye movements, and increased FHR variability. State 3F is another state of relative quiescence that includes continuous eye movements but without body movements or FHR accelerations. State 4F includes vigorous body movements, continuous eye movements, and accelerations of the fetal heart rate.[6] While useful to aid in the understanding of fetal physiology, fetal-state assessment in general is rarely used clinically.

As the fetus develops with advancing gestational age, the fetus acquires capability for more complex movements, including the ability to accelerate its heart rate in response to movements, breathing, flexion, and extension of limbs. These physiologic capabilities provide a basis for the interpretation and validation of most fetal-surveillance testing strategies, and in particular the fetal biophysical profile.

In 1972, Dawes and colleagues[7] originally described fetal-breathing movements in sheep and noted that there were two specific types of movements, including gasping/sighing and irregular bursts of diaphragmatic movements with paradoxic chest wall and abdominal wall movement. They found that inspiration corresponded to chest wall contraction and abdominal extension, while expiration corresponded to chest wall expansion and abdominal contraction.[7] Fetal breathing movements increase with advancing gestation, and may precede the ability of the fetus to accelerate its heart rate. The potential for breathing activity to be a reliable marker of fetal health is limited because many factors regulate fetal breathing activity.[6] For example, the absence of fetal breathing movements using sonographic evaluation may be because of fetal hypoxia, labor (term and preterm), hypoglycemia, sound stimuli, cigarette smoking, and fetal interventions, such as amniocentesis.[6] While fetal breathing movements may appear reassuring, the absence of fetal breathing is not a reliable predictor of fetal hypoxia and does not mandate immediate obstetric intervention.

TECHNIQUES AND DEFINITIONS

Electronic fetal monitoring is accomplished with the use of a specific monitor designed to record both fetal heart activity and maternal uterine contractions. For the practicing obstetric-care provider to appropriately assess the fetal condition, the fetus must be assessed in response to maternal stimuli, such as uterine contractions. To do this, the FHR monitor employs an electronic Doppler device that transmits an electronic signal from the fetus to a recording monitor that displays the FHR as it occurs from beat to beat. Typically, uterine activity is monitored simultaneously with the FHR and a waveform is produced that reflects uterine muscular tone. Deflections from the baseline of this waveform illustrate uterine contractions or activity. This information is recorded as the fetal tracing on paper or in an electronic medical record. Finally, the FHR tracing is interpreted visually by a physician or other provider familiar with the patient's current clinical situation. The FHR tracing, therefore, is different from electrocardiography in that a computer interpretation is not produced. While computerized algorithms for the interpretation of FHR tracings are in development, no such system has been validated by expert panels representing the ACOG or the Society for Maternal-Fetal Medicine (SMFM).

Aspects of FHR monitoring and interpretation have been debated since the inception of monitoring. A recent workshop sponsored by the National Institute of Child Health and Human Development (NICHD), SMFM, and the American Association of Women's Health and Obstetric Nursing revised the nomenclature and interpretation of FHR monitoring.[8] The following definitions are adapted from this workshop, as they provide common nomenclature for the interpretation of FHR monitoring. Importantly, this workshop recommended eliminating the use of the terms "hyperstimulation" and "hypercontractility" because these terms are ambiguous, ill-defined, subjective and should no longer be used clinically.[8]

A full description of a FHR tracing includes qualitative and quantitative analyses of uterine contractions, baseline FHR, FHR variability, presence of accelerations, presence of periodic or episodic decelerations, and changes or trends of FHR patterns over time. An interpretation of the overall FHR tracing is made, which should speak specifically to fetal well-being, and this interpretation should be documented in the patient's chart. These definitions are discussed using the latest NICHD recommendations.[8] Clinical examples are provided where appropriate.

Uterine Activity

One cannot interpret the FHR tracing completely unless the fetal heart tracing is assessed in relation to uterine activity. These definitions aid the practitioner and focus attention to the fetal response to maternal stimuli.

Uterine activity or contractions

Quantified as the number of contractions in a 10-minute window, uterine activity or contractions are averaged over 30 minutes. Contraction frequency, duration, intensity, and relaxation time in between should be assessed.

Normal uterine activity

Normal uterine activity is fewer than five contractions in 10 minutes, averaged over 30 minutes.

Tachysystole

Tachysystole is more than five contractions in 10 minutes, averaged over 30-minutes. Tachysystole, when noted, should be qualified as to the presence or absence associated FHR decelerations. Tachysystole may be present in spontaneous or stimulated labor and clinical management can differ, depending on the type of labor that is present. For example, if tachysystole with associated FHR decelerations is present in the context of oxytocin-stimulated labor during an induction, the clinical management should involve adjusting the oxytocin rate of administration. However, if tachysystole with associated FHR decelerations is seen in the context of spontaneous labor with a nonreassuring FHR tracing, immediate delivery may be indicated if in utero resuscitative efforts do not improve the fetal response.

Characteristics of Fetal Heart-Rate Tracings: The Baseline

Patterns of the fetal heart rate are defined by using four characteristics: baseline FHR, FHR variability, presence of accelerations, and presence and type of decelerations.

Considerations of the FHR baseline have incorporated many new definitions that are based on new insights into fetal physiology.

Baseline Fetal Heart Rate

Baseline FHR is the mean FHR rounded to increments of 5 beats per minute (bpm) during a 10-minute window. Accelerations, decelerations, and periods of marked variability are excluded when the baseline is being assessed. To calculate the baseline during a current 10-minute window, at least 2 minutes of a recorded FHR segment must be present or the baseline for that period is indeterminate. In such instances, the baseline is determined from the last 10-minute window that has been recorded in an acceptable manner.

Normal baseline

Normal baseline is a mean FHR of 110 to 160 bpm over 10 minutes. Note that this is a change from previous definitions of a normal baseline being between 120 to 160 bpm, reflecting new insight from clinical practice that many normally oxygenated fetuses have a baseline FHR from 110 to 120 bpm.

Bradycardia

Bradycardia is an abnormal baseline FHR that is less than 110 bpm over 10 minutes.

Tachycardia

Tachycardia is an abnormal baseline FHR that is greater than 160 bpm over 10 minutes.

Baseline change

Baseline change is an acceleration or deceleration that lasts for more than 10 minutes.

When considering changes in the fetal heart rate baseline, the obstetric care providers must take care to evaluate the entire FHR tracing, from the beginning of the monitoring period, as changes in the FHR baseline can provide important insights into changes in the maternal and fetal conditions.

Characteristics of the Fetal Heart-Rate Tracings: Variability

FHR variability is defined as irregular fluctuations in the baseline FHR frequency and amplitude over 10 minutes. The variability is visually quantitated as the amplitude of the peak-to-trough in beats per minute. Accelerations and decelerations are not included in this amplitude analysis. Variability can be described using four definitions: absent, minimal, moderate, and marked. In absent variability, the FHR amplitude range is undetectable. In minimal variability, the FHR amplitude range is detectable, but less than or equal to 5 bpm. In moderate variability, the FHR amplitude range is 6 to 25 bpm. In marked variability, the FHR amplitude range is greater than 25 bpm.

FHR variability can be difficult to adequately interpret when using external fetal monitoring, and more clinical information may be obtained when a fetal scalp electrode is placed as an internal monitor. Assessment of FHR variability is a critical first step in determining the overall health of a fetus. Poor variability may be an indicator of an acidotic or hypoxic fetus, but unfortunately, poor variability has poor sensitivity and a poor positive predictive value.

Characteristics of the Fetal Heart-Rate Tracing: Accelerations

Accelerations of the fetal heart rate are visually apparent and are characterized by an abrupt increase or upward deflection from the baseline of the FHR. Specifically, the time from the onset of the acceleration to the peak should be less than 30 seconds. The "15 × 15" rule is applied as the peak must be greater than or equal to 15 bpm and the time from onset to return to baseline should be greater than or equal to 15 seconds. Before 32 weeks gestation, a 10 × 10 rule applies, meaning that the peak must be greater than or equal to 10 bpm and the duration must be greater than or equal to 10 seconds. Prolongued acceleration is an acceleration in the FHR greater than or equal to 2 minutes but less than 10 minutes in duration. Baseline change is an acceleration lasting greater than or equal to 10 minutes. Accelerations of the FHR indicate fetal well being and are rarely seen in fetuses with acidosis or hypoxia. Noting FHR accelerations provides reassurance of a healthy fetus.

Characteristics of the Fetal Heart Rate: Early Versus Late Decelerations

Decelerations of the FHR are a visually apparent decrease or downward deflection from the baseline FHR. There are three types of decelerations, late, early, and variable, with each having specific characteristics (gradual or abrupt nature and relationship to a uterine contraction). Decelerations can vary in their severity with successive uterine contractions. Regardless of the type of deceleration, the decrease in FHR is calculated from the onset to the nadir of the contraction.

Early deceleration

Early deceleration is a decrease and return of the FHR to the baseline associated with a uterine contraction. The decrease is symmetric and gradual, meaning the time from the onset of the decrease to the nadir of the deceleration is greater than or equal to 30 seconds. An early deceleration has a nadir that mirrors the peak of the contraction; that is, the onset, nadir, and recovery of the deceleration correspond to the beginning, peak, and ending of the contraction, respectively.

Late deceleration

Late deceleration is similar to the early deceleration in that the decrease and return of the FHR to the baseline is associated with a uterine contraction. The decrease is symmetric and gradual, meaning the time from the onset of the decrease to the nadir of the deceleration is greater than or equal to 30 seconds.

A key and sometimes subtle difference between early and late decelerations is that the late deceleration is delayed in timing, with the nadir of the deceleration occurring after the peak of the contraction. Usually the onset, nadir, and recovery of the deceleration occur after the beginning, peak, and ending of the contraction, respectively. Although similar, these two decelerations have different implications. Early decelerations are thought to reflect head compression in a fetus with a normal oxygen status, whereas late decelerations are thought to represent a level of hypoxia in the fetus because of utero-placental insufficiency occurring secondary to various causes (eg, maternal hypovolemia, uterine tachysystole, placental abruption, uterine rupture). Late decelerations are a clue that the oxygen status of the fetus may be compromised and mandates a response from the obstetric care provider. Usually this involves efforts at fetal resuscitation in utero, but may lead to the need for immediate delivery.

Characteristics of the Fetal Heart Rate: Variable Decelerations

Variable decelerations are commonly seen during pregnancy, and particularly during labor. The impact of variable decelerations on the fetal conditions depends greatly on gestational age and the timing in the labor process. Preterm fetuses have less reserve for acid compared with term fetuses and so have less ability to tolerate variable decelerations over the course of the labor, often resulting in the need for immediate delivery.

Variable decelerations are defined as visually abrupt decreases in the FHR that have a "V" shape. Abrupt is defined as the onset of the decrease in the FHR to the nadir of the deceleration being less than 30 seconds. Furthermore, the decrease in FHR is greater than or equal to 15 bpm, lasts for greater than or equal to 15 seconds, but is less than 2 minutes in duration. These characteristics give the typical "V" shape of the deceleration. Usually variable decelerations denote umbilical cord compression. Often there are "upshoots" or "shoulders" of the FHR immediately preceding and following the deceleration as the FHR returns to the baseline. These "upshoots" are thought to represent the reflexive tachycardia as the fetus attempts to maintain cardiac output because of a decrease in venous return from compression of the umbilical cord.

Mild variable deceleration
Mild variable deceleration is a decrease in the FHR that is less than 60 bpm below the FHR baseline, lasts for less than 60 seconds, and has a nadir that is greater than 60 bpm.

Severe variable deceleration
Severe variable deceleration is a decrease in the FHR that is greater than 60 bpm below the FHR baseline, lasts for greater than or equal to 60 seconds, but less than 2 minutes, or has a nadir that is less than or equal to 60 bpm.

Prolonged deceleration
Prolonged deceration is a decrease in the FHR that is a visually apparent decrease in FHR from the baseline that is greater than or equal to 15 bpm, lasting greater than or equal to 2 minutes, but less than 10 minutes.

Baseline change
Baseline change is an FHR decrease lasting greater than 10 minutes.

Recurrent decelerations
Recurrent decelerations are if any type of FHR decrease occurs in greater than 50% of uterine contractions in any 20-minute time period.

Intermittent decelerations
Intermittent decelerations occur if any type of FHR decrease occurs in less than 50% of uterine contractions in any 20-minute time period.

Sinusoidal fetal heart-rate pattern
A sinusoidal FHR pattern is an FHR pattern with a sine wave-like undulating pattern of the FHR baseline that is visually apparent and smooth appearing. The so-called cycle frequency of this sine wave-like pattern has an amplitude of 3 to 5 bpms and typically does not have any variability that can be visualized. The pattern by definition should persist for greater than or equal to 20 minutes. This pattern has been associated with cases of severe fetal anemia or maternal narcotic ingestion.[8]

FHR decelerations often are inconsequential during labor, in particularly early or variable decelerations. However, late decelerations may indicate fetal hypoxia or academia. Unfortunately, late decelerations have poor sensitivity. In 50% of instances of late decelerations noted before labor, the fetus has no biochemical evidence of hypoxia. Interpretation of the FHR tracing requires obstetric judgment to optimize fetal and neonatal outcomes.

METHODS OF SURVEILLANCE AND THEIR CLINICAL IMPLICATIONS

Methods of fetal surveillance, and the gestational age at usual initiation of testing, are noted in **Table 1** and include maternal perception of fetal movements, nonstress

Table 1
Methods of fetal surveillance

Method	Gestational Age at Initiation
Fetal movement counting	20 weeks
Nonstress test (NST)	32 weeks
Biophysical profile	28 weeks
Modified biophysical profile (NST + amniotic fluid assessment)	32 weeks
Ultrasound assessment of fetal growth	24 weeks
Doppler velocimetry	24 weeks
Contraction stress test (CST)	36 weeks

testing (NST), various methods using real-time ultrasound, and contraction stress testing (CST). Ultrasound methods include assessment of the amniotic fluid volume, biophysical and modified biophysical profile testing, and umbilical artery Doppler velocimetry. Common indications for fetal surveillance and the level of evidence that supports the indication can be found in **Table 2**.[1] Typically, fetal testing begins at 32 to 34 weeks but can begin as early as 26 to 28 weeks in certain high-risk conditions (eg, early onset fetal growth restriction, multiple gestation, and medical complications of pregnancy, such as pregestational diabetes or systemic lupus erythematosus). The frequency of testing is at least weekly, but has been used as frequently as daily in certain high-risk conditions, such as severe fetal growth restriction or preterm premature rupture of the membranes.

Maternal Perception of Fetal Movement

With advancing gestation, especially in the late second and third trimesters, maternal perception of fetal movements can provide a sense of fetal well being both to clinicians and their patients alike. Quickening, or the first time fetal movements are perceived by

Table 2
Indications for antenatal fetal testing with level of evidence

Indication	Level of Evidence (Refs.)
Decreased fetal movement	12,16
Abnormal fetal growth (growth restriction)	1–10,13–15,17–37
Maternal disease (hypertension, thyroid dysfunction, diabetes, antiphospholipid syndrome, epilepsy, renal disease, hemoglobinopathy, systemic lupus erythematosus, cyanotic heart or lung disease)	1–10,13–15,17–37
Multiple gestation (with growth discordance)	1–10,13–15,17–37
Preterm premature rupture of membranes	1–10,13–15,17–37
Abnormalities of amniotic fluid (oligo- or poly-hydramnios)	1–10,13–15,17–37
Postterm pregnancy	1–10,13–15,17–37
Previous fetal demise	1–10,13–15,17–37
Alloimmunization	1–10,13–15,17–37
Maternal trauma	1–10,13–15,17–37
Unexplained vaginal bleeding	1–10,13–15,17–37
Preterm labor	1–10,13–15,17–37

the mother, typically occurs around 20-weeks gestation. These movements can be felt on a more routine basis as gestation advances. Each patient and her fetus serve as their own control and while the movements may change and become more discrete, the frequency of such movements usually does not decrease with advancing gestation.

In 1973, Sadovsky and colleagues reported cases in which fetal death was preceded by decreased fetal activity noted by the mother.[9] As a result, various protocols to quantify maternal perception of fetal movements or "fetal-kick counts" have been developed. However, a gold-standard protocol has yet to be defined. In 1989, Moore and Piacquadio described having mothers count up to 10 movements in a 24-hour period, and this was found to be reassuring in that study.[10] Using the mother's established baseline of acceptable fetal movement counts, Neldam in 1983 had patients count for 1 hour each day and reassurance was obtained if the baseline was surpassed.[11] Approximately 68,000 women were studied by Grant and colleagues[12] in a randomized fashion to test fetal-movement protocols where patients consciously counted the fetal movements at a particular time each day. Grant concluded that informal counting protocols, where the mother assessed fetal movement at routine prenatal visits, were just as effective as formal routine counting protocols.

Some form of fetal movement assessment is incorporated into contemporary obstetric care. Further testing (eg, NST, biophysical profile) is employed when maternal perception of fetal movement is decreased. Precautions to expectant mothers include recommendations to be evaluated should fetal movement be subjectively decreased. Although the positive predictive value of fetal-movement counting protocols is low because of the subjective nature of the test, some form of maternal perception of fetal movement is standard of care. Obstetricians are often prompted to induce labor for decreased fetal movement with normal fetal surveillance, even though there is little objective evidence to support this practice.

Nonstress Testing

Freeman first described the NST in 1975.[13] FHR accelerations in response to fetal movement in the absence of uterine contractions were noted to be a sign of fetal well being. The NST is easy to perform, requires no uterine stimulation, and is commonly employed as a first-line fetal surveillance technique. Autonomic influences mediated by sympathetic or parasympathetic impulses from the brainstem act to increase or decrease the FHR. As the parasympathetic nervous system develops, the FHR gradually decreases with advancing gestation.[6] The physiologic premise of the NST is that the nonhypoxic fetus that can temporarily accelerate its heart rate in reaction to a stimulus, such as its own movement.[6]

To perform an NST, the patient is placed in a lateral tilt position and the FHR and uterine activity are monitored with an external transducer.[1] During monitoring, the patient is asked to record by clicking a button that makes a mark on the tracing with each movement. Typically, the FHR is monitored for 20 minutes, but up to 40 minutes of monitoring may be required to account for variations in the fetal sleep-wake cycles. In some cases when the fetus is not reactive, acoustic stimulation is accomplished by placing an artificial larynx on the maternal abdomen and applying a sound stimulus for 1 to 2 seconds. The presence of accelerations in response to an acoustic stimulus is a sign of fetal well-being and does not appear to compromise the predictive value of the test.[14-16] The interpretation of the NST is the same as described above, but the overall result of the test is recorded as reactive or nonreactive. A reactive NST is the presence of two accelerations as defined above in a 20-minute time period with or without fetal movements.[17] A nonreactive NST is the absence of two accelerations in a 40-minute period with or without acoustic stimulation over a 40-minute period.

The ability of the fetus to accelerate its heart rate is gestational age-dependent, and so NST is not routinely started until 32-weeks gestation.[8] Up to 50% of NSTs will be reactive from 24- to 28-weeks gestation, while from 28 to 32 weeks of gestation 85% of NSTs are reactive.[18–20]

In up to 50% of NSTs variable decelerations may be observed. If the variable decelerations last for less than 30 seconds and there are fewer than two during a 20-minute period, they do not indicate fetal compromise and no intervention is required. If the variable decelerations suggest possible fetal compromise, further monitoring may be warranted as recurrent variable decelerations have been associated with an increased risk of fetal death.[21–25] With a reactive NST, the chance for fetal death within 1 week is 1.9 per 1,000, giving a negative predictive value of 99.8% after correction for lethal anomalies.[1,26] Thus, a reactive NST is reassuring, but a nonreactive NST is nonspecific and requires further evaluation. In most circumstances, obstetricians will perform a biophysical profile in the event of a nonreactive NST.

Biophysical Profile, Modified Biophysical Profile, and Assessment of Amniotic Fluid

The basis for the biophysical profile (BPP) is a compilation of five variables, including the NST, an assessment of the amniotic fluid volume, and three variables related to fetal movements visualized with real-time ultrasound. All of these variables reflect a fetus that can accelerate its heart rate, move appropriately, and is surrounded by a normal amount of amniotic fluid. These findings suggest that the fetus is not hypoxic or acidotic and the chance of fetal death is very low. When the BPP is interpreted, the variable either is present or not such that a total BPP score can be as high as 10 or as low as 0. By design, each of the five components receives a score of 0 or 2. If the variable is present, representing a reassuring finding, then a score of 2 out of 2 is assigned. If that variable is absent, then a score of 0 out of 2 is assigned and the total score is calculated. Some centers just use the ultrasound parameters and not the NST, as a score of 8 is just as reassuring as a 10, based on the relationship of umbilical venous pH and BPP score illustrated in **Fig. 1**.[27,28] Because FHR accelerations are one of the last of these variables to develop, some centers use the NST alone, assuming that if the NST is reactive, then the other variables should be present. Either approach is acceptable.

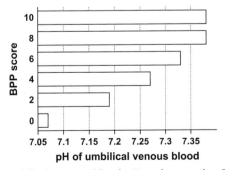

Fig. 1. Relationship of umbilical venous blood pH and respective BPP score. (*Data from* Manning FA, Snijders R, Harman CR, et al. Fetal biophysical profile score. VI. Correlation with antepartum umbilical venous fetal pH. Am J Obstet Gynecol 1993;169:755–63.)

The 5 variables of the BPP are the NST, amniotic fluid assessment, fetal breathing movements, fetal gross body movements, and fetal tone.[1] Real-time ultrasound is used to document the fluid assessment and movement variables, and a 30-minute time period is allowed if needed to visualize fetal behavior.

Reactive nonstress testing
Reactive NST is two accelerations in a 20- to 40-minute period and are scored 2 out of 2.

Amniotic fluid assessment
Amniotic fluid assessment is measurement of the depth of the largest vertical pocket of fluid free of fetal parts or cord. If this pocket is greater than 2-cm deep, the score is 2 out of 2, while a fluid pocket less than or equal to 2-cm deep is scored as 0.

Fetal breathing movements
If one or more episodes of rhythmic fetal breathing movements as described above is seen and lasts for greater than or equal to 30 seconds during the 30-minute observation period, a score of 2 out of 2 is given. If breathing movements are not seen or the duration of such movements is less than 30 seconds, then the score is 0 out of 2.

Gross body movements
Three or more discrete body or limb movements seen within the 30 minutes achieves a 2 out of 2 score. If fewer than three movements are seen, the score is 0 out of 2.

Fetal tone (flexion/extension)
If there are one or more episodes of extension of a fetal extremity and return to flexion within the 30 minutes, a score of 2 out of 2 is achieved. An episode of the hand opening and closing is also sufficient to score 2. If neither is present, 0 out of 2 is assigned.

When interpreting the results of the BPP, especially when the score is 6 or less, the attending obstetrician must assess the entire clinical situation. A simplified management scheme is illustrated in **Fig. 2**.[6,29,30] A score of 8 to 10 out of 10 is interpreted as normal and the chance for fetal death within 1 week of the test of normal singletons is less than 1 in a 1,000. Testing should be repeated weekly or as clinically indicated. In the setting of oligohydramnios before 37-weeks gestation, repeat testing is indicated. However, at term delivery is usually accomplished when oligohydramnios is noted. Oligohydramnios in the absence of ruptured fetal membranes may be a sign of placental insufficiency, mandating continued surveillance or potential delivery.

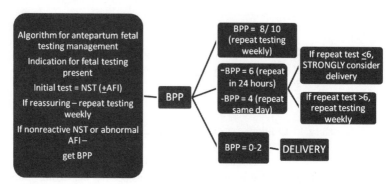

Fig. 2. Clinical algorithm for antepartum management of fetal testing. (*Data from* Refs.[6,29,30])

A BPP score of 6 out of 10 may indicate a lack of fetal well being, especially in the setting of oligohydramnios. Again, if the patient is term, delivery is recommended. If the patient is preterm with a 6 out of 10 score, the test is repeated in 24 hours and, if still 6 out of 10, delivery may be indicated, depending on the gestational age. If the repeat test is 8 to 10 out of 10, repeat testing should occur as clinically indicated. A score of 4 out of 10 is concerning for fetal compromise, with a high risk of fetal death, such that delivery may be indicated in most situations. In very preterm situations (<32 weeks) repeat testing the same day may be done and if the repeat test is 6 or less, then delivery should be strongly considered. A score of 0 to 2 out of 10 is an emergency and delivery should likely occur depending on the clinical circumstance. These recommendations are based on data comparing BPP scores and umbilical venous-blood pH values obtained via cordocentesis, illustrated in **Fig. 1**.[27] The lower the score, the lower the pH and greater chance for an adverse outcome.[27] An attending obstetrician familiar with testing protocols and the patient's clinical situation is critically important to accomplish optimal obstetric outcomes.

An abbreviated BPP, or a modified BPP, consists of a NST and an assessment of the amniotic fluid index (AFI). The AFI is the sum of the four largest vertical pockets of amniotic fluid noted in each quadrant of the uterus, measured in centimeters. The modified BPP is considered normal if the fluid volume is adequate (AFI greater than 5 cm) with a reactive NST. Further evaluation is warranted if the NST is nonreactive or the AFI less than 5 cm. Using the modified BPP is appealing because it takes less time to accomplish and is less subject to interobserver variability. Furthermore, the modified BPP has been studied in large series by different groups,[14,15,31] has been found to be a good predictor of pregnancy outcome, and is accepted by ACOG as an acceptable means of antepartum fetal surveillance.[1]

Umbilical Artery Velocimetry

Doppler ultrasonography is a noninvasive technique used to assess the hemodynamic components of vascular impedance[1] and is commonly used in cases of fetal growth restriction (FGR).[1,6] Various blood vessels have been investigated using Doppler velocimetry, including the maternal uterine artery, fetal middle cerebral artery, and fetal ductus venosus, in the evaluation of FGR. The hypoxia associated with FGR leads to a brain-sparing reflex similar to that seen in other cases of fetal hypoxemia. In this brain-sparing reflex, blood flow is shunted to the brain, heart, and adrenal glands at the expense of the placenta and peripheral circulation. Flow-velocity waveforms in various blood vessels can be different in cases of FGR because of increasing vascular resistance of placental vessels in the setting of worsening utero-placental insufficiency. In this circumstance, Doppler velocimetry of the umbilical artery is useful because of the vessel's accessibility and reproducibility. Commonly measured flow velocities include peak systolic-flow velocity and the diastolic flow velocity occurring at the end of the cardiac cycle.[1,6] Different indices can then be calculated, such as the systolic/diastolic ratio (S/D ratio), resistance index (systolic flow–diastolic flow/systolic flow), and pulsatility index (systolic flow–diastolic flow/frequency shift over entire cycle).[1,6]

With FGR, hypoxic fetuses have increased end-diastolic flow velocity (EDV) in the fetal middle-cerebral artery, whereas decreased, absent, or reversed EDV is evident in the umbilical artery. In addition, decreased cardiac function in the setting of chronic fetal hypoxia can lead to increased central-venous pressure that can be seen as reversed diastolic-blood flow in the ductus venosus and umbilical arteries, which may represent fetal cardiac decompensation.[32] Absent and reversed EDV have been associated with significant placental terminal villous obliteration, poor perinatal outcome, and high perinatal mortality.[32] The predictive value for fetal death and, more importantly, the timing of fetal death of absent EDV is limited.[32] The poor predictive value of Doppler velocimetry limits its utility primarily to the setting of fetal growth restriction.[1] A normal S/D ratio of less than 3 has a negative predictive value in the setting of growth restriction and can support continuing the pregnancy, especially in preterm cases.[1,6] However, detection of reversed EDV during FGR is predictive of a high risk of fetal death within 1 week, and has been used as a criterion to consider delivery, even of the preterm fetus.

Contraction Stress Test

Historically, the CST was the mainstay of fetal surveillance before the advent of other noninvasive tests. Developed in 1972 by Ray and colleagues,[33] the CST was originally termed the "oxytocin challenge test." During uterine contractions, placental blood flow is decreased. In pregnancies complicated by conditions that compromise uteroplacental blood flow, uterine contractions are associated with fetal hypoxia and the development of late decelerations.[6] As noted in the ACOG technical bulletin, "the CST is based on the response of the FHR to uterine contractions and it relies on the premise that fetal oxygenation will be transiently worsened by uterine contractions. Furthermore, in the suboptimally oxygenated fetus, the resultant intermittent worsening in oxygenation will, in turn, lead to late decelerations on the FHR tracing."[1]

The FHR is monitored as described above in the NST test. Uterine contractions are induced with oxytocin administration and, when three or more contractions (spontaneous or stimulated) lasting 40 or more seconds occur over a 10-minute period, the test can be interpreted.[1] The CST is interpreted as either negative or positive: negative (reassuring) has no late or significant variable decelerations visualized; positive (nonreassuring) has late or significant variable decelerations following 50% or more of contractions.

Disadvantages of the CST include the cost and complexity of the test, as well as the several relative contraindications of the test (eg, preterm gestation, bleeding, previous uterine surgery).[1] One laudable aspect of the CST is the negative predictive value, as the incidence of fetal death occurring within 1 week of the negative test result is 0.3 out of 1,000 in over 12,000 pregnancies studied.[34] However, the test is rarely used today because of the simplicity and ease of administration of the NST and BPP.

Umbilical Cord Blood Gas Analysis

Table 3 shows the umbilical cord blood gas analyses after normal labor and delivery.[35] Labor is a stressful event for the fetus, as evidenced by the low pH after a normal labor and delivery. In pregnancies complicated by conditions that further compromise uterine perfusion, even lower pH values may be noted. However, only very low pH

Table 3
Umbilical cord blood gas analysis after normal labor

Parameter ($n = 3,500$)	Arterial (Mean)	Venous (Mean)
pH	7.27	7.34
pCO_2 (partial pressure of carbon dioxide, mm Hg)	50	40
HCO_3 (bicarbonate, meq/L)	22	21
Base excess (meq/L)	−2.7	−2.4

Data from Weiner CP, Sipes SL, Wenstrom K. The effect of fetal age upon normal fetal laboratory values and venous pressure. Obstet Gynecol 1992;79(5Pt1):713–8.

values of 7.0 or less are associated with cerebral palsy.[36] One goal of current obstetric care, with the use of fetal surveillance, is to not only to prevent fetal death but also to identify those fetuses most at risk for fetal compromise that may lead to cerebral palsy. Unfortunately, the lack of specificity and positive predictive values of these fetal surveillance techniques limits the ability of the obstetrician to identify these fetuses most at risk.

NEW NICHD GUIDELINES FOR THE INTERPRETATION OF FHR MONITORING

The recent NICHD workshop on fetal monitoring recommended adoption of a three-tiered Fetal Heart Rate Interpretation System for the categorization of FHR patterns,[8] illustrated in **Table 4**. Category I FHR tracings are reassuring and fetal acidosis at the time of observation can be excluded, and no specific action is required. Category II FHR tracings are considered "indeterminate" and comprise the majority of FHR tracings. Category II tracings require further evaluation and monitoring, as they are not predictive of fetal acidosis, but there is not enough data to include them in either Category I or III. Category III tracings are abnormal and predictive of fetal acidosis when observed. Prompt evaluation is warranted and in utero resuscitative efforts should be considered, including maternal oxygen administration, changing the maternal position, discontinuation of labor stimulation, and addressing maternal hypotension.

Category II FHR tracings include indeterminate FHR tracings, such as bradycardia or tachycardia, with minimal variability. Other aspects of indeterminate tracings include minimal baseline variability with marked or no recurrent decelerations; no accelerations after fetal stimulation; periodic or episodic decelerations with recurrent variable decelerations and minimal or moderate baseline variability; prolonged decelerations, recurrent late decelerations with moderate baseline variability; or variable decelerations with other characteristics, such as a slow return to baseline, and "overshoots" or "shoulders." These findings are common during labor and require the obstetrician to be ever vigilant in monitoring labor progress and the fetal response to uterine activity.[8]

CLINICAL ALGORITHMS

The ACOG developed a pamphlet for patients to explain fetal testing, noting that, "If a test result suggests that there may be a problem, this does not always mean the baby is in trouble, it may simply mean that further testing may be necessary...."[37] The lack of improvement in perinatal outcomes with increased fetal surveillance

Table 4		
Three tier system for classifying fetal heart-rate tracings		
Category	**Description**	**Interpretation**
Category I	Baseline: 110–160; variability: moderate; decelerations: ± early, no late or variable; Accelerations ±	Normal
Category II	Those FHR tracings not included in Categories I or III. Includes a large portion of FHR tracings.	Indeterminate
Category III	Absent variability with recurrent late or variable decelerations or bradycardia. Sinusoid pattern	Abnormal

Data from Macones GA, Hankins GD, Spong CY, et al. The 2008 National Institute of Child Health and Human Development workshop report on electronic fetal monitoring: update on definitions, interpretation, and research guidelines. Obstet Gynecol 2008;112(3):661–6.

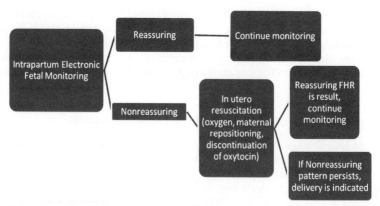

Fig. 3. Clinical algorithm for intrapartum management of fetal heart rate monitoring during spontaneous or stimulated labor.

testing in the recent decades indicates that randomized trials need to be performed to assess the effectiveness of fetal surveillance to improve outcomes. Despite the unproven value of antepartum fetal surveillance, fetal testing has been widely integrated into clinical practice in the developed world. Well-designed clinical trials with appropriate control populations are unlikely to be performed to determine the effectiveness of fetal surveillance.

Both providers and patients need to understand the limitations of fetal testing. Practitioners must fully evaluate in the clinical scenario to more rationally interpret fetal testing and make wise obstetric interventions based on the best available evidence. **Figs. 2** and **3** depict a brief overview of antepartum and intrapartum management schemes. For antepartum surveillance, the most common test employed is the NST. If the NST is nonreactive, a BPP is indicated. Should the BPP be 6 or less, then repeat testing, or perhaps delivery, is indicated. With intrapartum monitoring (see **Fig. 3**), the fetal tracing is assessed as being either reassuring or nonreassuring. Nonreassuring testing mandates a response for the obstetric care team, usually realized as in utero resuscitative efforts. If these efforts are not successful, then delivery is required.

These simplified and stylized algorithms do not account for the many clinical situations that fall outside these general guidelines. The obstetric care team has the responsibility to account for the many physiologic and pathophysiologic conditions that can affect the fetus and be reflected in the FHR tracings and biophysical parameters. With a complete assessment and wise insight to these conditions and how they affect the fetus, the obstetric care team can more rationally care for the mother and fetus.

SUMMARY

In many instances the results of fetal testing can be ambiguous. Because of the lack of sensitivity of fetal testing, the practicing obstetrician often has a low threshold to move to delivery with abnormal fetal surveillance in the term or near-term fetus to avert the potential for fetal death. Clear communication between the obstetric care team and the receiving pediatrician is imperative to ensure optimal obstetric and pediatric outcomes.

REFERENCES

1. American College of Obstetricians and Gynecologists, Practice Bulletin. Antepartum fetal surveillance in American College of Obstetricians and Gynecologists practice bulletin number 9. Int J Gynaecol Obstet 2000;68(2):175–85.
2. Boddy K, Dawes GS, Fisher R, et al. Fetal respiratory movements, electrocortical and cardiovascular responses to hypoxemia and hypercapnia in sheep. J Physiol 1974;243:599–618.
3. Manning FA, Platt LD. Maternal hypoxemia and fetal breathing movements. Obstet Gynecol 1979;53:758–60.
4. Seeds AE. Current concepts of amniotic fluid dynamics. Am J Obstet Gynecol 1980;138:575–86.
5. Nihjuis JG, van de Pas M, Jongsma HW. State transitions in uncomplicated pregnancies after term. Early Hum Dev 1998;52(2):125–32.
6. Cunningham FG, Leveno KL, Bloom SL, et al. Antepartum and intrapartum assessment. In: Cunningham FG, Leveno KL, Bloom SL, et al, editors. Williams Obstetrics. 22nd Edition. New York: McGraw-Hill; 2005. p. 374–86.
7. Dawes GS, Fox HE, Leduc BM, et al. Respiratory movements and rapid eye movement sleep in the fetal lamb. J Physiol 1972;220(1):119–43.
8. Macones GA, Hankins GD, Spong CY, et al. The 2008 National Institute of Child Health and Human Development workshop report on electronic fetal monitoring: update on definitions, interpretation, and research guidelines. Obstet Gynecol 2008;112(3):661–6.
9. Sadovsky E, Yaffe H. Daily fetal movement recording and fetal prognosis. Obstet Gynecol 1972;41(6):845–50.
10. Moore TR, Piacquadio K. A prospective evaluation of fetal movement screening to reduce the incidence of antepartum fetal death. Am J Obstet Gynecol 1989; 160(5Pt1):1075–80.
11. Neldam S. Fetal movements as an indicator of fetal well-being. Dan Med Bull 1983;30(4):274–8.
12. Grant A, Elbourne D, Valentin L, et al. Routine formal fetal movement counting and risk of antepartum late death in normally formed singletons. Lancet 1989; 2(8659):345–9.
13. Freeman RK. The use of the oxytocin challenge test for antepartum clinical evaluation of uteroplacental respiratory function. Am J Obstet Gynecol 1975;121:481–9.
14. Clark SL, Sabey P, Jolley K. Nonstress testing with acoustic stimulation and amniotic fluid volume assessment: 5973 tests without unexpected fetal death. Am J Obstet Gynecol 1989;160(3):694–7.
15. Miller DA, Rabello YA, Paul RH. The modified biophysical profile: antepartum testing in the 1990s. Am J Obstet Gynecol 1996;174(3):812–7.
16. Smith CV, Phelan JP, Platt LD, et al. Fetal acoustic stimulation testing. II A randomized clinical comparison with the nonstress test. Am J Obstet Gynecol 1986;155(1):131–4.
17. Evertson LR, Gauthier RJ, Schifrin BS, et al. Antepartum fetal heart rate testing. I Evolution of the nonstress test. Am J Obstet Gynecol 1979;133(1):29–33.
18. Bishop EH. Fetal acceleration test. Am J Obstet Gynecol 1981;141(8):905–9.
19. Lavin JP Jr, Miodovnik M, Barden TP. Relationship of nonstress test reactivity and gestational age. Obstet Gynecol 1984;63(3):338–44.
20. Druzin ML, Fox A, Kogut E, et al. The relationship of the nonstress test to gestational age. Am J Obstet Gynecol 1985;153(4):386–9.

21. Meis PJ, Ureda JR, Swain M, et al. Variable decelerations during nonstress tests are not a sign of fetal compromise. Am J Obstet Gynecol 1986;154(3):586–90.
22. O'Leary JA, Andrinopoulos GC, Giordano PC. Variable decelerations and the nonstress test: an indication of cord compromise. Am J Obstet Gynecol 1980; 137(6):704–6.
23. Bourgeois FJ, Thiagarajah S, Harbert GM Jr. The significance of fetal heart rate decelerations during nonstress testing. Am J Obstet Gynecol 1984;150:213–6.
24. Druzin ML, Gratacos J, Keegan KA, et al. Antepartum fetal heart rate testing. VII. The significance of fetal bradycardia. Am J Obstet Gynecol 1981;139:194–8.
25. Pazos R, Vuolo K, Aladjem S, et al. Association of spontaneous fetal heart rate decelerations during antepartum nonstress testing and intrauterine growth retardation. Am J Obstet Gynecol 1982;144:574–7.
26. Freeman RK, Anderson G, Dorchester W. A prospective multi-institutional study of antepartum fetal heart rate monitoring. I. Risk of perinatal mortality and morbidity according to antepartum fetal heart rate test results. Am J Obstet Gynecol 1982; 143:771–7.
27. Manning FA, Snijders R, Harman CR, et al. Fetal biophysical profile score. VI. Correlation with antepartum umbilical venous fetal pH. Am J Obstet Gynecol 1993;169:755–63.
28. Manning FA, Harman CR, Morrison I, et al. Fetal assessment based on fetal biophysical profile scoring. IV. An analysis of perinatal morbidity and mortality. Am J Obstet Gynecol 1990;162:703–9.
29. Manning FA, Morrison I, Harman CR, et al. Fetal assessment based on fetal biophysical profile scoring: experience in 19,221 referred high-risk pregnancies. II. An analysis of false-negative fetal deaths. Am J Obstet Gynecol 1987; 157(4Pt1):880–4.
30. Dayal AK, Manning FA, Berck DJ, et al. Fetal death after normal biophysical profile score: an eighteen-year experience. Am J Obstet Gynecol 1999; 181(5Pt1):1231–6.
31. Nageotte MP, Towers CV, Asrat T, et al. Perinatal outcome with the modified biophysical profile. Am J Obstet Gynecol 1994;170:1672–6.
32. Turan OM, Turan S, Gungor S, et al. Progression of Doppler abnormalities in intrauterine growth restriction. Ultrasound Obstet Gynecol 2008;32(2):160–7.
33. Ray M, Freeman R, Pine S, et al. Clinical experience with the oxytocin challenge test. Am J Obstet Gynecol 1972;114(1):1–9.
34. Freeman RK, Anderson G, Dorchester W. A prospective multi-institutional study of antepartum fetal heart rate monitoring. II. Contraction stress test versus nonstress test for primary surveillance. Am J Obstet Gynecol 1982;143(7):778–81.
35. Weiner CP, Sipes SL, Wenstrom K. The effect of fetal age upon normal fetal laboratory values and venous pressure. Obstet Gynecol 1992;79(5Pt1):713–8.
36. Hankins GD, Speer M. Defining the pathogenesis and pathophysiology of neonatal encephalopathy and cerebral palsy. Obstet Gynecol 2003;102:628–36.
37. American College of Obstetricians and Gynecologists. Patient education pamphlets. Special tests for monitoring fetal health. Washington DC: ACOG; 2006.

Newborn Screening for Genetic Disorders

Paul M. Fernhoff, MD, FAAP, FACMG[a,b],*

KEYWORDS

- Newborn metabolic screening • Newborn genetic screening
- Newborn filter paper card screening

Geneticists are often asked when universal genetic screening will be a reality.[1] My response is that universal genetic screening has been a reality for more than 45 years. Screening newborns for genetic disorders goes by several different names; many health care professionals simply call it the Newborn Screening (NBS) program. Others refer to it as the newborn metabolic screen, the newborn heel stick, or the newborn filter paper card screening program. Some still refer to it as "the PKU test," an outdated designation. Regardless of its name, the screen has become an integral part of the evaluation of more than 4 million newborns a year in the United States and of most newborns in industrialized countries and many in developing countries. NBS programs have saved thousands of children from disabilities and early death. NBS programs continue to grow because of innovative technologies and because of the concerns of parents, health care professionals, and advocates who understand the ability of NBS to prevent or reduce the effects of these devastating disorders. Because the term "newborn screening" refers to many procedures performed in a nursery such has screening for hearing loss or congenital heart disease, this discussion is limited to screening for genetic or congenital disorders with blood spotted on filter paper cards. This discussion reflects primarily the experiences and current status of NBS programs in the United States.

HISTORY OF NEWBORN SCREENING

The origins of the newborn screening for metabolic disorders are often traced back to 1934 when Professor Asbjorn Fölling, a Norwegian biochemist, was asked by one his former students, Dr. Harry Egland and his wife to examine two of their children. Unlike their other healthy children, both of these children had severe developmental delays, an unpleasant "wet fur" body, urine odor, and decreased skin pigmentation. After adding a small amount of ferric chloride, the urine of both children turned an unusual

a Division of Medical Genetics, Department of Human Genetics, Emory University School of Medicine, Atlanta, GA 30322, USA
b Department of Pediatrics, Emory University School of Medicine, Atlanta, GA 30322, USA
* Division of Medical Genetics, Department of Human Genetics, Emory University School of Medicine, Atlanta, GA 30322.
E-mail address: pfernhoff@genetics.emory.edu

Pediatr Clin N Am 56 (2009) 505–513
doi:10.1016/j.pcl.2009.03.002
0031-3955/09/$ – see front matter © 2009 Published by Elsevier Inc.

pediatric.theclinics.com

green color.[2] This observation led Fölling and others to recognize that the unusual color was caused by excess amounts of phenylketones, ie, by-products of phenylalanine, an essential amino acid found in nearly all natural protein sources.

These initial observations confirmed that phenylketonuria (PKU) was a classical inborn error of metabolism, caused by the inability of the affected child's body to convert phenylalanine to tyrosine owing to the lack of function of the hepatic enzyme phenylalanine hydroxylase. Subsequent observations found that when individuals with PKU were given a metabolic formula restricted in phenylalanine and enriched in tyrosine, their elevated blood phenylalanine levels could be reduced. If this formula and a diet restricted in natural proteins were instituted within the first few weeks of life, most of the devastating effects of the PKU were prevented.

Nearly 25 years after the Fölling observation, a phenylalanine-restricted infant formula became commercially available. Once available, pediatricians and other primary care providers needed to identify asymptomatic infants affected with PKU during the first few weeks of life before permanent brain damage was done. A solution to this problem and the technology that enabled newborn screening was the assay developed by Guthrie and Susi in 1963.[3] Robert Guthrie, who was the father of a child with intellectual disabilities and the uncle of a niece with PKU, recognized the need for a simple test that could be used on all infants to screen for this rare disorder. His solution was to use a card with a strip of filter paper that could be spotted with a few drops of blood obtained from a heel stick within the child's first 2 or 3 days of life. The dried blood spot could then be sent to a laboratory for relatively rapid analysis for elevated amounts of phenylalanine. Guthrie's original filter paper card and his bioassay for phenylalanine, along with the critical roles played by parents and advocates, helped establish and expand worldwide NBS programs.

After PKU screening programs began in the 1960s, advances in technologies spurred screening for other disorders that could be detected on the same filter paper card blood spot. As an example of the growth of screening for genetic disorders in one state's program, **Box 1** displays the history of the expansion of NBS in Georgia. Similarly, each state decides which disorders to include in its NBS panel and which laboratories (public or private, state or regional) will perform each screening test on their panel. In the United States, each state is responsible to fund and evaluate its own NBS program. In the early 2000s, significant media attention was directed at the difference in the disorders that were screened for by different states and regions in the United States. In 2006, as a result of collaborative efforts of public health and

---

Box 1
History of screening for genetic disorders in the state of Georgia

1969: Phenylketonuria (PKU)

1978: Maple Syrup Urine Disease, Homocystinuria, Tyrosinemia, Galactosemia, Congenital Hypothyroidism

1990: Congenital Adrenal Hyperplasia

1998: Sickle Cell Disease and hemoglobinopathies

2003: Biotinidase deficiency

2005: Medium Chain Acyl-CoA Dehydrogenase deficiency

2007: Cystic Fibrosis and Tandem Mass Spectrometry for Fatty Acid Oxidation Defects, Organic Acidemias, Aminoacidopathies.

professional pediatric and genetic organizations, recommendations were made to select which disorders to include in a "Uniform Screening Panel [USP]" for public health newborn screening programs.[4] These recommendations identified 29 conditions (including hearing loss) for which screening should be mandated in all newborns and an additional 25 conditions were identified because they were clinically significant and were revealed with screening technology, but lacked an efficacious treatment. Recommendations were included on how to propose and evaluate other disorders that could be added in the future to the USP. Recommendations for screening of congenital infections were not considered in these initial recommendations, but will undoubtedly be considered in the future. Most states currently screen for most of these disorders (see National Newborn Screening and Genetics Resouce Center: http://genes-r-us.uthscsa.edu).

NEWBORN SCREENING AS A PUBLIC HEALTH PROGRAM

In 1963, Massachusetts became the first state to institute mandatory, universal NBS for PKU. Since then, considerable debate has occurred whether NBS should be a core function of the public health system or should NBS be the responsibility of the primary care provider and family, as done in screening for neonatal jaundice. While some argue that the individual components of NBS are best provided completely by the private sector, most health care professionals agree that NBS is best kept as a public health program with participation of the private and commercial sectors to guarantee that all infants are screened for a core panel of disorders. When an infant screens positive for any disorder, a diagnosis needs to be quickly confirmed and affected infants rapidly treated to prevent death or disability.

NBS is a six-part public health program (**Box 2**).[5] The first component, education of parents and health care providers, is critical to the success of the NBS program, but is often overlooked and underfunded. Excellent online and print resources are available for parents and health care providers to understand the process of screening and how to act on abnormal screening results. (See the online resources at the end of the References section.) The second component of the NBS program, screening of the infant, begins in the hospital or birthing center after the child is at least 24 hours old. To ensure rapid analysis, the filter paper cards with the dried blood samples should be sent by a local or overnight courier to the designated screening laboratory. Many NBS programs experience unnecessary delayed results and are unable to track the filter paper cards because they still use the traditional postal services to transport the card from the place of birth to the screening laboratory. Because every state public laboratory does not have the technical expertise to perform the increasing array of analytic procedures, several states contract with commercial or academic center

---

Box 2
Six components of newborn screening as a public health program

1. Education of parents and health care providers

2. Filter paper card screening

3. Short-term follow-up of abnormal results

4. Confirmation of diagnosis

5. Case management and long-term follow-up

6. Program evaluation

laboratories to perform some or all of their NBS tests. Significant efforts and ongoing education of the staff of the birthing hospital or center ensure that the blood specimens are properly obtained and that each card has accurate and complete demographic information. Electronic data entry at the birthing site helps improve accuracy, lessens the likelihood for insufficient or inaccurate demographic information, and reduces delays in reporting. A comprehensive print and video resource for hospitals and birthing centers on the proper collection of blood on filter paper card is available from the Clinical and Laboratory Standards Institute (CLSI).[6]

An unsatisfactory NBS specimen results in the need to locate the infant, repeat the heel stick, and risk delays in diagnosis and treatment of an affected child. If a screening test is unsatisfactory or abnormal, immediate follow-up is needed. The submitting facility and clinician of record must be notified as quickly as possible about an unsatisfactory or abnormal test result. Short-term follow-up of abnormal results, the third component of the NBS program, is often performed by personnel in the screening laboratory or under contract by the state with a tertiary care provider. The infant must be quickly located (24/7) and a decision made based on the degree of abnormality of the screening result and the child's clinical status as to whether to simply repeat the filter paper screen or to proceed immediately to a diagnostic evaluation. The fourth component, diagnosis, often involves consultation with specialists in metabolic genetic disorders, pediatric endocrinologists, or pediatric hematologists. After a diagnosis is confirmed, case management and long-term case follow-up, the fifth component of the system, is usually performed by these same specialists along with the child's primary care provider. Long-term follow-up of affected children is critical to determine the outcome of the NBS program. Unfortunately long-term follow-up has been difficult because of inadequate funds and the difficulties of tracking affected children into adulthood.

The final component is NBS program evaluation. Each state is responsible to ensure that all infants are properly screened, that unsatisfactory specimens are kept to a minimum, that children with abnormal results are rapidly located and assessed for the disorder, and that affected children are rapidly diagnosed and treated and that their outcome is documented.

To monitor the success of the NBS program, most states have NBS advisory boards that consist of representatives of the state's public health program and laboratories, academic and private treatment centers, neonatologists and pediatric primary practitioners, advocacy and legal groups, and most important, members from families of affected children. Representatives of the advisory boards, parents, and advocates for children are essential to educate state and national legislators about the importance of NBS. Recent funding by the US Health Resources and Services Administration (HRSA) has helped to coordinate regional newborn screening activities and program evaluation.

NEWBORN SCREENING IN LOW BIRTH WEIGHT AND PRETERM INFANTS

Low birth weight (LBW) and preterm infants pose a special problem for NBS programs. Often LBW infants are critically ill, require parenteral nutrition and frequent transfusions, and most troublesome is that the reference ranges established for each NBS screen have usually been established in healthy full-term infants. During their protracted hospital stay, it is common for LBW infants to have multiple heel sticks to repeat abnormal metabolic screens and they need recurrent blood samples for diagnostic studies. In recognition of these difficulties, CLSI is scheduled to publish in 2009 guidelines for NBS in LBW infants that should help establish NBS protocols for special-care neonatal ICUs caring for LBW infants. One important goal of these guidelines is to optimize the timing and to minimize the number of blood spot collections that will be needed on LBW infants.

LONG-TERM ASSESSMENT OF PROGRAMS AND CONSEQUENCES

Many attempts have been made to assess the long-term outcome of NBS programs both in terms of medical outcome and financial costs and benefits. Most economic studies have found significant cost-effectiveness/benefit from NBS programs to save dollars for health care and educational costs.[7] Although many studies have documented the incidence of specific disorders detected by NBS and relatively short-term outcomes in affected children, few population-based long-term studies have evaluated the cost/effectiveness of NBS in preventing developmental disabilities. To determine whether NBS in Atlanta reduced the number of children with intellectual disabilities or less severe developmental delays from 1981 to1991, three independent federal, state, and university data sources were linked. Of an estimated 147 infants who screened positive for a metabolic or endocrine disorder (ie, were at risk for mental retardation if left untreated), only 3 children were identified with intellectual disabilities. Of an estimated 216 children who screened positive for a metabolic or endocrine disorder, 9 children were identified as having a developmental disability less severe than intellectual disabilities (eg, speech-language impairments).[8]

Despite the general successes of NBS programs, several unanticipated consequences of NBS have occurred. Initially, children with PKU were thought to only require a special diet during the first decade of life; however, as adolescents and young adults with PKU were removed from their phenylalanine-restricted diets or as they became less compliant with their diets, elevated blood phenylalanine levels proved deleterious to the function of their mature brains. In addition, women with PKU who conceived and carried children while not controlling their own blood phenylalanine levels were found to be at a significant risk for miscarriage or for having babies with congenital heart disease, microcephaly, and mental retardation. This situation is called maternal PKU.[9] Unfortunately, too many women with PKU were successfully treated as children but were unable to receive or stay on their PKU diet before and during their pregnancies. Many of these women have delivered multiple children with severe congenital impairments and long-term disabilities.

In a report of three states with well-organized metabolic services for care of PKU patients, only 8 (33%) of 24 women with PKU initiated the special diet before pregnancy. Of 22 medical records reviewed, only 12 (55%) indicated control of blood phenylalanine levels before 10 weeks' gestation. Risk factors for late dietary control included young age and belief that treatment costs complicated the diet. Although all of the women expressed confidence in their metabolic clinic staff, few perceived that their obstetricians were knowledgeable about the maternal PKU diet. Of 13 women enrolled in state-based assistance programs, 9 (69%) reported proof of pregnancy was required for eligibility. Many women using private insurance reported that their insurers were unwilling to pay for medical foods. When the data were stratified according to state of residence, differences were observed in the rate of live-born infants, prepregnancy medical food use, the average travel time to the metabolic clinic, and the gestational week when metabolic control was achieved. Studies that examined the long-term outcome of affected children found by NBS again emphasize the need to have lifetime access to experienced staff and resources and the ability to pay for expensive formula and low-protein medical foods, neither of which are routinely paid for by most third-party payers.

FUTURE OF NEWBORN SCREENING PROGRAMS

NBS programs grew slowly during their first 30 years by adding a few disorders to the screening panel. During the 1990s with the advent of new technologies, especially tandem mass spectrometry, it became possible to multiplex tests (ie, run many analyses) on one filter paper card specimen. Although DNA technology is currently too expensive to use in a primary newborn screen, it is used more frequently to confirm a diagnosis from dried blood spots when a primary metabolic screen is abnormal, such as molecular confirmation of the diagnosis of cystic fibrosis on a blood spot with elevated concentrations of immunoreactive trypsinogen.

Several disorders have been proposed to be added to the USP, including congenital infections such as cytomegalovirus and HIV, immunodeficiencies, lysosomal storage disorders, fragile X syndrome, Duchenne muscular dystrophy, and for chromosomal abnormalities such as common microdeletion and sex chromosome abnormalities Attempts have been made to agree on criteria for which disorders to add to a screening panel. Beginning with principles for screening for disease proposed by Wilson and Jungner,[10] these criteria have been modified for NBS to include those shown in **Box 3**. Surprisingly, the most difficult of the criteria used to evaluate each disorder is whether there is an available and effective treatment. For some disorders such as congenital hypothyroidism, early treatment with daily replacement doses of thyroid hormone prevents nearly all of the consequences of the mental and physical delays; however, for other disorders, early identification may simply mean a better long-term outcome.

For example, early detection and treatment of cystic fibrosis with pancreatic enzyme replacement therapy significantly improves children's early growth and nutrition. However, evidence is still limited that early detection improves long-term survival. For other disorders, such as Duchenne muscular dystrophy and fragile X syndrome, early detection may not always lead to an improved clinical outcome for the child. However, advocates argue that early detection of an affected, but presymptomatic child helps parents avoid a "diagnostic odyssey" and promotes entry into early intervention services. Also, early detection of these disorders gives parents and other family members important genetic information and reproductive options before having additional affected children. Opponents of screening for these disorders maintain that identification through NBS could interfere with the family's ability to emotionally bond with the affected child years before he or she becomes symptomatic. Another complicating issue is that filter paper screening can now be done for presymptomatic

---

Box 3
Modified criteria for inclusion of a disorder into the Newborn Screening uniform panel

Significant morbidity and/or mortality

Available and effective treatment

Time exists before onset of symptoms so that intervention can be effective

Clinical validity and clinical utility of screen

Economically "reasonable" and cost-beneficial

Natural history of the disease understood

Known and significant incidence in population to be screened

Data from Wilson JMG, Jungner G. Principles and practice of screening for disease. (Public Health Paper No. 34). Geneva: World Health Organization; 1968.

detection of disorders such as several of the lysosomal storage disorders, such as Gaucher disease and Fabry disease, where treatment may not be needed for several years. In some instances, the child's specific genotype may predict an early or late onset of symptoms, but in many cases either private mutations or those with insufficient data to predict phenotype make it impossible to predict the severity of the disorder and when to initiate therapy. Regardless, many advocates insist that the benefits of early detection outweigh any risk or negative consequences and that parents should be given this option.

LEGAL, ETHICAL, AND FINANCIAL CONCERNS

NBS has always been enmeshed in ethical and legal issues. A child with a disorder that should have been detected by NBS, but the diagnosis was delayed or missed raises many operational and legal concerns about where the system failed. **Box 4** lists several of the ethical concerns about NBS. Although very few programs require signed parental consent, most NBS programs use a policy of "informed dissent." Historically, parents have been given minimal information about the NBS test until shortly before their newborn is ready to be discharged from the hospital. They may be told that their baby "needs to have a PKU test or a heel stick" before discharge and the parents are asked whether they have any objections to the test. Most NBS programs allow parents to refuse the test for religious reasons. Fortunately, few parents refuse, but those who do risk that their child's diagnosis and treatment will be delayed or missed.

Although ample electronic and print information about NBS is available for parents, most receive little if any before the birth of their child. Thus they are ill prepared when they are called by their primary care provider or by an NBS coordinator that their child's NBS was abnormal. More information about NBS needs to be made available to parents during the last trimester of pregnancy, not immediately before their infant's hospital discharge. Why does my baby need a repeat study? How does a screening test differ from a diagnostic test, and how can parents obtain further information about the screening process and about specific disorders? Prospective parents need time to understand this important information about NBS, and the postpartum period is not the optimal time to learn about NBS.

As discussed previously, NBS has been proposed for disorders such as fragile X syndrome, sex chromosome abnormalities, and for chromosomal microdeletion syndromes. As yet there are no widely accepted medical or nutritional therapies for these disorders, but there are psychosocial and reproductive benefits for the family and society. Inclusion of such disorders in a mandatory newborn screen is unlikely. Until a treatment becomes available, NBS for these disorders may soon be available on a supplemental fee-for-service basis. An alternative approach would be to offer

---

Box 4
Several ethical and legal concerns associated with Newborn Screening

Consent of one or both parents needed

Storage and access to leftover dried blood spots

Linkage of NBS information and results to public health vital statistics

Screening for disorders where treatment is not necessary until later in life or supportive, but there is a significant recurrence risk and reproductive options in future pregnancies

Financial support for NBS

voluntary screening to parents of older, but still presymptomatic infants. Infant screening, which would be done at 6 to 12 months of age, still allows for presymptomatic diagnosis, ample time to educate the parents about the screening procedure, and prevents the "diagnostic odyssey." Infant screening would minimize potential interference with parent–infant bonding that could occur with newborn screening for these disorders. With advances in molecular technology, NBS for disorders that do not become symptomatic until late childhood or adulthood will be technically feasible but unlikely to be included in a USP unless a compelling argument can be made that presymptomatic treatment during infancy will significantly benefit the course of the disorder.

Another ethical and legal issue is that parents are poorly, if at all, informed about the storage and use of their child's leftover dried blood spot. Some NBS programs store dried blood spots for only a few months, whereas other NBS programs keep the dried spots for up to 21 years. Some blood spots are stored under ideal conditions; others are not. These spots are used for many purposes such as evaluation of new technologies, epidemiologic and forensic studies, and for program quality control. An important ethical concern is the ability to link demographic information and results of NBS with vital statistics such as birth and death records, referrals to early state developmental programs, and immunization records. Linking and tracking this information is extremely valuable to public health programs and to the primary care providers, but parents need to know how this information on their child will be used, who will have access to the information, and how it will be kept confidential. Privacy advocates have raised important concerns about how this information is stored, used, and retrieved. Some advise parents against newborn screening so that the "government" won't keep a sample of your child's blood and DNA.

Finally, as NBS programs have grown to screen for more disorders so have their costs. Most economic analyses of NBS programs have shown favorable cost–benefit/ratios.[7] Continuing programs and adding new disorders to the screening panel, increases costs to already financially strapped public health programs. Most state programs obtain partial reimbursement from hospitals and third party insurers, not just to support the efforts of the screening laboratory, but also to help finance all segments of the six-part NBS system. Additional funds usually have come from state and federal programs.

Several commercial laboratories now offer "expanded" NBS tests and have challenged the public health laboratories' exclusivity in courts and state legislatures. As new technology becomes available and additional disorders can be added to the screening panel, it is likely that commercial laboratories will offer these tests first directly to parents on a fee-for-service basis. Once screening for a specific disorder meets the acceptance for inclusion in the USP, it will be included in the "Uniform panel" along with those for the well-established disorders.

SUMMARY

Newborn filter paper card screening has been in existence for over 45 years, but it is no longer just "the PKU test." NBS is an essential component of a comprehensive public health program that touches nearly every newborn in the United States and many other countries. Parents and health care professionals have ready access to on-line resources (see http://www.savebabies.com or http://www.genes-r-us.uthscsa.edu). NBS programs have saved thousands of children from death and disability. With ongoing evaluation and input from a spectrum of health care professional and families, NBS will continue as a public health program that benefits the vast majority of infants to protect them from the consequences of an increasing number of devastating genetic, metabolic, and infectious disorders.

ONLINE RESOURCES

National Newborn Screening and Genetics Resouce Center. Available at: http://genes-r-us.uthscsa.edu.
Save Babies Through Screening Foundation, Inc. Available at: http://www.savebabies.org.
Star-G: Screening Technology and Research in Genetics. Available at: http://www.newbornscreening.info.

REFERENCES

1. Brown AS, Fernhoff PM, Waisbren SE, et al. Barriers to successful dietary control among pregnant women with phenylketonuria. Genet Med 2002;4(2):84–9.
2. Fölling A. Über Ausscheidung von Phenylbrenztraubensäure in den Harn als Stoffwecheselanomalie in Verbidung mit Imbezillitat. Z PhysiolChem 1934;277: 169–76.
3. Guthrie R, Susi A. A simple phenylalanine method for detecting phenylketonuria in large populations of newborn infants. Pediatrics 1963;32:338–43.
4. Watson AS, Mann MY, Lloyd-Puryear MA, et al. Newborn screening: toward a uniform panel and system. Executive summary. Genet Med 2006;8(1):1S–11S.
5. Pass KA, Lane PA, Fernhoff PM, et al. Second U.S. newborn screening system guidelines II: Follow-up of children, diagnosis, management, and evaluation: statement of the Council of Regional Networks for Genetic Services (CORN). J Pediatr 2000;137(4 Pt 2):S1–46.
6. Hannon WH, Whitley RJ, Davin B, et al. Blood collection on filter paper for newborn screening programs: approved standard-5th edition. CLSI document LA4-A5. Wayne, PA: Clinical and Laboratory Standards Institute; 2007.
7. Venditti AN, Venditti CP, Berry GT, et al. Newborn screening by tandem mass spectrometry of medium-chain Acyl-CoA dehydrogenase deficiency: a cost-effectiveness analysis. Pediatrics 2003;115:1005–15.
8. Van Naarden BK, Yeargin-Allsopp M, Schendel D, et al. Long-term developmental outcomes of children identified through a newborn screening program with a metabolic or endocrine disorder: a population-based approach. J Pediatr 2003;143(2):236–42.
9. Koch R, Hanley W, Levy H, et al. The maternal phenylketonuria international study: 1984–2002. Pediatrics 2003;112(6 Pt 2):1523–9.
10. Wilson JMG, Jungner G. Principles and practice of screening for disease. (Public Health Paper No. 34). Geneva: World Health Organization; 1968.

Delivery Room Management of the Newborn

Anand K. Rajani, MD*, Ritu Chitkara, MD, Louis P. Halamek, MD

KEYWORDS
- Resuscitation • Neonate • Cardiopulmonary resuscitation
- Cerebral resuscitation • Delivery room communication
- Simulation-based learning

PURPOSE OF RESUSCITATION

To resuscitate means to revive from unconsciousness or apparent death. Neonatal resuscitation is an attempt to facilitate the dynamic transition from fetal to extrauterine physiology. Although most births require little or no intervention, this definition should continue to remind pediatricians that the potential for a compromised newborn exists at every delivery. The level of support required by neonates varies widely, depending on factors such as gestational age, weight, presence of meconium in the amniotic fluid, and other issues. This article outlines the current practices in delivery room management of the neonate. Developments in cardiopulmonary resuscitation techniques and technology are discussed for term and preterm infants, and advances in the areas of cerebral resuscitation and thermoregulation are reviewed. Resuscitation in special circumstances (such as the presence of congenital anomalies) also is covered. The importance of communication with other members of the health care team and the family is discussed. Finally, future trends in neonatal resuscitation are explored.

MODERN NEONATAL RESUSCITATION

With the emergence of neonatal intensive care units (NICUs) in the 1970s, the National Institutes of Health funded five grants aimed at improving the care of newborns at the time of birth. One of these grants was awarded to Ronald Bloom, MD, and Catherine Cropley, RN, MN, at the Drew Postgraduate Medical School in Los Angeles, California. The work accomplished by Bloom and Cropley led to the creation of a training program in resuscitation of the newborn known as the Neonatal Educational Program,

Division of Neonatal and Developmental Medicine, Department of Pediatrics Stanford University School of Medicine, 750 Welch Road, Suite 315, Palo Alto, CA 94304, USA
* Corresponding author.
E-mail address: arajani@stanford.edu (A.K. Rajani).

Pediatr Clin N Am 56 (2009) 515–535
doi:10.1016/j.pcl.2009.03.003
0031-3955/09/$ – see front matter © 2009 Elsevier Inc. All rights reserved.

which consists of a series of educational modules, including readings, slides, and video. As the Neonatal Educational Program was completed, the American Academy of Pediatrics formed a task force led by George Peckham, MD, to standardize training in neonatal resuscitation. Using the Neonatal Educational Program as its basis, the Neonatal Resuscitation Program (NRP) was introduced in 1987 with a stated goal of ensuring the presence of a health care professional competent in neonatal resuscitation at every birth in the United States.[1] Over the past 20 years, more than 2 million US health care professionals have successfully completed the NRP.[2]

Management of the neonate in the delivery room focuses on airway, breathing, circulation, and drugs (the "ABCDs"). The algorithm developed by the NRP allows for a systematic, uniform approach to the newborn that encompasses term and preterm infants who require routine and extensive management in the delivery room. Conceptually, resuscitation of the newborn is similar to resuscitation of older children and adults. The resuscitation algorithm developed by the NRP standardizes the approach to the newborn in distress (**Fig. 1**). The newborn's airway should be assessed and cleared immediately after birth; the infant also should be dried and stimulated. The heart rate should be auscultated or palpated within 30 seconds of birth as a surrogate marker of cardiac output. Much of the NRP algorithm is predicated on the patient's heart rate; positive pressure ventilation (PPV) should be administered for heart rates between 60 and 100 beats per minute (bpm), whereas chest compressions are to be initiated after 30 seconds of PPV for heart rates of less than 60 bpm. If the heart rate continues to be less than 60 bpm after 30 seconds of ventilation and chest compressions, intravenous epinephrine should be administered.[3]

Most compromised neonates who require assistance in the transition from intrauterine to extrauterine life respond to effective PPV. Only 1% of all neonates require further intervention in the form of chest compressions or administration of intravenous fluids or medications.[3] Critically ill infants may have a multitude of problems that require attention, but not all of these problems can or should be addressed in the delivery room. Rather, in general the patient should be transported to a NICU once the airway is secured and the patient's heart rate is stabilized above 100 bpm.

RECENT CHANGES IN THE NEONATAL RESUSCITATION PROGRAM ALGORITHM: INTERNATIONAL LIAISON COMMITTEE ON RESUSCITATION AND THE EVIDENCE-BASED REVIEW PROCESS

The 1987 recommendations by the NRP were based primarily on expert opinion because there was little evidence-based treatment data available.[1] Since that time, the American Heart Association and the NRP have partnered with other national resuscitation councils working under the guidance of the International Liaison Committee on Resuscitation. Together, these bodies convene with international experts to review the most recent science in the fields of cardiopulmonary resuscitation and emergency cardiovascular care. These meetings result in the publication of a series of papers listing the consensus on science and guidelines for clinical care. The most recent guidelines for neonatal resuscitation were issued in 2005.[4]

CARDIOPULMONARY RESUSCITATION
Pulmonary Resuscitation

Immediately after birth, the infant should be placed on warm blankets under a radiant warmer. After drying and stimulation, the infant should be positioned with the neck slightly extended (the "sniffing position"). Such positioning is imperative to ensure proper alignment of the posterior pharynx, larynx, and trachea. In some cases,

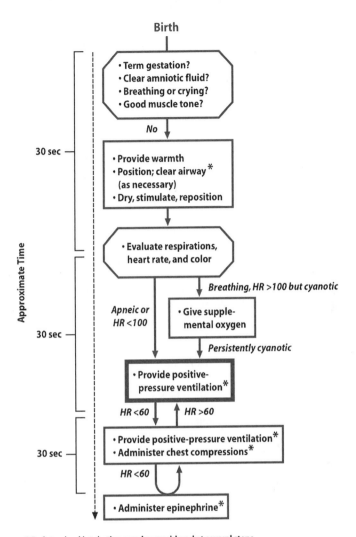

Birth

• Term gestation?
• Clear amniotic fluid?
• Breathing or crying?
• Good muscle tone?

No

• Provide warmth
• Position; clear airway*
  (as necessary)
• Dry, stimulate, reposition

• Evaluate respirations,
  heart rate, and color

Breathing, HR >100 but cyanotic

Apneic or HR <100

• Give supple-
  mental oxygen

Persistently cyanotic

• Provide positive-
  pressure ventilation*

HR <60   *HR >60*

• Provide positive-pressure ventilation*
• Administer chest compressions*

HR <60

• Administer epinephrine*

Approximate Time

30 sec

30 sec

30 sec

*Endotracheal intubation may be considered at several steps.

Fig. 1. NRP resuscitation flow diagram. (*From* Kattwinkel J, editor. Textbook of neonatal resuscitation. 5th edition. Elk Grove Village (IL): American Academy of Pediatrics and American Heart Association; 2006; with permission.)

elevation of the shoulders with a blanket may be helpful. After proper positioning, the initial approach to clearing the airway should include suctioning of the mouth followed by the nose (known as "M before N") because large particulate matter resides in the oropharynx rather than the nasopharynx.[3] Vigorous suctioning should be avoided because stimulation of the posterior pharynx may stimulate a vagal response, which can lead to bradycardia.

Along with the aforementioned interventions, an initial assessment of the patient's respiratory status should be made within the first 30 seconds. In some cases, the severity of respiratory distress improves over several minutes as retained fetal lung fluid is resorbed. Breath sounds should be auscultated to assess for equal air entry (asymmetric breath sounds may indicate a pneumothorax). In the preterm infant, substernal or subcostal retractions may indicate underlying lung immaturity and surfactant deficiency. Respiratory effort should be observed carefully to assess what degree of support is needed, because some preterm infants do not have sufficient respiratory drive. Grunting also may be noted on auscultation and may represent the preterm infant's attempt to create end-expiratory pressure to maintain lung inflation. Providing continuous positive airway pressure (CPAP) or positive end-expiratory pressure may help establish adequate functional residual capacity in the preterm population.

PPV should be initiated at rate of 40 to 60 breaths per minute. After 30 seconds of PPV, the infant should be reassessed. Clinical improvement after initiation of PPV is gauged by the onset of spontaneous breathing, improvement in muscle tone and color, and an increasing heart rate. The rate of PPV can be decreased and respiratory support weaned with improvement in these four areas. In case the patient does not improve, the airway should be assessed for obstruction, and the seal between the face and mask should be rechecked. If there is no physiologic improvement despite use of PPV, the provider should reposition the infant's head and suction his or her oropharynx. If there is poor chest movement after these steps are taken, the inspiratory pressure should be increased. In some cases, peak inspiratory pressure as high as 30 cm H_2O may be needed with initial breaths to establish the functional residual capacity.[3] Endotracheal intubation subsequently should be considered if there is no clinical improvement.

Modalities for administering positive-pressure ventilation

As noted in the NRP's "Textbook of Neonatal Resuscitation," there are several modalities for the administration of PPV, including the flow-inflating bag, self-inflating bag, T-piece resuscitator, and mechanical ventilator. The flow-inflating bag offers the advantage of providing tactile cues that may, in the hands of an experienced clinician, serve as a surrogate marker of pulmonary compliance. In contrast to the flow-inflating bag, the self-inflating bag does not require a compressed gas source, refills completely with each breath, and incorporates a pressure release valve to decrease the risk of barotrauma. The T-piece resuscitator allows the operator to preset the peak inspiratory pressure and positive end-expiratory pressure that is delivered. The operator has the ability to vary the inspiratory time and the ventilation rate by occluding the aperture at the end of the T-piece handle.[3] This advantage must be balanced by the possibility that persons who are inexperienced in its use may not be able to achieve consistent inspiratory times and rates.[5]

Bennett and colleagues evaluated each of these modalities using a mannequin and health care professionals with varying levels of experience and found using this model that the T-piece resuscitator delivered the preset peak inspiratory pressure most consistently but also took the longest amount of time to increase the peak inspiratory pressure from 20 to 40 cm H_2O. For a desired positive end-expiratory pressure of 5 cm H_2O, the investigators found that the self-inflating bag created significantly less positive end-expiratory pressure than the T-piece resuscitator or flow-inflating bag, but the flow-inflating bag required the most practice to operate correctly.[6] A full review of the specific advantages and disadvantages of each modality can be found in the "Textbook of Neonatal Resuscitation."[3]

Continuous positive airway pressure for preterm infants

Gregory and colleagues[7] initially described CPAP as a means of respiratory support for respiratory distress syndrome in 1971. Initially, CPAP was administered via endotracheal tube but currently is used frequently via mask or nasal prongs. In the delivery room, CPAP is frequently delivered via a facemask after an appropriate seal has been made with the infant's face. CPAP offers several advantages to the preterm infant during the initial transition from intrauterine to extrauterine life, including enhanced surfactant release, improved lung expansion, maintenance of functional residual capacity, and decreased atelectasis.[8]

In 1982, Drew[9] published a randomized controlled trial that investigated the mortality of very low birth weight infants who underwent elective intubation versus those who were managed with supplemental oxygen and selective intubation according to certain clinical criteria. Neonates who were electively intubated had a significantly better survival rate (77% versus 51%). Because infants assigned to the elective intubation group were managed by an attending neonatologist and infants in the selective intubation group were managed by a resident physician, it is possible that the level of experience of the practitioner influenced the outcomes. Despite these limitations, it became standard practice in many US NICUs to electively intubate infants of lower birth weights and gestational ages as a result of this study.[10]

In 1987, a study by Avery and colleagues[11] examined the respiratory outcomes of 1625 infants with birth weights of 700 to 1500 g at eight NICUs across the country. Among these NICUs, Columbia University Medical Center was found to have far lower rates of chronic lung disease, which prompted a closer look at their clinical practice. Several differences emerged during this analysis, including their use of CPAP and avoidance of mechanical ventilation in infants with respiratory distress, general tolerance of hypercarbia, avoidance of hyperventilation, and oversight by a single physician (rather than multiple physicians). Columbia's improved outcomes and noninvasive approach subsequently were embraced in many NICUs, sparking a renewed interest in the use of early CPAP in the management of the preterm infant.[10] As a result, several trials have been performed to compare the efficacy of CPAP to mechanical ventilation.

The Continuous Positive Airway Pressure or Intubation at Birth (COIN) trial attempted to examine whether early CPAP or mechanical ventilation affected an infant's risk of death or bronchopulmonary dysplasia. This international, prospective, randomized controlled trial investigated the use of nasal CPAP versus intubation in 610 infants born at 25 to 28 weeks' gestation. Infants in the nasal CPAP group required fewer days of mechanical ventilation and required less oxygen at 28 days of life, but there was no significant difference in the primary endpoint of death or bronchopulmonary dysplasia at 36 weeks' corrected gestational age. A subgroup analysis of infants born at 27 to 28 weeks' gestation did show a trend in favor of nasal CPAP (OR 0.72; 95% CI 0.47–1.11), but this difference was not found to be statistically significant.[12] This study made many contributions. First, it demonstrated that many infants who breathe spontaneously at birth can be treated successfully with nasal CPAP instead of intubation and mechanical ventilation. In contrast to the findings of Drew[9] the COIN trial reinforced the notion that this can be done without any increased risk of death, and data suggested that there may be a benefit in survival or bronchopulmonary dysplasia from infants of 27 to 28 weeks' gestation.

Monitoring

The use of end-tidal carbon dioxide detection devices is currently recommended by the NRP as a primary means of confirming endotracheal tube placement. Two modalities are available: (1) colorimetric devices display a change in color in the presence of CO_2, and (2) capnographs measure a specific CO_2 level via an electrode located at the endotracheal tube connector.[3] Readings from either of these devices should be interpreted with caution, because false-negative results can be seen with poor pulmonary blood flow, cardiac arrest, congenital heart disease.[13] Under these conditions, end-tidal carbon dioxide detection devices should be used in conjunction with auscultation and chest rise to ensure appropriate endotracheal tube placement.[3]

Oxygenation may be monitored by visual inspection of the color of the lips, tongue, and central thorax or through the use of an oximeter. A clinical assessment of color provides only a crude indicator of oxygenation; assessment of the patient's heart rate is more sensitive. Oximetry allows for a more precise measurement of the hemoglobin saturation (SaO_2), which results in more judicious use of oxygen. This device should be attached immediately after delivery. When a regular waveform is displayed with a heart rate that corroborates that which is auscultated, the SaO_2 should accurately reflect tissue oxygenation. In cases of poor cardiac output or excessive movement, a regular waveform may not result for several minutes, so resuscitation should not be delayed pending this information.[4]

Concentration of oxygen used during delivery room resuscitation

Much controversy exists around the issue of the optimal oxygen concentration to use for neonatal resuscitation in the delivery room. A meta-analysis performed by Saugstad and colleagues[14] in 2005 found a 5% reduction in neonatal mortality for infants resuscitated with 21% as opposed to 100% FiO_2. This analysis also showed a faster recovery (Apgar score at 5 minutes, heart rate at 90 seconds, time to first breath) in neonates resuscitated with 21% FiO_2. In 2007, Rabi and colleagues[15] performed a systematic review and meta-analysis of seven trials investigating newborns in need of resuscitation. Their analysis found that neonates resuscitated with 21% FiO_2 had lower mortality rates at 1 week and 1 month of life, and the authors concluded that 21% is superior to 100% FiO_2 as the initial choice for resuscitation of the term newborn.

Premature infants are more vulnerable to oxygen toxicity because of their diminished serum levels of antioxidant enzymes. Given the association of hyperoxia with morbidities such as bronchopulmonary dysplasia, retinopathy of prematurity, and necrotizing enterocolitis, in the premature infant, much attention has been paid to finding the optimal oxygen concentration to use when resuscitating premature neonates.[16–18] Wang and colleagues[19] performed a prospective, randomized, clinical trial investigating resuscitation of preterm neonates (23–32 weeks' gestation) using 21% versus 100% FiO_2. They found that all preterm infants resuscitated with 21% FiO_2 failed to achieve the preset target SaO_2 by 3 minutes of life. They concluded that resuscitation with 21% FiO_2 should not be recommended for resuscitation of preterm neonates. Recently, Escrig and colleagues[20] performed a prospective, randomized, clinical trial comparing the achievement of a targeted SaO_2 of 85% at 10 minutes of life in infants less than 28 weeks' gestation when resuscitation was initiated with low (30%) or high (90%) FiO_2. Levels were adjusted according to preductal SaO_2 values. They concluded that in extremely low gestational age neonates, resuscitation could be initiated safely with a low FiO_2 (approximately 30%).Oxygen concentration should then be adjusted to the infant's needs, thereby reducing the oxygen load and subsequent risk of oxygen toxicity.

Current NRP guidelines recommend that oxygen administration in preterm babies begin using a concentration between 21% and 100% FiO_2. A pulse oximeter should be applied to the preterm infant, and an oxygen blender should be used to adjust oxygen concentration in order to achieve a SaO_2 of approximately 90%. FiO_2 should be decreased subsequently as SaO_2 rises beyond 95%. For term babies, the NRP currently recommends using 100% oxygen when a baby is cyanotic or requires PPV. It does provide the caveat that "research suggests that resuscitation with something less than 100% oxygen may be just as successful."[3]

Management of the meconium-stained infant

Meconium stained amniotic fluid (MSAF) is encountered in approximately 7% to 20% of live births, with 2% to 9% of infants born through MSAF acquiring meconium aspiration syndrome (MAS).[21] The association between fetal bowel movements and increased neonatal morbidity and mortality has been noted since the time of Aristotle.[22] MAS is characterized by obstruction of the large airways (resulting in acute hypoxia) and chemically mediated inflammation of the small airways. There does not seem to be any difference in the rate of MAS based on the consistency (thick versus thin) of the meconium.[4] The recently published mortality rate of MAS was 2.5%,[23] in contrast to rates as high as 40% 25 years ago.[24] In the last century, the role of meconium in fetal and neonatal disease has been the subject of intense investigation and debate, and obstetricians and pediatricians have long pursued therapies for the prevention and treatment of meconium aspiration. Although we have come a long way in our understanding of meconium aspiration since the observations of Aristotle, many questions remain.

Many of the strategies for the prevention and treatment of MAS, although well intentioned, have been misguided. Intrapartum maternal opioid administration, cesarean section, cricoid pressure, epiglottal blockage, and thoracic compression have shown no positive benefit and actually may increase morbidity. Amnioinfusion, gastric suction, saline lavage, and chest physiotherapy are commonly practiced, but data from sufficiently powered, prospective, randomized trials confirming their efficacy are limited. Vain and colleagues[25] studied intrapartum (on the perineum) oropharyngeal suctioning of infants born through MSAF and determined that this procedure did not reduce the incidence of MAS, need for intubation, or mortality. In a multicenter, prospective, randomized, controlled trial, Wiswell and colleagues[26] answered the following question: Do intubation and suctioning of the trachea in vigorous, meconium-stained term neonates reduce the risk of MAS? Entry criteria included gestational age more than 37 weeks, birth through MSAF (regardless of consistency), and apparent vigor at delivery (defined as the presence of a heart rate > 100 bpm, spontaneous respirations, and normal muscle tone). They prospectively enrolled 2094 patients at 12 centers; 1051 were randomized to intubation with a standard meconium aspirator attached to the proximal end of the endotracheal tube. Suction, set at 80 mm Hg to 120 mm Hg, was applied for 1 to 5 seconds continuously and as the tube was withdrawn. If meconium was returned, the patient was reintubated and suctioning repeated until the fluid became clear. The randomized expectant management group included 1043 patients who did not receive suctioning at delivery; however, if neonates in this group later manifested respiratory distress, intubation and suctioning were permitted if clinically indicated.

The investigators also classified the consistency of meconium as thin (relatively clear and watery), moderately thick (opaque, no particles), and thick (opaque with particles, similar to pea soup). No significant difference was found between the two groups in the incidence of MAS: 2.7% of infants managed expectantly and 3.2% of infants intubated at delivery developed the disease. The thickness of meconium had no effect on outcome. No difference existed between groups in the incidence of respiratory distress due to other causes such as transient tachypnea of the newborn and pneumonia. The overall complication rate in the intubation group was low (3.8%), and all complications were transient and not serious. The authors concluded that intubation and suctioning of the term, vigorous, meconium-stained neonate do not reduce the incidence of respiratory distress, whether secondary to MAS or any other cause. They recommended that intubation and suctioning continue to be performed in meconium-stained neonates who are not vigorous, require PPV, or subsequently develop respiratory distress.[26]

Other studies of the postnatal management of the vigorous infant born through MSAF also demonstrated no significant improvement in the rate of MAS with intubation and tracheal suctioning.[27–29] Current management as prescribed by the NRP involves suctioning of the trachea only if the infant is not vigorous (as defined by a heart rate of < 100 bpm, decreased muscle tone, or ineffectual respirations).[3] Based on the current literature describing neonates delivered through MSAF, there are no data to support routine suctioning of the newborn's airway after the head is delivered on the perineum, nor are there data to support oropharyngeal suctioning once delivery is complete if the newborn is vigorous.[25] Arguably the most significant advance in the prevention of MAS has been improved estimation of gestational age and reduction in the incidence of postdate deliveries. Placental function steadily declines late in gestation, which increases the risk of impaired fetal substrate delivery, fetal stress, and passage of meconium. Avoiding post-date delivery has reduced the number of patients with classic postmaturity syndrome (eg, meconium passage, reduced subcutaneous body fat, peeling of the epidermis) and MAS.

MAS and persistent pulmonary hypertension of the newborn (PPHN) are relatively common conditions in sick full-term neonates and often occur concomitantly. It is important to understand that each disease also may exist independently and that appropriate therapy should be directed at the specific underlying pathophysiology. In utero, most fetal blood bypasses the lungs via the ductus arteriosus and foramen ovale. Pulmonary flow must increase at birth, however, as the liquid-breathing fetus becomes a gas-breathing neonate. This transition is normally accomplished by a fall in pulmonary arterial pressure, constriction of ductal tissue, and functional closure of the foramen. Pulmonary vasoregulation is achieved by a delicate balance of factors that produce constriction and dilatation, including endogenous mediators (eg, prostaglandins, bradykinin, leukotrienes, and thromboxanes) and mechanical forces involving alveolar inflation and vascular stretch.[30] Impaired fetal substrate delivery, secondary to declining placental function late in gestation or other factors, results in a redistribution of fetal blood flow to the brain and heart.

When delivery of substrates such as oxygen is impaired on a chronic (days to weeks) rather than acute (minutes to hours) basis, pulmonary vasoregulation is altered in several ways. Anatomically, hypertrophy of smooth muscle cells, extension of this hypertrophied musculature into distal vessels, and abnormal deposition of connective tissue have been described. Functionally, these vessels exhibit hyperresponsiveness to stimuli such as hypoxia and acidosis, which leads to intense vasospasm. It is important to understand that this underlying anatomic and functional predisposition to altered pulmonary vasoregulation is prenatal in origin and not secondary to some event occurring at or shortly after the time of birth.[31] PPHN, formerly known as persistent fetal circulation, is defined as a sustained elevation in pulmonary arterial pressure that results in persistent right-to-left shunting and impaired oxygenation. The incidence is approximately 0.1% of all term births.[32] It becomes manifest when a noxious stimulus such as hypoxemia, acidosis, or cold stress initiates a cycle of pulmonary vasospasm, right-to-left shunting, hypoxemia, anaerobic metabolism, acidosis, and increased vasospasm; death is likely if the cycle continues uninterrupted.

The distinction between hypoxemia secondary to pulmonary vascular disease and hypoxemia caused by parenchymal lung disease is clinically important. Term neonates with hypoxemia secondary to pure pulmonary vascular disease may have a normal chest radiograph at birth; in fact, it may be abnormally clear secondary to decreased pulmonary vascular markings indicative of reduced pulmonary blood flow. Neonates with PPHN often manifest a dynamic pH "setpoint" at which the pulmonary vasculature dilates and oxygenation greatly improves. This can be ascertained by reviewing serial arterial blood gasses. The presence of a clear chest radiograph and pH setpoint, together with evidence of right-to-left shunting on echocardiogram in the absence of structural heart disease, effectively establishes the clinical diagnosis of PPHN. Unlike the neonate with significant parenchymal lung disease (as in MAS), patients with pure PPHN have normal pulmonary compliance and low airway resistance and require minimal mean airway pressure to maintain adequate tidal volumes.

The use of excessive airway pressure serves only to increase intrathoracic pressure, decrease venous return, and reduce forward flow through the pulmonary arteries, which further reduces the oxygen content of the blood. Avoidance of unnecessarily high airway pressures also minimizes the risk of baro- and volutrauma and reduces the risk of iatrogenic lung injury. High-frequency oscillatory ventilation, especially when accompanied by suboptimal preload, actually may result in further compromise in oxygenation; conventional mechanical ventilation accompanied by continuous tidal volume monitoring may be more effective.[33] Not all neonates with PPHN also have MAS. Prompt recognition of this fact should prevent the implementation of potentially harmful therapies, avoid iatrogenic injury, and optimize patient outcome.

Naloxone for opioid-induced respiratory depression
Naloxone is no longer recommended for use in newborns in the delivery room but is described in this article because some health care professionals may choose to use it outside of the delivery room. An opioid antagonist, naloxone can be administered intravenously, intramuscularly, or via endotracheal tube. Should a newborn manifest respiratory depression in the delivery room, appropriate support of respirations should be undertaken and the newborn transported to the nursery for continued stabilization and evaluation. The half-life of naloxone is shorter than that of almost all opioids; as naloxone is metabolized and its ability to counteract the sedative effects of opioids wanes, respiratory depression and apnea may recur secondary to persistence of the opioid in the newborn's circulation.[3] Pharmacokinetic data suggest that peak levels are achieved much faster with the intravenous versus the intramuscular route (5–40 minutes versus 30–120 minutes).[34] Administration of naloxone should be undertaken in the postresuscitation period only after the mother's history can be reviewed and lack of longstanding prenatal exposure documented; administration of naloxone to neonates with chronic opioid exposure may produce acute withdrawal and seizures. No studies have examined the efficacy of naloxone in neonates at the currently recommended dose.[35]

Cardiac Resuscitation

Bradycardia
Hypoxia is the most common cause of bradycardia in the newborn; other less common causes include congenital heart block (usually as a result of maternal autoantibodies, anti-SSA or -SSB) and congenital structural heart disease (arteriovenous septal defects, ventricular inversion, heterotaxy syndrome, and other defects that disrupt electrical conduction).[36]

Treatment of bradycardia

Most of the interventions described in the NRP algorithm are based on the neonate's heart rate. This heart rate is used as a surrogate marker of the patient's cardiac output. The initial heart rate is assessed along with the patient's tone, color, and breathing at 30 seconds of life. If the heart rate is less than 100 bpm, PPV is initiated and the heart rate is rechecked at 1 minute of life. For any heart rate less than 60 bpm, chest compressions and PPV are to be initiated synchronously with a ratio of three compressions to every ventilation. The quality of the chest compressions is the most important determinant of restoration of adequate cardiac output. The chest should be compressed to one-third the depth in the anteroposterior diameter.[3]

Epinephrine is the drug of choice for refractory neonatal bradycardia. The administration of epinephrine leads to increased end-diastolic pressure and improved coronary artery perfusion, resulting in increased blood flow to the myocardium and resumption of spontaneous circulation.[37] Intravenous epinephrine administration (via the umbilical vein or other central route) is preferred in a dose of 0.1 to 0.3 mL/kg of a 1:10,000 solution (0.01–0.03 mg/kg) given every 3 to 5 minutes.[38] Although intravenous access should not be delayed, it is acceptable to deliver epinephrine via the endotracheal tube in a dose of 0.3 to 1.0 mL/kg of 1:10,000 solution (0.03–0.1 mg/kg).[3]

The optimal route of epinephrine delivery remains under investigation. Numerous questions have been raised about the efficacy of endotracheal epinephrine administration, including the effects on efficacy of dilution in alveolar fluid, poor blood flow to the lungs during bradycardia/asystole, and pulmonary vasoconstriction secondary to acidosis.[39] Studies of endotracheal epinephrine in anesthetized dogs have shown a measurable increase in heart rate and blood pressure at doses ten times higher than currently recommended by the NRP.[40] To date, no prospective, randomized, controlled studies of endotracheal epinephrine have been conducted in the human neonatal population.[37]

Tachycardia

Tachycardia in the newborn can be a result of intrapartum processes such as infection or acute blood loss or as a result of an underlying tachydysrhythmia. Most cases of tachydysrhythmias in the fetus are supraventricular in nature. These tachydysrhythmias are usually well tolerated when intermittent. Sustained fetal tachydysrhythmias or persistent tachycardias are more likely to lead to fetal hydrops, a potentially lethal condition.[41] If a sinus tachycardia is appreciated at birth, an assessment should be made of the infant's core temperature because fever secondary to maternal temperature elevation—as in chorioamnionitis—is often the cause. The antepartum history should be reviewed for evidence of hemorrhage as in placental abruption. Any infant who presents with the combination of edema and sustained tachycardia should be evaluated for hydrops fetalis secondary to a supraventricular tachycardia.

Treatment of tachycardia

If the perfusion of vital organs seems compromised, cardiopulmonary resuscitation should be undertaken to support cardiac output, and intravenous access should be established rapidly (via the umbilical vein). If a supraventricular tachydysrhythmia is suspected and the patient is hemodynamically stable, a nasogastric tube may be inserted to stimulate the vagus nerve and break the tachycardia. In the case of hydrops fetalis or acute blood loss, volume resuscitation with crystalloid or colloid solutions should be undertaken because the intravascular volume in these patients is frequently depleted. In the case of hydrops in an infant, an electrocardiogram should be performed and a pediatric cardiologist should be consulted for guidance regarding cardioversion.[41]

SPECIAL CARDIOPULMONARY RESUSCITATION CIRCUMSTANCES
Pierre Robin Sequence

Infants born with Pierre Robin sequence should be placed in the prone position, which allows the tongue to fall forward and open the airway; the supine position is to be avoided. If simple positioning of the newborn does not allow adequate respirations, a jaw thrust may be performed until a more stable and permanent mode of maintaining airway patency is possible. Placement of an oral airway, a nasopharyngeal airway, or an endotracheal tube often alleviates or lessens the obstruction.[3] In addition to these devices, the laryngeal mask airway offers another option. It is placed in the supraglottic space and allows for positive pressure to be delivered above the laryngeal inlet.[42]

Pneumothorax

A pneumothorax should be suspected in the presence of diminished breath sounds on one side of the infant's chest. In many cases there is a history of CPAP or PPV administration. A tension pneumothorax occurs when the pleural space fills with enough gas to produce severe compression of the ipsilateral lung and shift the mediastinal contents to the contralateral side. This results in diminished venous return and pulmonary blood flow, which lead to cyanosis and bradycardia. Transillumination of the chest may be helpful in making the diagnosis, but a chest radiograph provides definitive answers. A tension pneumothorax is a potentially life-threatening condition and should be treated in the delivery room if the patient remains bradycardic. If evacuation of the pneumothorax is to be attempted, the infant should be placed on his or her side, with the affected side in the superior position in preparation for a needle thoracostomy. An 18- or 20-gauge catheter-over-needle is then inserted into the pleural space at the fourth intercostal space in the anterior axillary line. The needle is removed, leaving the overlying catheter in the pleural space. The catheter is then attached to one hub of a three-way stopcock while a 20-mL syringe is attached to one of the remaining hubs. By closing the stopcock to the atmosphere and pulling back on the syringe, any air within the pleural space is drawn into the syringe and can be evacuated to the atmosphere. If the pneumothorax requires continuous drainage, placement of a chest tube should be considered. A chest radiograph should be obtained to look for residual pneumothorax after any attempts at drainage.[3]

Congenital Diaphragmatic Hernia

The incidence of congenital diaphragmatic hernia is approximately 1 in 3000 live births.[42] Approximately 84% are left-sided, 13% are right-sided, and 2% are bilateral; most cases involve the posterolateral aspect of the diaphragm.[43] Although prenatal ultrasonography often results in the early detection of these anomalies, some cases still go undiagnosed and present challenges to personnel charged with resuscitation of newborns in the delivery room.

The classic presentation at birth of a newborn with a significant congenital diaphragmatic hernia is marked by the presence of respiratory distress, a scaphoid abdomen, and bowel sounds in the chest. Because the herniated intestine and other abdominal organs compress the lungs and shift the mediastinal structures, compromise of oxygenation, ventilation, and cardiac output is often immediate. In the case of a known or suspected congenital diaphragmatic hernia, the duration of PPV with bag and mask should be minimized and intubation undertaken quickly to avoid gastrointestinal distension and further compromise of lung expansion and function. An orogastric tube also should be placed to allow ongoing decompression of the gastrointestinal tract.[3] Consultation with a neonatologist and pediatric surgeon should take place immediately.

Congenital Heart Disease

As a result of recent advances in fetal ultrasonography and echocardiography, pediatricians are frequently asked to attend deliveries for infants with suspected congenital heart disease.[44] Several studies that examined the accuracy of fetal echocardiography suggested that these studies provide correct diagnoses in approximately 90% of cases.[45–47] Because of this degree of accuracy and the frequency with which these patients require intervention in the delivery room, pediatricians need to be aware of how the presence of fetal congenital heart disease may alter the normal flow of neonatal resuscitation.[48] Although studies suggest that infants with certain forms of congenital heart disease can be stabilized and transported to a cardiac center uneventfully,[49] others with particular lesions may decompensate quickly and require urgent evaluation by a pediatric cardiologist and possible treatment by a cardiothoracic surgeon. Transposition of the great arteries with intact ventricular septum and restrictive atrial septal defect, hypoplastic left heart syndrome with intact atrial septum, and obstructed total anomalous pulmonary venous return all can present with profound hypoxemia secondary to their inability to provide adequate pulmonary venous blood flow to the systemic circulation. In these instances, delivery in a specialized cardiac center may be beneficial because the patient can receive immediate life-saving treatments such as balloon atrial septostomy.[44]

Pulse oximetry may be helpful in caring for infants with suspected congenital heart disease. Whereas healthy full-term infants reach preductal SaO_2 levels of more than 95% by 12 minutes of life,[50] goals for SaO_2 in newborns with congenital heart disease, in whom there is mixing of oxygenated and deoxygenated blood, are typically in the 75% to 85% range. In this population, systemic blood flow largely depends on the relative resistances of the pulmonary and systemic circulations; oxygen should be used cautiously in these infants. In cases in which systemic output depends on blood flow through the ductus arteriosus, prostaglandin E_1 should be delivered via continuous infusion at a dose of 25 to 100 ng/kg/min to maintain ductal patency (**Box 1**). Apnea, vasodilation, hypotension, and fever are all common side effects of prostaglandin E_1. Significant desaturation and apnea should be treated with intubation and mechanical ventilation.[44]

Gastroschisis and Omphalocele

Gastroschisis and omphaloceles are congenital defects of the abdominal wall. Gastroschisis typically occurs as an isolated defect with an incidence of 2.6 in 10,000 live births.[51] Omphaloceles more frequently present as one component of a multiple

---

Box 1
Common defects that require prostaglandin E_1 infusion

Transposition of the great arteries

Tetralogy of Fallot

Single ventricle physiology with ductal-dependent systemic blood flow

Single ventricle physiology with ductal-dependent pulmonary blood flow

malformation syndrome, and their presence should initiate an extensive evaluation for associated anomalies involving the heart, kidneys, and other organs and a karyotype to determine the presence of chromosomal abnormalities, such as trisomy 13.[52] Immediately after delivery, the infant should be placed in a sterile, clear plastic bag that is drawn up over the feet to the chest—effectively covering the defect—to limit physical trauma, insensible water loss, and heat loss. An orogastric tube should be placed to minimize gastrointestinal distention, and a neonatologist and pediatric surgeon should be consulted immediately for further management.

Myelomeningocele

Myelomeningocele is an open defect of the spinal cord that results from a failure of closure of the neural tube. As a result, there is maldevelopment of the neural tube and secondary neural damage after prolonged exposure to amniotic fluid.[53] Treatment of a myelomeningocele in the delivery room includes decubitus positioning of the newborn to avoid direct pressure and application of a sterile plastic covering or bag to protect the lesion from infection, desiccation, and direct trauma. Any resuscitative measures should be carried out with the neonate in the decubitus position. Consultation with a neonatologist and pediatric neurosurgeon should be sought immediately.

THERMOREGULATION
Term Infants

In 1979, Hammarlund and colleagues[54] examined the properties of evaporative, conductive, and radiant heat loss in term infants. All of the infants weighed more than 3.2 kg and were estimated to have total losses as high as 155 W/m^2, translating to declines of body temperature of 0.9°C in 15 minutes. Because of the risk of hypothermia, the NRP recommends that all newborns be dried with warm blankets and kept under a radiant warmer during resuscitation in the delivery room.[3] Heat loss also may be limited by relatively simple measures such as hats and skin-to-skin contact with the mother.[55,56]

Preterm Infants

Preterm infants face numerous challenges in an attempt to maintain body temperature after birth. Compared to term infants, their relatively thin skin and higher body-surface-area-to-mass ratio increases their rate and degree of heat loss. Several recent studies correlated low body temperatures upon admission to the nursery in the preterm population with increased rates of mortality. Deriving rates of heat loss from the initial findings of Hammarland and colleagues,[54] Watkinson[57] calculated that a radiant warmer alone is insufficient for maintaining thermal homeostasis in the preterm infant. For this reason, several additional methods of limiting heat loss in preterm neonates' thermal regulation have been introduced. Vohra and colleagues[58] investigated the efficacy of polyethylene wraps in 59 preterm infants. Although there was no significant difference in the rectal admission temperatures of the infants of 28 to 31 weeks' gestation, the 18 infants younger than 28 weeks' gestation who were covered in polyethylene wraps had a rectal temperature that was 1.9°C higher (P < 0.001) than infants who were openly exposed to the environment.

A subsequent prospective, randomized, controlled study of infants younger than 28 weeks' gestation also demonstrated a benefit with polyethylene occlusive wrap versus nonwrapped controls; infants in the intervention group had an admission temperature of 36.5°C versus 35.6°C in the control group (P < 0.002).[59] Heated mattresses initially were used for thermoregulation during the transport of preterm infants[60,61] and later were used to maintain body temperature after transport.[57,62] Twenty-four preterm infants ranging from 24 to 32 weeks' gestation and weighing 531 to 1498 g were randomized to be warmed with a heated mattress or receive standard care in the delivery room. The infants treated with the heated mattress had a mean admission temperature of 36.6°C (1.6°C higher than the control group) and a statistically significant decrease in the relative risk of hypothermia, as defined by a body temperature of less than 36.5°C or skin temperature of 36.5°C (RR 0.3, 95% CI 0.11–0.83).[62] Concerns with this means of warming include the potential for hyperthermia or even burns, because the mattress temperatures can be higher than desired depending on the preactivation temperature. Kangaroo care is another effective method of maintaining thermoregulation in larger preterm infants with spontaneous breathing and adequate oxygenation.[63]

CEREBRAL RESUSCITATION

Historically the term "resuscitation" has been interpreted as restoration of the function of the heart and lungs. Despite its importance to human beings, the brain has not been the focus of resuscitative techniques. With the advent of interventions carrying the promise of protecting the brain from injury during periods of suboptimal oxygen delivery, the field of resuscitation medicine recently began to consider the concept of "cerebral" resuscitation. The current NRP guidelines outline several strategies for limiting brain injury in the preterm infant, with many of these strategies specifically aimed at preventing intraventricular hemorrhage. Gentle handling and proper positioning (avoidance of the head-down position) and minimizing intrathoracic pressure (as with PPV) are advocated as means of preventing obstruction of cephalic venous drainage and reducing the risk of intraventricular hemorrhage. Rapid changes in $PaCO_2$ are also to be avoided, because the corresponding changes in cerebral blood flow in infants without mature cerebral vasoregulatory ability also at increased risk for intraventricular hemorrhage. Finally, hypertonic intravenous fluids should not be delivered to preterm newborns, nor should any crystalloid or colloid solution be infused at a rapid rate. Currently, the NRP has no formal recommendations on the use of hypothermia in term infants for neuroprotection after perinatal depression. (See the section on hypothermia for infants with hypoxic-ischemic encephalopathy [HIE].) Hyperthermia, however, is to be avoided in infants of all gestations, as is hypoglycemia. Seizures may be another manifestation of perinatal depression, and anticonvulsant therapy may be needed for control.[3]

Overview and Examination Findings in Hypoxic-ischemic Encephalopathy

HIE occurs in approximately 2 to 3 in 1000 infants in the United States and is a leading cause of neonatal morbidity and mortality around the world.[64] According to criteria set forth by the American Academy of Pediatrics, the term "asphyxia" should be used only to describe infants with a fetal pH of less than 7, evidence of multiorgan dysfunction, neurologic dysfunction, and Apgar scores of 0 to 3 at longer than 5 minutes.[65] Alternate causes for neonatal encephalopathy should be considered, because the neonate who experiences an overwhelming infection may present in a similar fashion. Information regarding intrapartum events should be documented; uteroplacental insufficiency, uterine rupture, cord prolapse, cord avulsion, significant decelerations of the fetal heart rate, or any event that limits blood flow or placental gas exchange is a potential cause of the encephalopathy.[64] Three clinical levels of HIE were originally described by Sarnat and Sarnat[66] and have been used in assessing the level of postanoxic injury. Decreased level of consciousness, decreased spontaneous activity, decerebrate or decorticate posturing, decreased tone, weak or absent primitive reflexes, and generalized dysfunction of the autonomic nervous system are signs seen with more severe HIE.

Hypothermia for Infants with Hypoxic-ischemic Encephalopathy

After a hypoxic insult, several metabolic pathways are activated that may have deleterious effects on the brain. Release of excitatory neurotransmitters, production of nitric oxide,[67] and alterations in cerebral blood flow and metabolism[68] have been implicated as causes of brain injury seen with HIE. Hypoxic-ischemic animal models have demonstrated benefits in decreasing brain injury by reducing brain temperatures by 2° to 5°C for up to 72 hours with minimal physiologic effects.[69,70] Two human studies explored this therapeutic option in term infants. The Cool Cap Trial used selective head cooling with mild systemic hypothermia in infants with moderate to severe HIE treated within 6 hours of birth. This prospective, randomized, controlled trial enrolled infants of 36 weeks' gestation or older with a diagnosis of HIE based on clinical criteria. Amplitude-integrated electroencephalograms performed 1 hour or more after birth were also performed to stratify patients with moderate or severe HIE. Subjects underwent selective head cooling for 72 hours while body temperatures were maintained at 34° to 35°C. This study revealed a reduction in the incidence of moderate to severe disability at 18 months in patients with moderate HIE. Infants with severe encephalopathy or seizures noted on amplitude-integrated electroencephalograms at the time of enrollment received no benefit from selective head cooling.[71]

A prospective, randomized, controlled study of whole-body hypothermia in infants of 36 weeks' gestation or older initiated within 6 hours of birth for moderate to severe HIE based on clinical criteria was reported by Shankaran and colleagues.[69] This study used whole-body hypothermia to produce a core esophageal temperature of 33.5°C for 72 hours prior to gradual rewarming to normal body temperature. The rate of death or moderate to severe disability at 18 to 22 months of age was reduced in the intervention (whole-body cooling) group; there was no difference, however, in the rate of cerebral palsy between the intervention and control groups. The authors of this study hypothesized that whole-body hypothermia produced consistent cooling of deeper brain structures that are frequently affected in HIE, representing a potential advantage over selective head cooling.[72] Because the classification criteria and primary outcomes were defined differently in each study, no conclusions can be drawn regarding which intervention is optimal. It remains controversial as to whether hypothermia should be considered the standard of care.

COMMUNICATION IN THE DELIVERY ROOM
Communication with Parents Regarding Resuscitation

Parents act as the surrogate decision makers for their children. In all situations involving newborns in whom the prognosis is uncertain, the survival rate is borderline, or the morbidity rate is high, the parents' views on initiating, continuing, or discontinuing resuscitation should be respected. Given current outcome data, it is reasonable to consider noninitiation of resuscitative efforts for any infant who is less than 23 completed weeks' gestation, has a birth weight less than 400 g, or has lethal anomalies such as anencephaly. Discontinuation of aggressive resuscitative efforts is considered ethically equivalent to noninitiation of such care. In cases in which the chances of survival with acceptable neurologic function are low or there are no signs of life after

10 minutes of continuous, technically correct cardiopulmonary resuscitation, it is reasonable to discontinue resuscitative efforts.[73]

Communication with Colleagues

In 2004, the Joint Commission issued a Sentinel Event Alert describing 47 cases of neonatal death or severe disability that were reported to that agency since 1996. Sixty-two additional cases were added to the series by December 2005. Root cause analyses of these cases indicated that problems with communication played a major role in the outcome of more than 70% of these cases. As a result, the Joint Commission recommended that health care organizations responsible for the delivery of newborns "conduct team training in perinatal areas to teach staff to work together and communicate more effectively."[74] This effective communication is characterized by clear, audible instructions that are professional, directed at specific individuals, and acknowledged (either verbally or nonverbally) by the recipients. Effective communication is one of ten important behavioral skills adapted from the crew resource management program of commercial aviation for use in the delivery room.[75]

NEW DEVELOPMENTS IN NEONATAL RESUSCITATION
Delivery Room Intensive Care Units

In a recent commentary on the integration of intensive care technology into the delivery room, Vento and colleagues[76] described the apparent dichotomy in practice and technology between the NICU and the delivery room. Although care in the NICU typically includes the application of highly sophisticated monitoring and therapeutic technologies and procedures, care in the delivery room usually involves the pediatrician's eyes, ears, and hands as monitoring devices and therapeutic interventions. Examining the unchanged rates in neonatal survival or survival rate without major morbidity (including necrotizing enterocolitis, bronchopulmonary dysplasia, and intraventricular hemorrhage) in the past 10 years, the authors posit that applying the more sophisticated technologies already used in the NICU to delivery room practice may have a pivotal effect on the outcomes of the sickest infants. Coining the phrase "delivery room ICU," the authors propose that the use of continuous heart rate monitoring, oximetry, oxygen blenders, T-piece resuscitators, and neonatal ventilators will improve outcomes for the most critically ill patients.[76,77]

Simulation-based Learning Methodologies

The Joint Commission recommended in 2004 that clinical drills followed by debriefings be conducted for high-risk events such as neonatal resuscitation to "evaluate team performance and identify areas for improvement."[74] Simulation-based learning affords trainees the opportunity to work through clinically challenging situations without risk to real patients, practice the incorporation of cognitive, technical, and behavioral skills, and reflect on their performance during constructive debriefing sessions.[78] The emergence of simulation as a form of active, trainee-centered learning also caught the attention of the NRP of the American Academy of Pediatrics. The NRP is evolving from a biennial training experience based on lectures and skills stations to a career-long series of simulation-based learning opportunities.[1] This transition undoubtedly will have a profound impact on its 2.2 million trainees[2] as they care for neonates in delivery rooms across the United States.

SUMMARY

Neonatal resuscitation remains a cornerstone of pediatric care because a health care professional skilled in its techniques must be immediately available for each of the 4 million newborns delivered annually in the United States. As the evidence behind the clinical guidelines and the learning methodologies underlying its techniques continues to grow, so too does the quantity of expertise and the level of sophistication required to perform safe and effective neonatal resuscitation. Given the large number of newborns and the wide range of clinical presentations, mastering resuscitation of the neonate remains essential.

REFERENCES

1. Halamek LP. Educational perspectives: the genesis, adaptation and evolution of the neonatal resuscitation program. NeoReviews 2008;9:e142–9.
2. Escobedo M. Moving from experience to evidence: changes in US Neonatal Resuscitation Program based on International Liaison Committee on Resuscitation Review. J Perinatol 2008;28:S35–40.
3. Kattwinkel J, editor. Textbook of neonatal resuscitation. 5th edition. Elk Grove Village (IL): American Academy of Pediatrics and American Heart Association; 2006.
4. Perlman JM, Kattwinkel J. Delivery room resuscitation past, present, and the future. Clin Perinatol 2006;33:1–9.
5. McHale S, Thomas M, Hayden E, et al. Variation in inspiratory time and tidal volume with T-piece neonatal resuscitator: association with operator experience and distraction. Resuscitation 2008;79:230–3.
6. Bennett S, Finer NN, Rich W, et al. A comparison of three neonatal resuscitation devices. Resuscitation 2005;67:113–8.
7. Gregory GA, Kitterman JA, Phibbs RH, et al. Treatment of idiopathic respiratory distress syndrome with continuous positive airway pressure. N Engl J Med 1971;284:1333–40.
8. Halamek LP, Morley C. Continuous positive airway pressure during neonatal resuscitation. Clin Perinatol 2006;33:83–98.
9. Drew H. Immediate intubation at birth of the very low birthweight baby. Am J Dis Child 1982;38:207–10.
10. Dunn MS, Reilly MC. Approaches to the initial respiratory management of preterm neonates. Paediatr Respir Rev 2003;4:2–8.
11. Avery ME, Tooley WH, Kelley JB. Is chronic lung disease in low birth weight infants preventable? A survey of eight centres. Pediatrics 1987;79:6–30.
12. Morley CJ, David PG, Doyle LW, et al. Coin trial investigators: nasal CPAP or intubation at birth for very preterm infants. N Engl J Med 2008;358:700–8.
13. 2005 American Heart Association (AHA) guidelines for cardiopulmonary pesuscitation (CPR) and emergency cardiovascular care (ECC) of pediatric and neonatal patients: neonatal resuscitation guidelines. Pediatrics 2006;115:e1–10.
14. Saugstad OD, Ramji S, Vento M, et al. Resuscitation of depressed newborn infants with ambient air or pure oxygen: a meta-analysis. Biol Neonate 2005;87:27–34.
15. Rabi Y, Rabi D, Yee W. Room air resuscitation of the depressed newborn: a systematic review and meta-analysis. Resuscitation 2007;72:353–63.
16. Tin W, Milligan DW, Pennefather P, et al. Pulse oximetry, severe retinopathy, and outcome at one year in babies of less than 28 weeks gestation. Arch Dis Child Fetal Neonatal Ed 2001;84(2):F106–10.

17. Saugstad OD. Bronchopulmonary dysplasia and oxidative stress: are we closer to an understanding of the pathogenesis of BPD? Acta Paediatr 1997;86(12): 1277–82.
18. Bell EF. Preventing necrotizing enterocolitis: what works and how safe? Pediatrics 2005;115(1):173–4.
19. Wang CL, Anderson C, Leone TA, et al. Resuscitation of preterm neonates by using room air or 100% oxygen. Pediatrics 2008;121:1083–9.
20. Escrig R, Arruza L, Izquierdo I, et al. Achievement of targeted saturation values in extremely low gestational age neonates resuscitated with low or high oxygen concentrations: a prospective, randomized trial. Pediatrics 2008;121:875–81.
21. Velaphi S, Vidyasagar D. Intrapartun and postdelivery management of infants born to mothers with meconium-stained aminotic fluid: evidence-based recommendations. Clin Perinatol 2006;33:29–42.
22. Antonowicz I, Schwachman H. Meconium in health and disease. Adv Pediatr 1979;26:275–310.
23. Dargaville PA, Copnell BC. The epidemiology of meconium aspiration syndrome: incidence, risk factors, therapies, and outcome. Pediatrics 2006;117:1712–21.
24. Vidyasagar D, Harris V, Pildes RS. Assisted ventilation in infants with meconium aspiration syndrome. Pediatrics 1975;56:208–13.
25. Vain NE, Szyld EG, Prudent LM, et al. Oropharyngeal and nasopharyngeal suctioning of meconium-stained neonates before delivery of their shoulders: multicentre, randomised controlled trial. Lancet 2004;364:597–602.
26. Wiswell TE, Gannon CM, Jacob J, et al. Delivery room management of the apparently vigorous meconium-stained neonate: results of the multicenter, international collaborative trial. Pediatrics 2000;105:1–7.
27. Liu WF, Harrington T. The need for delivery room intubation of thin meconium in the low-risk newborn: a clinical trial. Am J Perinatol 1998;15:657–82.
28. Daga SR, Dave K, Mehta V, et al. Tracheal suction in meconium stained infants: a randomized controlled study. J Trop Pediatr 1994;40:198–200.
29. Halliday H, Sweet D. Endotracheal intubation at birth for preventing morbidity and mortality in vigorous meconium-stained infants born at term. Cochrane Database Syst Rev 2001;1:CD000500.
30. Gibbons GH, Dzau VJ. The emerging concept of vascular remodeling. N Engl J Med 1994;330:1431–8.
31. Morin FC, Stenmark KR. Persistent pulmonary hypertension of the newborn. Am J Respir Crit Care Med 1995;151:2010–32.
32. Yu VYH. Persistent pulmonary hypertension of the newborn. Early Hum Dev 1993; 33:163–75.
33. Simma B, Fritz M, Fink C, et al. Conventional ventilation versus high-frequency oscillation: hemodynamic effects in newborn babies. Crit Care Med 2000;28: 227–31.
34. Moreland TA, Brice JE, Walker CH, et al. Naloxone pharmacokinetics in the newborn. Br J Clin Pharmacol 1980;9:609–12.
35. Guinsburg R, Wyckhoff MH. Naloxone during neonatal resuscitation: acknowledging the unknown. Clin Perinatol 2006;33:121–32.
36. Buyon JP. Autoimmune-associated congenital heart block: demographics, mortality, morbidity, and recurrence rates obtained from a national neonatal lupus registry. J Am Coll Cardiol 1998;31:1658–66.
37. Wyckhoff MH, Wyllie J. Endotracheal delivery of medications during neonatal resuscitation. Clin Perinatol 2006;33:153–60.

38. Kattwinkel J, Niermeyer S, Nadkarni V, et al. Resuscitation of the newly born infants: an advisory statement from the pediatric working group of the international liaison committee on resuscitation. Resuscitation 1999;40:71–88.
39. Wyckhoff MH, Perlman J, Niermeyer S. Medications during resuscitation: what is the evidence? Semin Neonatol 2001;6:251–9.
40. Manisterski Y, Vakin Z, et al. Endotracheal epinephrine: a call for larger doses. Anesth Analg 2002;95:1037–41.
41. Skinner JR, Sharland G. Detection and management of life threatening arrhythmias in the perinatal period. Early Hum Dev 2008;84:161–72.
42. Torfs CP, Curry CJ, Bateson TF, et al. A population-based study of congenital diaphragmatic hernia. Teratology 1992;46:555–65.
43. Enns GM, Cox VA, Goldstein RB, et al. Congenital diaphragmatic defects and associated syndromes, malformations, and chromosome anomalies: a retrospective study of 60 patients and literature review. Am J Med Genet 1998;79: 215–25.
44. Johnson BA, Ades A. Delivery room and early postnatal management of neonates who have prenatally diagnosed congenital heart disease. Clin Perinatol 2005;25: 921–46.
45. Forbus GA, Atz AM, Shirali GS. Implications and limitations of an abnormal fetal echocardiogram. Am J Cardiol 2004;94:688–9.
46. Perolo A, Prandstraller D, Ghi T, et al. Diagnosis and management of fetal cardiac anomalies: 10 years experience at a single institution. Ultrasound Obstet Gynecol 2001;18:615–8.
47. Rychik J, Tian ZY, Fogel MA, et al. The single ventricle heart in the fetus: accuracy of prenatal diagnosis and outcome. J Perinatol 1997;17:183–8.
48. Mirlesse V, Cruz A, Le Bidois J, et al. Perinatal management of fetal cardiac anomalies in a specialized obstetric-pediatrics center. Am J Perinatol 2001;18: 363–71.
49. Kelsall A, Yates R, Sullivan I. Antenatally diagnosed cardiac disease: where to deliver. Arch Dis Child 2000;82:A33–4.
50. Toth B, Becker A, Seelback-Gobel B. Oxygen saturation in healthy newborn infants immediately after birth measured by pulse oximetry. Arch Gynecol Obstet 2002;266:105–7.
51. Vu LT, Nobuhara KK, Laurent C, et al. Increasing prevalence of gastroschisis: population-based study in California. J Pediatr 2008;152:807–11.
52. Stoll C, Alembik Y, Dott B, Roth M-P. Omphalocele and gastroschisis and associated malformations. Am J Med Genet A 2008;146A:1280–5.
53. Kaufman B. Neural tube defects. Pediatr Clin North Am 2004;51:389–419.
54. Hammarlund K, Nilsson GE, Oberg PA, et al. Transepidermal water loss in newborn infants. V. Evaporation from the skin and heat exchange during the first hours of life. Acta Paediatr Scand 1980;69:385–92.
55. Anderson GC, Moore E, Hepworth J, et al. Early skin-to-skin contact for mothers and their healthy newborn infants. Cochrane Database Syst Rev 2003;2: CD003519.
56. Fardig JA. A comparison of skin-to-skin contact and radiant heaters in promoting neonatal thermoregulation. J Nurse Midwifery 1980;25:19–20.
57. Watkinson M. Temperature control of premature infants in the delivery room. Clin Perinatol 2006;33:43–53.
58. Vohra S, Frent G, Campbell V, et al. Effect of polyethylene occlusive skin wrapping on heat loss in very low birth weight infants at delivery. J Pediatr 1999; 134:547–51.

59. Vohra S, Roberts RS, Zhang B, et al. Heat loss prevention (HeLP) in the delivery room: a randomized controlled trial of polyethylene occlusive skin wrapping in very preterm infants. J Pediatr 2004;145:750–3.
60. Nielsen HC, Jung AL, Atherton SO. Evaluation of the Porta-Warm mattress as a source of heat for neonatal transport. An Pediatr (Barc) 1976;58:500–4.
61. L'Herault J, Petroff L, Jeffrey J. The effectiveness of a thermal mattress in stabilizing and maintaining body temperature during the transport of very low birth weight newborns. Appl Nurs Res 2001;14:210–9.
62. Brennan AB. Effect of sodium acetate transport mattress on admission temperatures of infants <1500 g [master's thesis]. Gainesville (FL): University of Florida; 1996.
63. Bergman N, Linley LL, Fawcus SR. Randomized controlled trial of skin-to-skin contact from birth versus conventional incubator for physiological stabilization in 1200- to 2199-gram newborns. Acta Paediatr 2004;93:779–85.
64. Shankaran S, Laptook AR. Hypothermia as a treatment for birth asphyxia. Clin Obstet Gynecol 2007;50:624–35.
65. American Academy of Pediatrics and American College of Obstetricians and Gynecologists. Care of the neonate. In: Gilstrap LC, Oh W, editors. Guidelines of perinatal care. 5th edition. Elk Grove Village (IL): American Academy of Pediatrics; 2002. p. 187–235.
66. Sarnat HB, Sarnat MS. Neonatal encephalopathy following fetal distress: a clinical and electroencephalographic study. Arch Neurol 1976;33:696–705.
67. Thoresen M, Satas S, Puka-Sundvall M, et al. Post-hypoxic hypothermia reduces cerebrocortical release of NO and excitotoxins. Neuroreport 1997;8:3359–62.
68. Baldwin WA, Kirsch JR, Hurn PD, et al. Hypothermic cerebral reperfusion and recovery from ischemia. Am J Physiol 1991;261:H774–81.
69. Laptook AR, Corbett RJT, Sterett R, et al. Modest hypothermia provides partial neuroprotection when used for immediate resuscitation after brain ischemia. Pediatr Res 1997;42:17–23.
70. Gunn AJ, Gunn TR, Gunning MJ, et al. Neuroprotection with prolonged head cooling started before postischemic seizures in fetal sheep. Pediatrics 1998; 102:1098–106.
71. Gluckman PD, Wyatt JS, Azzopardi D, et al. Selective head cooling with mild systemic hypothermia after neonatal encephalopathy: multicentre randomised trial. Lancet 2005;365:663–70.
72. Shakaran S, Laptook AR, Ehrenkranz RA, et al. Whole-body hypothermia for neonates with hypoxic-ischemic encephalopathy. N Engl J Med 2005;353: 1574–84.
73. International Liaison Committee on Resuscitation. The International Committee on Resuscitation (ILCOR) consensus on science with treatment recommendations for pediatric and neonatal patients: neonatal resuscitation. Pediatrics 2006;117: e978–88.
74. Available at: http://www.jointcommission.org/SentinelEvents/SentinelEventAlert/sea_30.htm. Accessed December 10, 2008.
75. Halamek LP, Kaegi DM, Gaba DM, et al. Time for a new paradigm in pediatric medical education: teaching neonatal resuscitation in a simulated delivery room environment. Pediatrics 2000;106:e45.
76. Vento M, Aguar M, Leone TA, et al. Using intensive care technology in the delivery room: a new concept for the resuscitation of extremely preterm neonates. Pediatrics 2008;122:1113–6.

77. Halamek LP. The simulated delivery-room environment as the future modality for acquiring and maintaining skills in fetal and neonatal resuscitation. Semin Fetal Neonatal Med 2008;13:448–53.

78. Halamek LP. Simulation-based training: opportunities for the acquisition of unique skills. Virtual Mentor 2006;8:84–7. Available at: http://virtualmentor.ama-assn.org/2006/02/medu1-0602.html.

Goals and Strategies for Prevention of Preterm Birth: An Obstetric Perspective

Christopher T. Lang, MD[a,b,*], Jay D. Iams, MD[a]

KEYWORDS

- Spontaneous preterm birth • Prevention
- Indicated preterm birth • Perinatal mortality
- Neonatal outcomes

When all the sequelae of preterm birth are considered, complications of prematurity surpass congenital malformations as the leading cause of infant mortality in the United States, accounting for 34% of infant deaths in 2004, with 95% of these deaths occurring in neonates born before 32 weeks' gestation.[1] In 2005, 12.7% of all infants were born before 37 completed weeks of gestation, continuing a steady rise in preterm birth since 1990.[2] The increase in the leading cause of infant mortality has alarmed health professionals from all disciplines. This review from a prenatal perspective confirms those concerns and describes risks and opportunities that may attend efforts to improve the health of fetuses, newborns, and infants. Notably, the authors include fetal and live-born outcomes and seek to convince their pediatric colleagues of the value of this perspective.

PREVENTION OF PRETERM BIRTH

Obstetric efforts to prevent preterm birth have targeted the reduction or elimination of specific risk factors, with the expectation that the preterm birth rate would fall according to the contribution of that factor to the overall prematurity rate. The failure of this approach has contributed to the current concept of preterm birth as a syndrome in which multiple factors interact to promote preterm parturition.[3,4] Despite general acceptance of preterm parturition as syndromic, conceptual impediments to preterm birth prevention remain strong. For example, obstetric taxonomy still reflects the traditional belief that the clinical presentation (ie, uterine contractions, ruptured membranes, bleeding, or cervical dilation) defines the etiology of preterm delivery,

[a] Department of Obstetrics and Gynecology, Division of Maternal–Fetal medicine, The Ohio State University College of Medicine, 395 West 12th Avenue, Columbus, OH 43210, USA
[b] Mount Carmel St. Ann's Hospital, 500 South Cleveland Avenue, Westerville, OH 43081, USA
* Corresponding author.
E-mail address: ctlmed1@aol.com (C.T. Lang).

Pediatr Clin N Am 56 (2009) 537–563
doi:10.1016/j.pcl.2009.03.006
0031-3955/09/$ – see front matter © 2009 Elsevier Inc. All rights reserved.
pediatric.theclinics.com

a construct analogous to asserting that the pathophysiology of myocardial infarction is distinct from that of angina. The common educational diagram[5] showing four collaborative causal pathways (inflammation, decidual hemorrhage, stress-induced endocrine activation, and uterine stretch) to preterm birth is still interpreted in practice to represent four distinct pathways. Births before and after 20 weeks' gestation are still often considered as having separate etiologies, an error that is perpetuated by the manner in which pregnancy outcome data are recorded. Ideally, prevention should be based on knowledge of how these interactions occur. Until then, progress toward prevention will continue to be slow and inefficient.

Preventive strategies applied to preterm birth may be primary, secondary, or tertiary:

Primary strategies are directed to all women who are or will enter their reproductive years.
Secondary strategies target women who have increased risk for preterm birth.
Tertiary strategies are employed in women in whom preterm parturition has begun, to prevent fetal, infant, and maternal morbidity and mortality.

RISKS VERSUS BENEFITS OF PREVENTION

Most reviews of efforts to prevent preterm birth begin by assessing the efficacy of the interventions employed, but it is increasingly recognized that prevention efforts, even when successful, may have adverse as well as salutary results. The causes of preterm parturition include conditions that may jeopardize maternal or fetal health if the pregnancy continues. In developed countries, about one fourth to one third of preterm births are preceded by overt maternal or fetal pathology, most commonly preeclampsia/hypertension, bleeding from placental abruption or previa, or fetal growth restriction, and are classified after delivery as "indicated" preterm births.[6] The remaining preterm births, called "spontaneous," present clinically as preterm labor, ruptured membranes, cervical "insufficiency," or a combination thereof.[4] Intrauterine inflammation related to microbial colonization, uterine vascular compromise, or decidual hemorrhage, however, may exist for many weeks before becoming clinically apparent as preterm cervical effacement, membrane rupture, labor, or vaginal bleeding. Tertiary or secondary interventions to prevent or delay preterm delivery must therefore include consideration of the possibility that prolongation of pregnancy intended to promote maturation may instead allow continued exposure to a suboptimal intrauterine environment. This concern increases as gestational age advances. Primary prevention strategies avoid this concern.

There are several examples that reveal the potential risks of strategies intended to prevent prematurity. Maternal treatment with antenatal corticosteroids (ANCS), and intrapartum antibiotic prophylaxis for women colonized with group B streptococcus or who present with preterm prelabor rupture of membranes (PROM) are tertiary interventions that are generally considered effective in reducing neonatal morbidity and mortality; however, both have potential risks. ANCS are unquestionably the single most helpful perinatal intervention available, but the selection of candidates and the timing of treatment are still matters of debate because prediction of imminent preterm delivery is not optimal. The current recommendation for a single course of ANCS before preterm delivery[7] is based on animal and human data showing fetal and neonatal growth restriction when multiple antenatal courses are given.[8–10] The effect of this recommendation is that obstetricians currently wait until delivery is expected within hours, risking an incomplete or missed course of ANCS, or they treat more aggressively and confront the uncertain risks of multiple courses. Antenatal antibiotics may prolong latency and reduce perinatal morbidity[11,12] yet offer another example of the risks that may accompany effective perinatal interventions. More specifically, with the increasing use of antibiotic prophylaxis for neonatal group B streptococcal sepsis, there has come a change in the pathogens causing early-onset sepsis, with gram-negative organisms (eg, *Escherichia coli*) becoming more common, at least in very low birth weight infants.[13] In 2001, Kenyon and colleagues[12,14] reported companion trials of antibiotic (erythromycin with or without amoxicillin clavulanate) treatment for women who had preterm PROM and for women who had preterm labor. There was short-term benefit for infants born to antibiotic-treated mothers who had preterm PROM but no advantage for those born to women who had spontaneous preterm labor, many of whom did not deliver preterm. The investigators recently reported outcomes at 7 years for infants born to mothers in both studies.[15,16] Infants born to mothers who had preterm PROM who were treated with antibiotics had neither benefit nor harm compared with infants of placebo-treated mothers, but "the prescription of erythromycin for women in spontaneous preterm labor with intact membranes was associated with an increase in functional impairment among their children at 7 years of age. The risk of cerebral palsy was increased by either antibiotic." In an accompanying editorial, Bedford Russell and Steer[17] speculated that antibiotic suppression of infection might prolong fetal in utero exposure to a damaging environment.

Given the potential fetal contribution to the onset of preterm parturition, and the considerable role of inflammation in causing preterm delivery and its neonatal sequelae,[18–20] the safety of the intrauterine environment for the fetus is always an issue. For example, an oft-cited report relating indomethacin tocolysis to necrotizing enterocolitis and intraventricular hemorrhage is likely the result of the "success" of this treatment in prolonging fetal exposure to in utero inflammation. In this study, indomethacin was used only after other agents had failed and without limit on the duration or gestational age of treatment.[21] No such associations have since been reported when current protocols that limit the duration and gestational age of exposure are used.[22–24] Similar concerns attend the secondary prevention strategy of prophylactic use of antibiotics in the second trimester. Increased rates of preterm birth have been reported in pregnant women screened and treated with antibiotics for *Trichomonas vaginalis*[25] or for a positive fetal fibronectin screen.[26,27]

More recently, prophylaxis of spontaneous preterm birth with supplemental progestins such as 17α-hydroxyprogesterone caproate has been studied to reduce the risk of recurrent preterm birth[28,29] and in women who have a short cervix.[30] Questions about the wisdom of this strategy[31] demonstrate the conundrum created by any effective tertiary or secondary measure intended to prevent preterm birth: How does it work? Does it reduce in utero inflammation or uterine blood flow, and if so, does that also reduce the risk for the fetus or instead allow prolonged exposure to an adverse environment? Against these concerns, primary preventive strategies applied before or after pregnancy (eg, preconceptional folate supplementation or prolongation of the interpregnancy interval for at-risk women), are much more appealing.

Because prematurity prevention strategies are understood to have risks in addition to benefits, the need for improved measures of perinatal outcome has become apparent.[32] Specifically, antenatal assessment of fetal versus neonatal risk must be improved. Condition-specific risk profiles of the maternal and fetal disorders that precede preterm birth are needed. Which pregnancy problems have the highest and lowest likelihood of causing fetal or neonatal death? Which are more or less "predictable" in their progression from mild to severe disease? What factors do obstetricians weigh when deciding to continue or end a complicated pregnancy? The literature that addresses these questions is limited, which compromises accurate communication between pediatricians and obstetricians around these births. Deficits in the literature are most apparent in the ongoing evaluation of the rising rate of preterm birth, for which positive and negative effects on fetal and neonatal outcomes have been reported.

THE RISING RATE OF PRETERM BIRTH—WHAT DOES IT MEAN FOR PERINATAL AND INFANT MORTALITY AND MORBIDITY?

Traditional measures of infant health include the rates of low birth weight, preterm birth, and infant mortality. All are reported annually by the National Center for Health Statistics (NCHS) relative to the number of live births. The infant mortality rate declined steadily from 10.1 per 1000 live births in 1987 until a recent plateau between 6.85 and 6.97, the first interruption of the sustained decline since the 1950s.[33] The rate is estimated from preliminary 2006 data to be 6.71, a 2% decline from 6.87 in 2005.[34,35] The plateau between 2000 and 2005 was attributed to a slight increase in very preterm births and an increase in late preterm births (34–36 weeks' gestation) (**Table 1**). The final NCHS report for 2005 observed a low birth weight rate of 8.2%, 22% higher than the 1984 rate of 6.7%, and 8% over the rate in 2000, when it was 7.6%. Similarly, the preterm birth rate has increased to 12.7% for 2005, a 9% increase since 2000 and a 20% increase since 1990 (see **Table 1**).

These increases are the result of three concurrent trends, two of which are well known: the rise in multifetal gestations[36,37] and the marked increase in indicated late preterm births between 32 and 36 weeks' gestation.[38,39] The third trend—equally important but often ignored as arcane—is an adjustment in the reported rate of preterm birth caused by the increased use between 1990 and 2000 of ultrasound to determine gestational age.[40–43] This practice has resulted in far fewer pregnancies identified as being postterm and has shifted the reported distribution of births to the left (**Fig. 1**). Thus, some fraction of the apparent increase in preterm births is the result of improved gestational dating.

Regardless of the methods used to determine gestational age, the true incidence of preterm birth has clearly increased. The increase conveys a worrisome message about the health of infants in the United States that has sparked renewed efforts to prevent preterm birth, a seemingly logical goal. But is it? Our review of methods to prevent preterm birth begins by asking whether prevention of preterm birth is the appropriate goal.

Table 1
Percentage distribution of gestational age for all births and for singleton births only in the United States, 1990, 2000, 2004, and 2005

Gestational Age	All Births				Singleton Births			
	2005	2004	2000	1990	2005	2004	2000	1990
<28 wk	0.77	0.75	0.72	0.71	0.61	0.61	0.59	0.61
28–31 wk	1.26	1.25	1.21	1.21	1.02	1.01	0.99	1.08
32–33 wk	1.60	1.59	1.49	1.40	1.28	1.28	1.22	1.24
Total <34 wk	3.63	3.60	3.42	3.32	2.91	2.89	2.80	2.93
34–36 wk	9.09	8.90	8.22	7.30	8.09	7.88	7.33	6.77
Total <37 wk	12.73	12.49	11.64	10.61	11.00	10.78	10.12	9.70
37–39 wk	53.54	52.36	48.83	41.38	54.26	53.03	49.27	41.42
≥40 wk	33.73	35.15	39.54	48.00	34.74	36.20	40.61	48.88

Data from Martin JA, Hamilton BE, Sutton PD, et al. Births: final data for 2005. Natl Vital Stat Rep 2007;56:1–103.

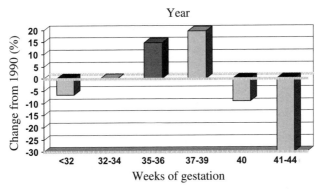

Fig. 1. Changes in distribution of singleton preterm births in the United States, 1990–2002. (*Data from* Davidoff MJ, Dias T, Damus K, et al. Changes in gestational age distribution among US singleton births: impact on rates of later preterm birth, 1992 to 2002. Sem Perinatol 2006;30:8–15.)

WHAT IS THE APPROPRIATE MEASURE OF PERINATAL HEALTH?

Unlike the infant mortality rate, the preterm birth rate is not itself a health outcome but rather a surrogate marker of the increased mortality and morbidity experienced by preterm infants compared with infants born alive at term. Despite their unquestioned standing as benchmarks, the rates of delivery for preterm and low birth weight infants do not provide a complete picture of infant health; missing is an assessment of fetal and infant health as measured by the perinatal mortality rate, defined by the NCHS in two ways:[44]

Definition I is defined narrowly as early neonatal deaths before 7 days of age plus fetal deaths after a stated or presumed period of gestation of 28 weeks or more per 1000 live births and fetal deaths.
Definition II is defined more inclusively as neonatal deaths before 28 days of age plus fetal deaths after a stated or presumed period of gestation of 20 weeks or more.

Unlike the preterm and infant mortality rates, the denominator for the perinatal mortality rate is the total number of births: live-born plus stillborn. The perinatal mortality rate thus measures the effects of prenatal, intrapartum, and neonatal care. In contrast to the infant mortality rate,[44] the perinatal mortality rate improved substantially between 1990 and 2004 (**Fig. 2**). The improvement (**Fig. 3**) is explained in part by fewer fetal deaths after 28 weeks' gestation (there was no change in fetal deaths before 28 weeks' gestation between 1990 and 2004). Could the decline in late fetal deaths have caused the plateau in the infant mortality rate by transferring the location of death from in utero to the neonatal ICU? If so, neonatal deaths before 7 or 28 days might have increased as the fetal death rate fell, but that did not occur: the number of infant deaths before 7 and 28 days in 1999 (14,874 and 18,700, respectively) were approximately the same in 2004 (14,836 and 18,602, respectively).[44]

Of interest, the decline in the fetal death rate between 1990 and 2005 was coincident with the increase in late preterm births between 34 and 36 weeks' gestation (**Fig. 4**).

Late preterm births account for essentially all of the rise in the overall preterm birth rate (**Fig. 5**), and the increase in late preterm birth is almost entirely the result of an

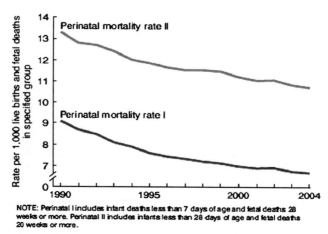

Fig. 2. Perinatal mortality rates in the United States, 1990–2004. (*Data from* Mathews TJ, MacDorman MF. Infant mortality from the 2005 period linked birth/infant death data set. Natl Vital Stat Rep 2008;57:1–32.)

increase in indicated late preterm births—those that occur in conjunction with perceived risk to the mother, the fetus, or both if the pregnancy continues (eg, preeclampsia, fetal growth restriction, maternal diabetes, or significant bleeding) (**Fig. 6**).

Some of these births are inevitable—the result of labor brought on by placental abruption, preeclampsia, or other complications; others follow a decision by the obstetrician to initiate labor or perform a cesarean birth for maternal or fetal indications. The trends displayed in **Fig. 4** suggest that many of these decisions are apparently well founded: the perinatal mortality rate has declined as late preterm birth has increased. The increased willingness of obstetricians to choose delivery over expectant management for complicated pregnancies appears to have created an environment of obstetric intervention that has had an opposite effect. Many hospitals are reporting increased deliveries of late (34–36 weeks) and near-term (36–38 weeks) infants in which the indication for scheduled birth is marginal or absent.[45] These

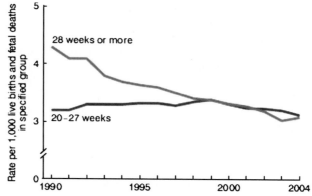

Fig. 3. Fetal mortality rates by period of gestation in the United States, 1990–2004. (*Data from* Mathews TJ, MacDorman MF. Infant mortality from the 2005 period linked birth/infant death data set. Natl Vital Stat Rep 2008;57:1–32.)

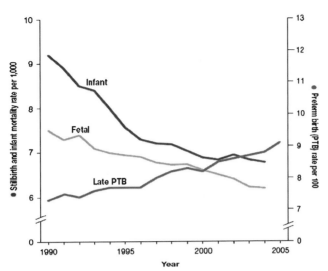

Fig. 4. Trends in late preterm birth, stillbirth, and infant mortality in the United States, 1990–2004. (*From* Ananth CV, Gyamfi C, Jain L. Characterizing risk profiles of infants who are delivered at late preterm gestations: does it matter? Am J Obstet Gynecol 2008;199:329–31; with permission.)

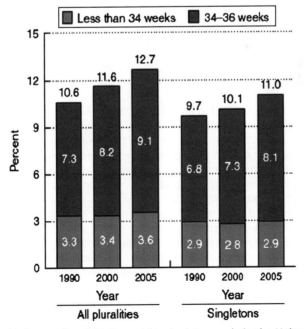

Fig. 5. Preterm birth rates for all births and for singletons only in the United States, 1990, 2000, and 2005. (*Data from* Hamilton BE, Martin JA, Sutton PD, et al. Births: final data for 2005. Natl Vital Stat Rep 2007;56.)

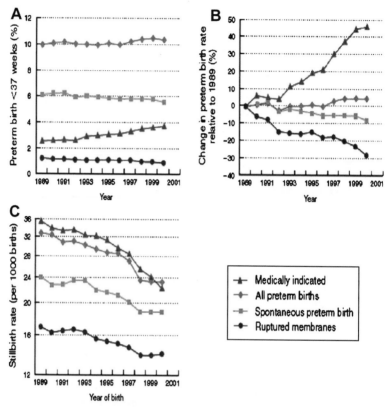

Fig. 6. Temporal changes in singleton preterm births (<37 weeks) (*A*), relative temporal changes in pretem birth since 1989 (*B*), and temporal changes in stillbirth among preterm births (*C*), each according to preterm birth category. (*From* Ananth CV, Joseph KS, Oyelese Y, et al. Trends in preterm birth and perinatal mortality among singletons: United States, 1989 through 2000. Obstet Gynecol 2005;105:1084–91; with permission.)

scheduled births have resulted in admission of the neonate to a special or intensive care nursery—a necessary result when delivery is the safer choice for the mother or fetus but one that is totally unacceptable without clear documentation of risks. In the current environment, examples at the extremes are abundant: from the mother who has diabetes or hypertension whose complaint of decreased fetal movement prompts tests that reveal fetal compromise, to the opposite scenario whereby a birth is scheduled around an upcoming business or social event. There are many more examples in which the data to inform decisions about the wisdom of prolonging pregnancy versus the risks of preterm delivery are not as clear. For example, efforts to prevent indicated preterm births are traditionally regarded separately from those for spontaneous preterm birth (those that follow spontaneous preterm labor or preterm PROM). The distinction is somewhat artificial, however, and can even be misleading because intrauterine inflammation related to microbial infection, uterine vascular compromise, or decidual hemorrhage can exist for days, weeks, or longer before becoming clinically apparent as preterm cervical effacement, membrane rupture, labor, or vaginal bleeding. Thus, the possibility that maintaining a pregnancy might confer increased fetal or neonatal risk must be considered regardless of the clinical presentation.

EFFORTS TO PREVENT PREMATURITY

With this preface, the following sections review interventions intended to prevent preterm birth. **Table 2** summarizes primary, secondary, and tertiary interventions for preterm birth taken from the obstetric and pediatric literature,[159] whereas **Table 3** displays pediatric efforts to reduce the incidence and effects of preterm birth, including programs to prolong the interpregnancy interval, to increase birth weight, and to reduce risk factors for preterm birth.

Pre- and Interconceptional Interventions

Preconceptional interventions for all women

Preconceptional interventions to reduce or eliminate risk factors are attractive because concerns about fetal risk are avoided and because as many as 50% of preterm births occur in women who do not have known risk factors.[174] Smoking cessation, optimal nutrition, and periodontal care are commonly recommended, but evidence of their effect on preterm birth risk is limited. Interventions specifically targeted to reproductive-age women include improved public awareness of the lifetime consequences of preterm birth in general[175] and the increased risk of preterm birth that accompanies singleton and multifetal gestations conceived after assisted reproductive technology.[176] Policies intended to reduce the risk of multiple gestation can be expected to result in a lower risk of preterm birth.[177,178]

Table 2
Preterm birth prevention strategies from the obstetric and pediatric literature

Category of Prevention	Intervention	References
Primary (preconceptional)	Public and professional policy	46–50
	Nutritional supplements	51
	Smoking cessation	52–54
Primary (postconceptional)	Nutritional supplements	55–60
	Smoking cessation	61,62
	Prenatal care	63,64
	Periodontal care	65–70
	Screening	71–90
Secondary (preconceptional)	Uterine "repair"	91
	Home visits	92
	Antibiotics	93,94
Secondary (postconceptional)	Preeclampsia prevention	58,95–101
	Reducing activity	102–104
	Nutritional supplements	98,99
	Intensive prenatal care	105–113
	Antibiotics	27,78,114–116
	Progesterone	28,29,117–121
	Cerclage	87,88,122–140
Tertiary	Early diagnosis	109,112,113,141–144
	Acute tocolysis	145–151
	Corticosteroids	152
	Group B streptococcus prophylaxis	153
	Preterm PROM management	11,12
	"Maintenance" tocolysis	154,155
	Routine cesarean delivery	156–158

Table 3
Preterm birth prevention strategies from the pediatric literature

Category/Outcome	Intervention or Variable	Reference
Primary/preterm birth	Prevention programs	160
	Young adult education	161
Secondary/preterm birth	Home visits	105,110
	Establishing prenatal care	162
	Patient education	163
Secondary/interpregnancy interval	Home visits	164–167
	Interpregnancy care	168
Secondary/birth weight	Home visits	105,110
	Interpregnancy care	168
	Comprehensive prenatal care	169
Tertiary/neonatal morbidity and mortality	Corticosteroids	170
Association/preterm birth	Occupational factors	171
	Delayed childbearing	172
	Serum cholesterol	173

Women considering a pregnancy are routinely advised to initiate prenatal vitamins prior to conception and to avoid known risk factors such as cigarette smoking.[179] Because most pregnancies are unplanned, these recommendations have limited opportunity to affect the preterm birth rate. A randomized trial of vitamin supplementation that enrolled women before conception and continued through the first 2 months of pregnancy found no effect on the rate of preterm birth.[51] A recent report claimed a 50% to 70% reduction in spontaneous preterm births among women who reported taking prenatal vitamins with folate for more than 1 year prior to conception,[180] but there was no effect in women who reported taking vitamins with folate for less than 12 months before pregnancy. Prospective studies of prolonged vitamin and folate supplements have not been reported.

Preconceptional interventions for women who have a prior preterm birth

Women who have a prior preterm birth have an increased risk of recurrence[181,182] regardless of whether their prior preterm birth was spontaneous or indicated.[183,184] A review of records from prior pregnancies may identify opportunities to eliminate or reduce risks, including some that require preconceptional intervention such as correction of Müllerian anomalies[91] or that could influence prenatal care such as prophylactic progesterone or cerclage. One study found that 40% of preterm births were related to prepregnancy risk factors[185] and suggested that women who have increased medical risks for preterm birth might benefit from preconceptional interventions such as control of medical disorders (eg, diabetes, seizures, asthma, or hypertension); however, evidence that these steps affect the preterm birth rate is lacking. In fact, this model has been the de facto approach for several decades while the preterm birth rate has risen.

Because genital tract infection is associated with preterm birth, interconceptional antimicrobial treatment was studied in a randomized trial[93] in which women who had a prior early preterm birth received metronidazole plus azithromycin or placebo at 3-month intervals between pregnancies. The rate of recurrent preterm birth was unaffected by treatment arm.

There are several studies from the pediatric literature that attempted to reduce the incidence of preterm birth directly[105,110] or indirectly by increasing the interpregnancy interval.[162,164–168] One randomized controlled trial of home nurse visitation found an increased length of gestation among women younger than 17 years,[105] whereas another trial found no benefit among primarily African American women who were unmarried, had less education, or were unemployed.[110] In two additional randomized controlled trials of home visitations, interpregnancy intervals were increased among young, socioeconomically disadvantaged women. Long-term follow-up of up to 15 years confirmed these findings, along with improved stability at home and a reduction in criminal activity.[165,167] A pilot evaluation of coordinated primary health care and social support for African American women following the birth of a very low birth weight infant resulted in a greater likelihood of achieving an 18-month interpregnancy interval.[168]

Postconceptional Interventions to Prevent Preterm Birth

Medical prophylaxis of indicated preterm birth

A large literature describes postconceptional interventions to prevent or reduce the risk of indicated and spontaneous preterm birth. Studies aimed at prevention of indicated preterm births include trials of low-dose aspirin,[95,96] calcium,[57] and antioxidant vitamins C and E[59,97,186] to prevent preeclampsia in low- and high-risk women—all of which reported no effect on the rates of preeclampsia or preterm birth.

Medical prophylaxis of spontaneous preterm birth

Absent a clear understanding of pathways leading to preterm birth, efforts directed at the prevention of spontaneous preterm birth most commonly involve interventional trials that address a specific clinical question (eg, Does an intervention aimed at a risk factor associated with preterm birth reduce the rate of preterm birth in women known or suspected to have that risk factor?). Women who have a risk factor such as prior preterm birth, multiple gestation, or a positive screening test are most commonly enrolled. Such trials have rarely found benefit for the intervention studied and are often criticized post hoc for having chosen the wrong intervention or study population. An alternate strategy evaluates comprehensive prenatal or preconceptional interventions in a service model of care. These studies more often report success but are also subject to post hoc critique for their less rigorous study design and inability to identify the exact mechanism of benefit.[47,48,64,105–111,160,187]

Prenatal care and social support

The association between early registry for prenatal care and low rates of preterm birth has led to promotion of improved access to care as a way to decrease prematurity. It is unfortunate that this relationship is related more to the high preterm birth rate for women who receive no prenatal care than to the content of care for those who receive it (**Table 4**).

Early access to care did not reduce preterm birth in African American women in a study limited to women who received early prenatal care.[63] Although perhaps beneficial in adolescents,[105,106] enhanced prenatal care including social support, home visits, and preterm birth education has not reduced preterm birth in larger studies.[107–111] These conclusions did not change when data from multiple trials were subjected to meta-analysis.[113] The aforementioned studies from Olds and colleagues,[164–167] however, were more successful at yielding increased interpregnancy intervals.

Table 4
Rate of preterm birth by maternal race and trimester of first prenatal visit

Trimester of First Prenatal Visit	NHB	NHW	Asian Pacific	Native American	Hispanic
First	14.7	8.3	8.6	10.4	9.7
Second	17.6	10.2	10.8	12.7	11.0
Third	16.0	10.0	9.5	12.3	10.0
None	33.4	21.7	19.4	24.0	19.8

Abbreviations: NHB, non-Hispanic black; NHW, non-Hispanic white.
Data from Behrman RE, Stith Butler A, editors. Committee on understanding premature birth and assuring healthy outcomes. Washington, DC: National Academies Press; 2006. p. 129–46.

Modification of maternal activity

Bed rest is frequently recommended for women whose pregnancies are at risk for spontaneous or indicated preterm birth, but there is no evidence that it is beneficial.[102,103] Limitation of work and sexual activity is commonly recommended despite a lack of supporting evidence.[104] Bed rest and limitation of sexual activity, however, have not been studied specifically in women who are most likely to benefit, such as those who have a short cervix.

Nutritional supplements

Observational studies suggesting improved rates of preterm birth in women taking dietary supplements[55] have not been confirmed by prospective trials. Protein and calorie supplementation have no apparent effect on preterm birth rates.[56] Calcium supplementation did not reduce the rate of preeclampsia or preterm birth in a large National Institute of Child Health and Human Development (NICHD) trial;[57] a Cochrane Review that included this trial and others for a total of almost 15,000 women found that calcium supplementation did not influence the rate of preterm birth (relative risk, 0.81; 95% confidence interval: 0.64–1.03).[58] Increased intake of the antioxidant vitamins C and E had no effect on the preterm birth rate in recent large placebo-controlled trials of these vitamins intended to assess their effect on the rate of preeclampsia.[59,97]

Trials of supplemental omega-3 polyunsaturated fatty acids (PUFAs) have been performed on the basis of low rates of preterm birth in populations that have a high dietary intake. These low rates are postulated to occur because omega-3 PUFAs reduce levels of proinflammatory cytokines. Dietary supplementation has been associated with reduced production of inflammatory mediators, and two randomized trials of omega-3 supplements conducted in women at risk for preterm birth found a decrease in preterm birth.[98] A third trial in women who had a prior preterm birth and received progesterone supplementation found no difference in the rate of recurrent preterm birth in those given supplemental omega-3 PUFAs.[188]

Periodontal care

The risk of preterm birth rises with increased severity of periodontal disease and when periodontal disease progresses in pregnancy,[65] but the basis for this association is uncertain. Although postulated to arise from hematogenous transmission of oral microbial pathogens to the genital tract, it is more likely the result of shared variations in the inflammatory response[66] to resident microflora. Periodontal care has been advocated as an intervention to reduce preterm birth, but recent studies do not support treatment of periodontal disease to reduce preterm birth.[68–70,189,190] Studies of the effect of preconceptional periodontal care on preterm birth risk have not been reported.

Antibiotic treatment

Antibiotic treatment has been studied to reduce the risk of preterm delivery because of the strong and consistent association of preterm birth with genitourinary tract colonization and infection. Treatment of asymptomatic bacteriuria reduces the rate of preterm birth,[71,72,191] but the value of antibiotic treatment to reduce the risk of preterm birth in women who have genital colonization or infection is uncertain. In previous studies, women were enrolled on the basis of obstetric history,[27,192–194] detection of bacterial vaginosis (BV; an alteration in the vaginal ecosystem),[195–204] colonization with a specific microorganism (*T vaginalis*,[25] group B streptococcus,[75] or *Ureaplasma urealyticum*[74]) or after a positive test for cervicovaginal fetal fibronectin, a marker for disturbance of the fetal–maternal interface.[26,27]

Trials of treatment for BV-positive women vary in timing, dosage, and choice of antibiotic treatment and show conflicting results. None of these trials directly tested the hypothesis that antibiotic treatment in women who had a prior preterm birth and are BV-positive can reduce the rate of preterm birth or its morbidity and mortality. Rather, secondary analyses[192,196] suggest that such a reduction may be the case and are supported by data summarized by Lamont and colleagues[202] that emphasize the need for treatment before 20 weeks of pregnancy and the selection of clindamycin as the preferred antibiotic. These data are countered by other secondary analyses that found increased rates of preterm birth in women who received antibiotics compared with placebo-treated women in controlled trials.[25–27,93,194] The current consensus is that symptomatic vaginal infections with BV, *T vaginalis*, and yeast should be treated but that screening and prophylaxis is not recommended.[205]

Progesterone supplementation

Progesterone supplementation for women at risk for preterm birth has been investigated on the basis of several potential mechanisms of action, including reduced gap junction formation and oxytocin antagonism leading to relaxation of smooth muscle, maintenance of cervical integrity, and anti-inflammatory effects. A 1990 review[117] suggesting benefit led to two randomized trials reported in 2003 that found a significant reduction in the risk of recurrent preterm birth in women treated with progesterone prophylaxis.[8,29] Subsequent meta-analyses of these studies and others concluded that the risk of recurrent preterm birth could be reduced by as much as 40% to 55%.[118,119] These studies were not powered to evaluate an effect on neonatal morbidity.

Subsequent randomized trials have evaluated progesterone prophylaxis in other at-risk groups. Women who have a short cervix (<15 mm) had a reduced rate of preterm birth when treated with prophylactic progesterone,[30] but progesterone supplementation had no effect on the rate of preterm birth in twin pregnancies.[206] Trials in women who have other risk factors such as a positive fibronectin, bleeding, or current preterm labor have not been reported. The mechanism of action is uncertain at this point. The effect of supplemental progesterone compounds is not universally seen in women who have a prior preterm birth, indicating that some pathways to preterm birth are not influenced by this therapy. The absence of benefit in twin pregnancy compared with the benefit in women who have historical risk and short cervix (a condition strongly linked to recurrent preterm birth[73,83]) suggests that the action of progesterone may be related to its effects on inflammation rather than to suppression of uterine contractility. This idea is intriguing but raises questions about fetal and maternal safety if progesterone prophylaxis were to prolong pregnancy in the presence of intrauterine inflammation. Although there is no evidence from trials in humans that this prolongation in a potentiallly inflammatory milieu has occurred—rates of fetal morbidity are reduced or unchanged in progesterone-treated women, and outcomes at 4 years of age are similar to those in placebo-treated control subjects[207]—the trials reported to date have not been powered to detect fetal morbidity or mortality. The safety of progesterone supplementation is supported by a review of outcomes of pregnancies treated before 1990,[208] by a review of animal studies,[209] and more recently by a thorough neurodevelopmental evaluation of children at 4 years of age who were born to women treated in the NICHD trial.[207] Nevertheless, the potential risks remain a concern.[31] The Food and Drug Administration (FDA) has acted very slowly in response to a new drug application despite the favorable recommendations of an expert advisory panel. The medication is available from compounding pharmacies, but lack of FDA approval has limited its use.

The economic benefit of widespread use of progesterone supplementation is uncertain. Although the rate of preterm birth may not decline appreciably if treatment is limited to those who have a prior preterm birth,[210] the cost savings of treating only these women has been estimated at more than $2 billion dollars annually in the United States.[211,212]

Cervical cerclage

Studies of the appearance of the cervix using endovaginal ultrasound have observed that the process of cervical effacement precedes clinical symptoms such as contractions and ruptured membranes by many weeks in most instances. Of importance, preterm cervical effacement or shortening seen by ultrasound does not always or even usually progress to preterm birth, so a "short" cervix may be interpreted as evidence that preterm parturition has begun but not as evidence that preterm birth will occur. The finding of a short cervix was initially attributed to cervical insufficiency or occult labor but is now understood to be more commonly the result of biochemical influences of paracrine, endocrine, or inflammatory origin. The appropriate intervention to arrest preterm cervical effacement is uncertain. It will progress to preterm birth in less than 50% of women, and the rate of progression is variable. Cerclage would seem to be appropriate only when there is a structural defect or deficiency to be repaired, but identification of the appropriate candidate is difficult. The efficacy of cerclage likely varies according to the cause but, at present, there is not a diagnostic algorithm to select those who will benefit versus those who will not. The view emerging from existing studies is that cerclage will ultimately be found to have benefit only when preterm cervical effacement or shortening can be determined to have occurred in the absence of inflammation. Until that is possible, clinical judgment must be based on that expectation rather than on history of early delivery or sonographic findings alone, reserving cerclage for those women thought to have anatomic insufficiency.

SUMMARY

Preterm birth remains a tremendous challenge for modern-day medicine. Numerous primary, secondary, and tertiary means of prevention have been studied, of which some have proved effective in certain circumstances and in specific patients and others have been associated with negative outcomes. The recent trend of increasing preterm birth secondary to an indicated intervention on behalf of the obstetrician (and the resulting debate) has illustrated a fundamental difference between obstetric and pediatric responsibility and measures of success (eg, prevention of stillbirth and optimizing neonatal maturity, respectively).

An especially poignant and recent illustration of these competing interests comes from Shapiro-Mendoza and colleagues[213] in a retrospective pediatric vital statistics review from 1998 to 2003 in Massachusetts to determine the relative and joint contributions to newborn morbidity made by late preterm birth and selected maternal medical conditions. The most significant finding from this study was the greater-than-additive effect in the adjusted relative risk for neonatal morbidity with the combination of late preterm birth and underlying medical conditions, especially true for antepartum hemorrhage and hypertensive disease of pregnancy. The study made two logical conclusions: (1) the importance of anticipating management issues following the birth of a late preterm infant, and (2) (addressing obstetricians) "because some maternal medical conditions are potentially preventable and/or amenable to treatment, early recognition and better treatment of women with chronic and pregnancy-related health conditions may decrease rates of newborn morbidity in all infants but especially in late-preterm infants." The first conclusion can be reconciled with the obstetric end point of perinatal mortality, in that, especially for significant antepartum hemorrhage and hypertensive disorders of pregnancy, late preterm birth not only is indicated but is also the standard of care for the fetus and mother. Supportive care for antepartum hemorrhage and hypertension may prolong pregnancy for a short time. Control of chronic hypertension reduces maternal risk of stroke but curiously does not reduce the rate of abruption, fetal growth restriction, or indicated preterm birth.[214,215] The next step in the process then falls on the shoulders of the neonatologist and the resuscitation team. The second conclusion is more difficult to reconcile. Careful control of maternal diabetes with diet and medication can reduce the risk of fetal death, but aggressive pregnancy management of other chronic conditions such as lung disease, maternal infection, cardiac disease, renal disease, or genital herpes has not been definitively associated with a reduction in preterm birth or late preterm birth. Therefore, until we as obstetricians are able to consistently predict and manage these two conditions without having to deliver the fetus, our end point remains not only perinatal mortality but also maternal mortality. A greater-than-additive effect with the combination of antepartum hemorrhage with or without hypertensive disease of pregnancy along with late preterm birth in terms of neonatal morbidity may appear a disingenuous finding in the eyes of the obstetrician, because for the infants in this study to experience morbidity, they must first have had to be born alive.

Obstetrics is faced with the unique situation of having responsibility for two patients simultaneously at any given time. The maternal mortality rate has plateaued since 1982 despite advances in diagnosis and critical care medicine, with hemorrhage and preeclampsia/eclampsia remaining major causes, along with thromboembolic disease, infection, and complications related to maternal obesity.[216] Given the "Healthy People 2010" goal of less than 3.3 maternal deaths per 100,000 live births[217] and the current overall maternity mortality rate of 11.8,[216] delivery to prevent any excess mortality (especially secondary to hemorrhage and hypertensive disorders[213]) remains prudent.

To some degree, the decision to proceed with an indicated preterm birth may be based on a distrust of fetal monitoring in the prevention of stillbirth, especially when the obstetrician is convinced of underlying pathology that perhaps has not yet manifested itself. The major forms of fetal monitoring—nonstress testing, stress testing, biophysical profile scoring, and maternal fetal movement counts—all share a common benefit, and that is to reliably exclude the presence of fetal acidosis and stillbirth within 1 week following reassuring testing.[218] These forms of fetal monitoring also suffer from the same limitation—that of an inability to predict unforeseen adverse events such as an acute placental abruption, for example, when the original indication for monitoring was mild preeclampsia or preterm PROM. Three other examples that illustrate the limitations of obstetrics include placenta previa, prior classical cesarean delivery, and cholestasis of pregnancy. In all three, the optimal timing of delivery is debatable, and no monitoring exists that allows for the prediction of potentially catastrophic events (acute hemorrhage and sudden fetal demise) secondary to placental trauma, uterine rupture, and presumed direct fetal cardiotoxicity,[219–223] respectively. Despite this underlying concern, many obstetricians still rely on fetal lung maturity testing to determine timing of delivery; however, even one case of a stillbirth (not to mention a potentially grave maternal outcome) while awaiting fetal lung maturity can leave a lifelong impression on the obstetrician and result in a much more aggressive approach in future cases.

REFERENCES

1. Callaghan WM, MacDorman MF, Rasmussen SA, et al. The contribution of preterm birth to infant mortality in the United States. Pediatrics 2006;118: 1566–73.
2. Martin JA, Hamilton BE, Sutton PD, et al. Births: final data for 2004. Natl Vital Stat Rep 2006;55:1–101.
3. Romero R, Espinoza J, Mazor M, et al. The preterm parturition syndrome. In: Critchley H, Bennett P, Thornton S, editors. Preterm birth. London: RCOG Press; 2004. p. 28–60.
4. Goldenberg RL, Culhane JF, Iams JD, et al. Epidemiology and causes of preterm birth. Lancet 2007;371:73–82.
5. Lockwood CJ, Iams JD. Preterm labor and delivery. In: Berens PD, Bukowski RK, Clark SL, editors. Precis: obstetrics. Danvers (MA): ACOG; 2005. p. 59.
6. Meis PJ, Michielutte R, Peters TJ, et al. Factors associated with preterm birth in Cardiff Wales: II. Indicated and spontaneous preterm birth. Am J Obstet Gynecol 1995;173:597–602.
7. American College of Obstetricians and Gynecologists. Management of preterm labor. ACOG Practice Bulletin number 43. Obstet Gynecol 2003;101:1039–47.
8. Murphy KE, Hannah ME, WIllan AR, et al. Multiple courses of antenatal corticosteroids for preterm birth (MACS): a randomised trial. Lancet 2008;372:2143–51.
9. Wapner RJ, Sorokin Y, Thom EA, et al. Single vs. weekly courses of antenatal corticosteroids: evaluation of safety and efficacy. Am J Obstet Gynecol 2006; 195:633–42.
10. Wapner RJ, Sorokin Y, Mele L, et al. Long term outcomes after repeat doses of antenatal corticosteroids. N Engl J Med 2007;357:1190–8.
11. Mercer BM, Miodovnik M, Thurnau GR, et al. Antibiotic therapy for reduction of infant morbidity after preterm premature rupture of the membranes. A randomized controlled trial. National Institute of Child Health and Human Development Maternal-Fetal Medicine Units Network. JAMA 1997;278:989–95.
12. Kenyon SL, Taylor DJ, Tarnow-Mordi W, for the ORACLE Collaborative Group. Broad spectrum antibiotics for preterm, prelabour rupture of the fetal membranes: the ORACLE I randomised trial. Lancet 2001;357:979–88.
13. Stoll BJ, Hansen N, Fanaroff AA, et al. Changes in pathogens causing early-onset sepsis in very-low-birth-weight infants. N Engl J Med 2002;347:240–7.
14. Kenyon SL, Taylor DJ, Tarnow-Mordi W, for the ORACLE Collaborative Group. Broad spectrum antibiotics for spontaneous preterm labour: the ORACLE II randomised trial. Lancet 2001;357:989–94.

15. Kenyon SL, Pike K, Jones DR, et al. Childhood outcomes after prescription of antibiotics to pregnant women with preterm rupture of the membranes: 7-year follow-up of the ORACLE I trial. Lancet 2008;372:1310–8.
16. Kenyon SL, Pike K, Jones DR, et al. Childhood outcomes after prescription of antibiotics to pregnant women with spontaneous preterm labour: 7-year follow-up of the ORACLE II trial. Lancet 2008;372:1319–27.
17. Bedford Russell AR, Steer PJ. Antibiotics in preterm labour—the ORACLE speaks. Lancet 2008;372:1276–8.
18. Romero R, Espinoza J, Kusanovic JP, et al. The preterm parturition syndrome. BJOG 2006;113(Suppl 3):118–35.
19. Jobe AH. Glucocorticoids, inflammation, and the perinatal lung. Semin Neonatol 2001;6:331–42.
20. Dammann O, Leviton A. Inflammation, brain damage, and visual dysfunction in preterm infants. Semin Fetal Neonatal Med 2006;11:363–8.
21. Norton ME, Merrill J, Cooper BA, et al. Neonatal complications after the administration of indomethacin for preterm labor. N Engl J Med 1993;329:1602–7.
22. Vermillion ST, Newman RB. Recent indomethacin tocolysis is not associated with neonatal complications in preterm infants. Am J Obstet Gynecol 1999;181:1083–6.
23. Loe SM, Sanchez-Ramos L, Kaunitz AM. Assessing the neonatal safety of indomethacin tocolysis: a systematic review with meta-analysis. Obstet Gynecol 2005;106:173–9.
24. Suarez RD, Grobman WA, Parilla BV. Indomethacin tocolysis and intraventricular hemorrhage. Obstet Gynecol 2001;97:921–5.
25. Klebanoff MA, Carey JC, Hauth JC, et al. Failure of metronidazole to prevent preterm delivery among pregnant women with asymptomatic Trichomonas vaginalis infection. N Engl J Med 2001;345:487–93.
26. Andrews WW, Sibai BM, Thom EA, et al. Randomized clinical trial of metronidazole plus erythromycin to prevent spontaneous preterm delivery in fetal fibronectin-positive women. Obstet Gynecol 2003;101:847–55.
27. Shennan A, Crawshaw S, Briley A, et al. A randomised controlled trial of metronidazole for the prevention of preterm birth in women positive for cervicovaginal fetal fibronectin: the PREMET Study. BJOG 2006;113:65–74.
28. da Fonseca EB, Bittar RE, Carvalho MH, et al. Prophylactic administration of progesterone by vaginal suppository to reduce the incidence of spontaneous preterm birth in women at increased risk: a randomized placebo-controlled double-blind study. Am J Obstet Gynecol 2003;188:419–24.
29. Meis PJ, Klebanoff M, Thom E, et al. Prevention of recurrent preterm delivery by 17-alpha-hydroxyprogesterone caproate. N Engl J Med 2003;348:2379–85.
30. Fonseca EB, Celik E, Parra M, et al. Progesterone and the risk of preterm birth among women with a short cervix. N Engl J Med 2007;357:462–9.
31. Elovitz MA, Mrinalini C. The use of progestational agents for preterm birth: lessons from a mouse model. Am J Obstet Gynecol 2006;195:1004–10.
32. Consequences of preterm birth. In: Behrman RE, Stith Butler A, editors. Preterm birth: causes, consequences, and prevention (Institute of Medicine). Washington, DC: National Academies Press; 2007. p. 311–45.
33. Kung HC, Hoyert DL, Xu JQ, et al. Deaths: final data for 2005. Natl Vital Stat Rep 2008;56:1–120.
34. MacDorman MF, Mathews TJ. Recent trends in infant mortality in the United States. NCHS data brief, no 9. Hyattsville (MD): National Center for Health Statistics; 2008.

35. Martin JA, Hamilton BE, Sutton PD, et al. Births: final data for 2005. Natl Vital Stat Rep 2007;56:1–103.
36. CDC. Preliminary births for 2004. Available at: http://www.cdc.gov/nchs/products/pubs/pubd/hestats/prelim_births/prelim_births04.htm.
37. Martin JA, Hamilton BE, Ventura SJ, et al. Births: final data for 2001. Natl Vital Stat Rep 2002;51:1–102.
38. Ananth CV, Vintzileos AM. Medically indicated preterm birth: recognizing the importance of the problem. Clin Perinatol 2008;35:53–67.
39. Fuchs K, Gyamfi C. The influence of obstetric practices on late prematurity. Clin Perinatol 2008;35:343–60.
40. Alexander GR, De Caunes F, Hulsey TC, et al. Validity of postnatal assessments of gestational age: a comparison of the method of Ballard, et al and early ultrasonography. Am J Obstet Gynecol 1992;166:891–5.
41. Savitz DA, Terry JW Jr, Dole N, et al. Comparison of pregnancy dating by last menstrual period, ultrasound scanning, and their combination. Am J Obstet Gynecol 2002;187:1660–6.
42. Yang CY, Kramer MS, Platt RW, et al. How does early ultrasound scan estimation of gestational age lead to higher rates of preterm birth? Am J Obstet Gynecol 2002;186:433–7.
43. Davidoff MJ, Dias T, Damus K, et al. Changes in gestational age distribution among US singleton births: impact on rates of later preterm birth, 1992 to 2002. Semin Perinatol 2006;30:8–15.
44. MacDorman MF, Munson ML, Kirmeyer S, et al. Fetal and perinatal mortality, United States, 2004. Natl Vital Stat Rep 2007;56:1–19.
45. Engle WA, Kominiarek MA. Late preterm infants, early term infants, and timing of elective deliveries. Clin Perinatol 2008;35:325–41.
46. Jain T, Missmer SA, Hornstein MD. Trends in embryo-transfer practice and in outcomes of the use of assisted reproductive technology in the United States. N Engl J Med 2004;350:1639–45.
47. Di Renzo GC, Moscioni P, Perazzi A, et al. Social policies in relation to employment and pregnancy in European countries. Prenat Neonatal Med 1998;3:147–56.
48. Saurel-Cubizolles MJ, Zeitlin J, Lelong N, et al. for the Europop Group. Employment, working conditions, and preterm birth: results from the Europop case-control survey. J Epidemiol Community Health 2004;58:395–401.
49. Launer LJ, Villar J, Kestler E, et al. The effect of maternal work on fetal growth and duration of pregnancy: a prospective study. BJOG 1990;97:62–70.
50. Pompeii LA, Savitz DA, Evenson KR, et al. Physical exertion at work and the risk of preterm delivery and small-for-gestational-age birth. Obstet Gynecol 2005;106:1279–88.
51. Czeizel AE, Dudas I, Metnecki J. Pregnancy outcomes in a randomized controlled trial of periconceptional multivitamin supplementation. Final report. Arch Gynecol Obstet 1994;255:131–9.
52. Burguet A, Kaminski M, Abraham-Lerat L, et al. The complex relationship between smoking in pregnancy and very preterm delivery: results of the Epipage study. BJOG 2004;111:258–65.
53. Shah NR, Bracken MB. A systematic review and meta-analysis of prospective studies in the association between maternal cigarette smoking and preterm delivery. Am J Obstet Gynecol 2000;182:465–72.
54. Salihu HM, Pierre-Louis BJ, Alexander GR. Levels of excess infant deaths attributable to maternal smoking during pregnancy in the United States. Matern Child Health J 2003;7:219–27.

55. Vahratian A, Siega-Riz AM, Savitz DA, et al. Multivitamin use and the risk of preterm birth. Am J Epidemiol 2004;160:886–92.

56. Kramer MS, Kakuma R. Energy and protein intake in pregnancy. Cochrane Database Syst Rev 2003;4:CD000032.

57. Levine RJ, Hauth JC, Curet LB, et al. Trial of calcium to prevent preeclampsia. N Engl J Med 1997;337:69–76.

58. Hofmeyr GJ, Atallah AN, Duley L. Calcium supplementation during pregnancy for preventing hypertensive disorders and related problems. Cochrane Database Syst Rev 2006;3:CD001059.

59. Rumbold AR, Crowther CA, Haslam RR, et al. Vitamins C and E and the risks of preeclampsia and perinatal complications. N Engl J Med 2006;354:1796–806.

60. Smuts CM, Huang M, Mundy D, et al. A randomized trial of docosahexanoic acid supplementation during the third trimester of pregnancy. Obstet Gynecol 2003; 101:469–79.

61. Ricketts SA, Murray EK, Schwalberg R. Reducing low birth weight by resolving risks: results from Colorado's prenatal plus program. Am J Public Health 2005; 95:1952–7.

62. Lumley J, Oliver SS, Chamberlain C, et al. Interventions for promoting smoking cessation during pregnancy. Cochrane Database Syst Rev 2004;4:CD001055.

63. Healy AJ, Malone FD, Sullivan LM, et al. Early access to prenatal care: implications for racial disparity in perinatal mortality. Obstet Gynecol 2006;107:625–31.

64. Papiernik E, Bouyer J, Dreyfus J, et al. Prevention of preterm births: a perinatal study in Haguenau, France. Pediatrics 1985;76:154–8.

65. Offenbacher S, Boggess KA, Murtha AP, et al. Progressive periodontal disease and risk of very preterm delivery. Obstet Gynecol 2006;107:29–36.

66. Stamilio DM, Chang JJ, Macones GA. Periodontal disease and preterm birth: do the data have enough teeth to recommend screening and preventative treatment? Am J Obstet Gynecol 2007;196:93–4.

67. Pretorius C, Jagatt A, Lamont RF. The relationship between periodontal disease, bacterial vaginosis, and preterm birth. J Perinat Med 2007;35:93–9.

68. Moore S, Ide M, Coward PY, et al. A prospective study to investigate the relationship between periodontal diseases and adverse pregnancy outcome. Br Dent J 2004;197:251–8.

69. Michalowicz BS, Hodges JS, Di Angelis AJ, et al. Treatment of periodontal disease and the risk of preterm birth. N Engl J Med 2006;355:1885–94.

70. Vergnes J-N, Sixou M. Preterm low birthweight and paternal periodontal status: a meta-analysis. Am J Obstet Gynecol 2007;196:135. e1–7.

71. Elder HA, Santamarina BA, Smith S, et al. The natural history of asymptomatic bacteriuria during pregnancy: the effect of tetracycline on the clinical course and the outcome of pregnancy. Am J Obstet Gynecol 1971;111:441–6.

72. Romero R, Oyarzun E, Mazor M, et al. Meta-analysis of the relationship between asymptomatic bacteriuria and preterm delivery/low birth weight. Obstet Gynecol 1989;73:576–82.

73. Goldenberg RL, Iams JD, Mercer BM, et al. The preterm prediction study: the value of new vs. standard risk factors in predicting early and all spontaneous preterm births. NICHD MFMU Network. Am J Public Health 1998;88:233–8.

74. Eschenbach DA, Nugent RP, Rao VR, et al. A randomized placebo-controlled trial of erythromycin for the treatment of U. urealyticum to prevent premature delivery. Am J Obstet Gynecol 1991;164:734–42.

75. Klebanoff MA, Regan JA, Rao VR, et al. Outcome of the vaginal infections and prematurity study: results of a clinical trial of erythromycin among pregnant

women colonized with group B streptococci. Am J Obstet Gynecol 1995;172: 1540–5.

76. Kigozi GG, Brahmbhatt H, Wabwire-Mangen F, et al. Treatment of trichomonas in pregnancy. Am J Obstet Gynecol 2003;189:1398–400.

77. Riggs MA, Klebanoff MA. Treatment of vaginal infections to prevent preterm birth: a meta-analysis. Clin Obstet Gynecol 2004;47:796–807.

78. McDonald HM, Brocklehurst P, Gordon A. Antibiotics for treating bacterial vaginosis in pregnancy. Cochrane Database Syst Rev 2007;1:CD000262.

79. ACOG Practice Bulletin 31. Assessment of risk factors for preterm birth. Obstet Gynecol 2001;98:708–16.

80. CDC. Sexually transmitted diseases treatment guidelines 2006. Available at: http://www.cdc.gov/std/treatment/.

81. Leveno KJ, Cox K, Roark ML. Cervical dilatation and prematurity revisited. Obstet Gynecol 1986;68:434–5.

82. Andersen HF, Nugent CE, Wanty SD, et al. Prediction of risk for preterm delivery by ultrasonographic measurement of cervical length. Am J Obstet Gynecol 1990;163:859–67.

83. Iams JD, Goldenberg RL, Meis PJ, et al. The length of the cervix and the risk of spontaneous preterm delivery. N Engl J Med 1996;334:567–73.

84. Taipale P, Hiilesmaa V. Sonographic measurement of uterine cervix at 18–22 weeks' gestation and the risk of preterm delivery. Obstet Gynecol 1998;92:902–7.

85. Heath VC, Southall TR, Souka AP, et al. Cervical length at 23 weeks of gestation: prediction of spontaneous preterm delivery. Ultrasound Obstet Gynecol 1998; 12:312–7.

86. Matijevic R, Grgic O, Vasili O. Is sonographic assessment of cervical length better than digital examination in screening for preterm delivery in a low-risk population? Acta Obstet Gynecol Scand 2006;85:1342–7.

87. To MS, Alfirevic Z, Hauth VC, et al. Cervical cerclage for prevention of preterm delivery in women with short cervix: randomized controlled trial. Lancet 2004; 363:1849–53.

88. Berghella V, Odibo A, To MS, et al. Cerclage for short cervix on ultrasonography; meta-analysis of trials using individual patient data. Obstet Gynecol 2005;106: 181–9.

89. Iams JD, Goldenberg RL, Mercer BM, et al. The Preterm Prediction Study: can low risk women destined for spontaneous preterm birth be identified? Am J Obstet Gynecol 2001;184:652–5.

90. Goldenberg RL, Iams JD, Mercer BM, et al. The Preterm Prediction Study: toward a multiple-marker test for spontaneous preterm birth. Am J Obstet Gynecol 2001;185:643–51.

91. Patton PE, Novy MJ, Lee DM, et al. The diagnosis and reproductive outcome after surgical treatment of the complete septate uterus, duplicated cervix and vaginal septum. Am J Obstet Gynecol 2004;190:1669–75.

92. Lumley J, Donohue L. Aiming to increase birth weight: a randomized trial of prepregnancy information, advice and counseling in inner-urban Melbourne. BMC Public Health 2006;6:299.

93. Andrews WW, Goldenberg RL, Hauth JC, et al. Inter-conceptional antibiotics to prevent spontaneous preterm birth: a randomized trial. Am J Obstet Gynecol 2006;194:617–23.

94. Espinoza J, Erez O, Romero R. Preconceptional antibiotic treatment to prevent preterm birth in women with a previous preterm delivery. Am J Obstet Gynecol 2006;194:630–7.

95. Sibai BM, Caritis SN, Thom E, et al. Prevention of preeclampsia with low-dose aspirin in healthy, nulliparous pregnant women. N Engl J Med 1993;329: 1213–8.
96. Caritis S, Sibai B, Hauth J, et al. Low-dose aspirin to prevent preeclampsia in women at high risk. N Engl J Med 1998;338:701–5.
97. Poston L, Briley AL, Seed PT, et al. Vitamins in Pre-eclampsia (VIP) Trial Consortium. Vitamin C and vitamin E in pregnant women at risk for pre-eclampsia (VIP trial): randomized placebo-controlled trial. Lancet 2006;367:1145–54.
98. Olsen SF, Sorenson JD, Secher NJ, et al. Randomized controlled trial of effect of fish-oil supplementation on pregnancy duration. Lancet 1992;339:1003–7.
99. Olsen SF, Secher NJ, Tabor A, et al. Randomized controlled trials of fish oil supplementation in high risk pregnancies. Fish Oil Trials in Pregnancy (FOTIP) Team. BJOG 2000;107:382–95.
100. Duley L, Henderson-Smart DJ, Meher S, et al. Antiplatelet agents for preventing pre-eclampsia and its complications. Cochrane Database Syst Rev 2007;2: CD004659.
101. Rumbold A, Duley L, Crowther C, et al. Antioxidants for preventing pre-eclampsia. Cochrane Database Syst Rev 2005;4:CD004227.
102. Goldenberg RL, Cliver SP, Bronstein J, et al. Bed rest in pregnancy. Obstet Gynecol 1994;84:131–6.
103. Sosa C, Althabe F, Belizan J, et al. Bed rest in singleton pregnancies for preventing preterm birth. Cochrane Database Syst Rev 2004;1:CD003581.
104. Yost NP, Owen J, Berghella V, et al. Effect of coitus on recurrent preterm birth. Obstet Gynecol 2006;107:793–7.
105. Olds DL, Henderson CR Jr, Tatelbaum R, et al. Improving delivery of prenatal care and outcomes of pregnancy: a randomized trial of nurse home visitation. Pediatrics 1986;77:16–28.
106. Quinlivan JA, Evans SF. Teenage antenatal clinics may reduce the rate of preterm birth: a prospective study. BJOG 2004;111:571–8.
107. Bryce RL, Stanley FJ, Garner RB. Randomized controlled trial of antenatal social support to prevent preterm birth. BJOG 1991;98:1001–8.
108. Villar J, Farnot U, Barros F, et al. A randomized trial of psychosocial support during high risk pregnancies. N Engl J Med 1992;327:1266–71.
109. Collaborative Working Group on Prematurity. Multicenter randomized controlled trial of a preterm birth prevention trial. Am J Obstet Gynecol 1993;169:352–66.
110. Kitzman H, Olds DL, Henderson CR Jr, et al. Effect of prenatal and home visitation by nurses on pregnancy outcomes, childhood injuries, and repeated childbearing. A randomized study. JAMA 1997;278:644–52.
111. Klerman LV, Ramey SL, Goldenberg RL, et al. A randomized trial of augmented prenatal care for multiple-risk, Medicaid-eligible African American women. Am J Public Health 2001;91:105–11.
112. Dyson DC, Danbe KH, Bamber JA, et al. Monitoring women at risk for preterm birth. N Engl J Med 1998;338:15–9.
113. Hodnett ED, Fredericks S. Support during pregnancy for women at increased risk of low birth weight babies. Cochrane Database Syst Rev 2003;3:CD000198.
114. Lamont RF. Can antibiotics prevent preterm birth—the pro and con debate. BJOG 2005;112(Suppl 1):67–73.
115. Goldenberg RL, Mwatha A, Read JS, et al. The HPTN 024 study: the efficacy of antibiotics to prevent chorioamnionitis and preterm birth. Am J Obstet Gynecol 2006;194:650–61.

116. Ugwumadu A, Reid F, Hay P, et al. Oral clindamycin and histologic chorioamnionitis in women with abnormal vaginal flora. Obstet Gynecol 2006;107:863–8.
117. Keirse MJ. Progestogen administration in pregnancy may prevent preterm delivery. BJOG 1990;97:149–54.
118. Sanchez-Ramos L, Kaunitz AM, Delke I. Progestational agents to prevent preterm birth: a meta-analysis of randomized controlled trials. Obstet Gynecol 2005;10:273–9.
119. Dodd JM, Flenady V, Cincotta R, et al. Prenatal administration of progesterone for preventing preterm birth. Cochrane Database Syst Rev 2006;1:CD004947.
120. Mackenzie R, Walker M, Armson A, et al. Progesterone for the prevention of preterm birth among women at increased risk. A systematic review and meta-analysis of randomized controlled trials. Am J Obstet Gynecol 2006;194:1234–42.
121. Pouse DJ, Caritis SN, Peaceman AM, et al. A trial of 17 alpha-hydroxyprogesterone caproate to prevent prematurity in twins. N Engl J Med 2007;357:454–61.
122. Althusius SM, Dekker GA, Hummel P, et al. Final results of the Cervical Incompetence Prevention Randomized Cerclage Trial (CIPRACT): therapeutic cerclage with bed rest versus bed rest alone. Am J Obstet Gynecol 2001;185:1106–12.
123. Rust OA, Atlas RO, Reed J, et al. Revisiting the short cervix detected by transvaginal ultrasound in the second trimester: why cerclage therapy may not help. Am J Obstet Gynecol 2001;185:1098–105.
124. Guzman ER, Forster JK, Vintzileos AM, et al. Pregnancy outcomes in women treated with elective versus ultrasound-indicated cervical cerclage. Ultrasound Obstet Gynecol 1998;12:323–7.
125. Hassan SS, Romero R, Maymon E, et al. Does cervical cerclage prevent preterm delivery in patients with a short cervix? Am J Obstet Gynecol 2001;184:1325–9.
126. Berghella V, Haas S, Chervoneva I, et al. Patients with prior second-trimester loss: prophylactic cerclage or serial transvaginal sonograms? Am J Obstet Gynecol 2002;187:747–51.
127. To MS, Palaniappan V, Skentou C, et al. Elective cerclage vs. ultrasound-indicated cerclage in high-risk pregnancies. Ultrasound Obstet Gynecol 2002;19:475–7.
128. Kurup M, Goldkrand JW. Cervical incompetence: elective, emergent, or urgent cerclage. Am J Obstet Gynecol 1999;181:240–6.
129. Guzman ER, Ananth CV. Cervical length and spontaneous prematurity: laying the foundation for future interventional randomized trials for the short cervix. Ultrasound Obstet Gynecol 2001;18:195–9.
130. Althusius SM, Dekker GA, van Geijn HP, et al. Cervical incompetence prevention randomized cerclage trial (CIPRACT): study design and preliminary results. Am J Obstet Gynecol 2000;183:823–9.
131. Althuisius S, Dekker G, Hummel P, et al. Cervical Incompetence Prevention Randomized Cerclage Trial (CIPRACT): effect of therapeutic cerclage with bed rest vs. bed rest only on cervical length. Ultrasound Obstet Gynecol 2002;20:163–7.
132. Berghella V, Odibo AO, Tolosa JE. Cerclage for prevention of preterm birth in women with a short cervix found on transvaginal ultrasound examination: a randomized trial. Am J Obstet Gynecol 2004;191:1311–7.
133. Lazar P, Gueguen S, Dreyfus J, et al. Multicentred controlled trial of cervical cerclage in women at moderate risk of preterm delivery. BJOG 1984;91:731–5.

134. Rush RW, Isaacs S, McPherson K, et al. A randomized controlled trial of cervical cerclage in women at high risk of spontaneous preterm delivery. BJOG 1984;91: 724–30.

135. Final Report of the Medical Research Council/Royal College of Obstetricians and Gynaecologists multicentre randomized trial of cervical cerclage. MRC/RCOG Working Party on Cervical Cerclage. BJOG 1993;100:516–23.

136. Althusius SM, Dekker GA, Hummel P, et al. Cervical Incompetence Prevention Randomized Cerclage Trial: emergency cerclage with bed rest versus bed rest alone. Am J Obstet Gynecol 2003;189:907–10.

137. Berghella V, Daly SF, Tolosa JE, et al. Prediction of preterm delivery with transvaginal ultrasonography of the cervix in patients with high-risk pregnancies: does cerclage prevent prematurity? Am J Obstet Gynecol 1999;181:809–15.

138. Groom KM, Bennett PR, Golara M, et al. Elective cervical cerclage versus serial ultrasound surveillance of cervical length in a population at high risk for preterm delivery. Eur J Obstet Gynecol Reprod Biol 2004;112:158–61.

139. Higgins SP, Kornman LH, Bell RJ, et al. Cervical surveillance as an alternative to elective cervical cerclage for pregnancy management of suspected cervical incompetence. Aust N Z J Obstet Gynaecol 2004;44:228–32.

140. Sakai M, Shiozaki A, Tabata A, et al. Evaluation of effectiveness of prophylactic cerclage of a short cervix according to interleukin-8 in cervical mucus. Am J Obstet Gynecol 2006;194:14–9.

141. Mueller-Heubach E, Reddick D, Barnett B, et al. Preterm birth prevention: evaluation of a prospective controlled randomized trial. Am J Obstet Gynecol 1989; 160:1172–8.

142. Hueston WA, Knox MA, Eilers G, et al. The effectiveness of preterm birth educational programs for high-risk women. Obstet Gynecol 1995;86:705–12.

143. A multicenter randomized controlled trial of home uterine monitoring: active versus sham device. The Collaborative Home Uterine Monitoring Study (CHUMS) Group. Am J Obstet Gynecol 1995;173:1120–7.

144. Towers CV, Bonebrake R, Padilla G, et al. The effect of transport on the rate of severe intraventricular hemorrhage in very low birth weight infants. Obstet Gynecol 2000;95:291–5.

145. Smith GN, Walker MC, Ohlsson A, et al. Canadian Preterm Labour Nitroglycerin Trial Group. Randomized double blind placebo controlled trial of transdermal nitroglycerin for preterm labor. Am J Obstet Gynecol 2007;196:37 e1–8.

146. King JF, Flenady VJ, Papatsonis DNM, et al. Calcium channel blockers for inhibiting preterm labour. Cochrane Database Syst Rev 2003;1:CD002255.

147. Papatsonis D, Flenady V, Cole S, et al. Oxytocin receptor antagonists for inhibiting preterm labour. Cochrane Database Syst Rev 2005;3:CD004452.

148. Anotayanonth S, Subhedar NV, Neilson JP, et al. Betamimetics for inhibiting preterm labour. Cochrane Database Syst Rev 2004;4:CD004352.

149. Crowther CA, Hiller JE, Doyle LW. Magnesium sulphate for preventing preterm birth in threatened preterm labour. Cochrane Database Syst Rev 2002;4: CD001060.

150. Mittendorf R, Covert R, Boman J, et al. Is tocolytic magnesium sulphate associated with increased total paediatric mortality? Lancet 1997;350:1517–8.

151. King J, Flenady V, Cole S, et al. Cyclo-oxygenase (COX) inhibitors for treating preterm labour. Cochrane Database Syst Rev 2005;2:CD001992.

152. Roberts D, Dalziel S. Antenatal corticosteroids for accelerating fetal lung maturation for women at risk of preterm birth. Cochrane Database Syst Rev 2006;3: CD004454.

153. Schrag S, Gorwitz R, Fultz-Butts K, et al. Prevention of perinatal group B strepto-coccal disease. Revised guidelines from CDC. MMWR Recomm Rep 2002;51:1–22.
154. Nanda K, Cook LA, Gallo MF, et al. Terbutaline pump maintenance therapy after threatened preterm labor for preventing preterm birth. Cochrane Database Syst Rev 2002;4:CD003933.
155. Dodd JM, Crowther CA, Dare MR, et al. Oral betamimetics for maintenance therapy after threatened preterm labour. Cochrane Database Syst Rev 2006;1:CD003927.
156. Grant A, Penn ZJ, Steer PJ. Elective or selective caesarean delivery of the small baby? A systematic review of the controlled trials. BJOG 1996;103:1197–200.
157. Deulofeut R, Sola A, Lee B, et al. The impact of vaginal delivery in premature infants weighing less than 1251 grams. Obstet Gynecol 2005;105:525–31.
158. Riskin A, Riksin-Mashiah S, Lusky A, et al. The relationship between delivery mode and mortality in very low birthweight singleton vertex-presenting infants. BJOG 2004;111:1365–71.
159. Iams JD, Romero R, Culhane JF, et al. Primary, secondary, and tertiary interventions to reduce the morbidity and mortality of preterm birth. Lancet 2008;371:164–75.
160. Papiernik E. Preventing preterm birth—is it really impossible? A comment on the IOM report on preterm birth. Matern Child Health J 2007;11:407–10.
161. Hall RT. Prevention of premature birth: do pediatricians have a role? Pediatrics 2000;105:1137–40.
162. Tyson J, Guzick D, Rosenfeld CR, et al. Prenatal care evaluation and cohort analyses. Pediatrics 1990;85:195–204.
163. Maloni JA, Damato EG. Reducing the risk for preterm birth: evidence and impli-cations for neonatal nurses. Adv Neonatal Care 2004;4:166–74.
164. Olds DL, Henderson CR Jr, Tatelbaum R, et al. Improving the life-course devel-opment of socially disadvantaged mothers: a randomized trial of nurse home visitation. Am J Public Health 1988;78:1436–45.
165. Olds DL, Eckenrode J, Henderson CR Jr, et al. Long-term effects of home visitation on maternal life course and child abuse and neglect. Fifteen-year follow-up of a randomized trial. JAMA 1997;278:637–43.
166. Olds DL, Robinson J, O'Brien R, et al. Home visiting by paraprofessionals and by nurses: a randomized, controlled trial. Pediatrics 2002;110:486–96.
167. Olds DL, Kitzman H, Hanks C, et al. Effects of nurse home visiting on maternal and child functioning: age-9 follow-up of a randomized trial. Pediatrics 2007; 120:e832–845.
168. Dunlop AL, Dubin C, Raynor BD, et al. Interpregnancy primary care and social support for African-American women at risk for recurrent very-low-birthweight delivery: a pilot evaluation. Matern Child Health J 2008;12:461–8.
169. McLaughlin FJ, Altemeier WA, Christensen MJ, et al. Randomized trial of comprehensive prenatal care for low-income women: effect on infant birth weight. Pediatrics 1992;89:128–32.
170. Peltoniemi OM, Kari MA, Tammela O, et al. Randomized trial of a single repeat dose of prenatal betamethasone treatment in imminent preterm birth. Pediatrics 2007;119:290–8.
171. Luke B, Marmelle M, Keith L, et al. The association between occupational factors and preterm birth: a United States nurses' study. Research Committee of the Association for Women's Health, Obstetric, and Neonatal Nurses. Am J Obstet Gynecol 1995;173:849–62.
172. Tough SC, Newburn-Cook C, Johnston DW, et al. Delayed childbearing and its impact on population rate changes in lower birth weight, multiple birth, and preterm delivery. Pediatrics 2002;109:399–403.

173. Edison RJ, Berg K, Remaley A, et al. Adverse birth outcome among mothers with low serum cholesterol. Pediatrics 2007;120:723–33.
174. Mercer B, Milluzzi C, Collin M. Periviable birth at 20 to 26 weeks of gestation: proximate causes, previous obstetric history and recurrence risk. Am J Obstet Gynecol 2005;193:1175–80.
175. Massett HA, Greenup M, Ryan CE, et al. Public perceptions about prematurity: a national survey. Am J Prev Med. 2003;24:120–7.
176. ACOG Committee Opinion #324. Perinatal risks associated with assisted reproductive technology. Obstet Gynecol 2005;106:1143–6.
177. Behrman RE, Stith Butler A, editors. Committee on understanding premature birth and assuring healthy outcomes. Washington, DC: National Academies Press; 2006.
178. Min JK, Claman P, Hughes E, et al. Guidelines for the number of embryos to transfer following in vitro fertilization. J Obstet Gynaecol Can 2006;28:799–813.
179. ACOG Committee Opinion # 313. The importance of preconception care in the continuum of women's health care. Obstet Gynecol 2005;106:665–6.
180. Bukowski R, Malone FD, Porter F, et al. Preconceptional folate prevents preterm delivery. Am J Obstet Gynecol 2007;197:S3 [abstract], 2008 Society for Maternal Fetal Medicine.
181. Bakketeig LS, Hoffman HJ. Epidemiology of preterm birth: results from a longitudinal study in Norway. In: Elder MG, Hendricks CH, editors. Preterm labor. London: Butterworths; 1981. p. 17.
182. Adams MM, Elam-Evans LD, Wilson HG, et al. Rates of and factors associated with recurrence of preterm delivery. JAMA 2000;283:1591–6.
183. Goldenberg RL, Andrews WW, Faye-Peterson O, et al. The Alabama preterm birth project: placental histology in recurrent spontaneous and indicated preterm birth. Am J Obstet Gynecol 2006;195:792–6.
184. Ananth CV, Getahun D, Peltier MR, et al. Recurrence of spontaneous versus medically indicated preterm birth. Am J Obstet Gynecol 2006;195:643–50.
185. Haas JS, Fuentes-Afflick E, Stewart AL, et al. Pre-pregnancy health status and the risk of preterm delivery. Arch Pediatr Adolesc Med 2005;159:58–63.
186. Roberts JM, for the NICHD MFMU Network. A randomized controlled trial of antioxidant vitamins to prevent serious complications associated with pregnancy related hypertension in low risk nulliparous women. Am J Obstet Gynecol 2008;199:S4 [abstract], 2009 Society for Maternal Fetal Medicine.
187. Biermann J, Dunlop AL, Brady C, et al. Promising practices in preconception care for women at risk for poor health and pregnancy outcomes. Matern Child Health J 2006;10:S21–8.
188. Harper M. Randomized controlled trial of omega-3 fatty acid supplementation for recurrent preterm birth prevention [abstract]. Presented at the International Society for the Study of Fatty Acids and Lipids 2008.
189. Offenbacher S, Beck J, Jared H, et al. Maternal oral therapy to reduce obstetric risk (MOTOR): a report of a multicentered periodontal therapy randomized controlled trial on rate of preterm delivery [abstract]. Am J Obstet Gynecol 2008;199:52.
190. Macones G, Jeffcoat M, Parry S, et al. Screening and treating periodontal disease in pregnancy does not reduce the incidence of preterm birth: results from the PIPS Study [abstract]. Am J Obstet Gynecol 2008;199:53.
191. Smaill F. Antibiotics for asymptomatic bacteriuria in pregnancy. Cochrane Database Syst Rev 2001;2:CD000490.

192. Hauth JC, Goldenberg RL, Andrews WW, et al. Reduced incidence of preterm delivery with metronidazole and erythromycin in women with bacterial vaginosis. N Engl J Med 1995;333:1732–6.
193. Gichangi PB, Ndinya-Achola JO, Ombete J, et al. Antimicrobial prophylaxis in pregnancy: a randomized, placebo-controlled trial with cefetamet-pivoxil in pregnant women with a poor obstetric history. Am J Obstet Gynecol 1997; 177:680–4.
194. Vermeulen GM, Bruinse HW. Prophylactic administration of clindamycin 2% vaginal cream to reduce the incidence of spontaneous preterm birth in women with an increased recurrence risk: a randomised placebo-controlled double-blind trial. Br J Obstet Gynaecol 1999;106:652–7.
195. Joesoef MR, Hillier SL, Wiknjosastro G, et al. Intravaginal clindamycin treatment for bacterial vaginosis: effects on preterm delivery and low birth weight. Am J Obstet Gynecol 1995;173:1527–31.
196. McDonald HM, O'Loughlin JA, Vigneswaran R, et al. Impact of metronidazole therapy on preterm birth in women with bacterial vaginosis flora (*Gardnerella vaginalis*): a randomized, placebo controlled trial. BJOG 1997;104:1391–7.
197. Carey JC, Klebanoff M, Hauth JC. Metronidazole to prevent preterm delivery in pregnant women with asymptomatic bacterial vaginosis. National Institute of Child Health and Human Development Network of Maternal-Fetal Medicine Units. N Engl J Med 2000;342:534–40.
198. Rosenstein IJ, Morgan DJ, Lamont RF, et al. Effect of intravaginal clindamycin cream on pregnancy outcome and on abnormal vaginal microbial flora of pregnant women. Infect Dis Obstet Gynecol 2000;8:158–65.
199. Kurkinen-Raty M, Vuopala S, Koskela M, et al. A randomized controlled trial of vaginal clindamycin for early pregnancy bacterial vaginosis. BJOG 2000;107: 1427–32.
200. Kekki M, Kurki T, Pelkonen J, et al. Vaginal clindamycin in preventing preterm birth and peripartal infections in asymptomatic women with bacterial vaginosis. Obstet Gynecol 2001;97:643.
201. Ugwumadu A, Manyonda I, Reid F, et al. Effect of early oral clindamycin on late miscarriage and preterm delivery in asymptomatic women with abnormal vaginal flora and bacterial vaginosis: a randomised controlled trial. Lancet 2003;361:983–8.
202. Lamont RF, Duncan SLB, Mandal D, et al. Intravaginal clindamycin to reduce preterm birth in women with abnormal genital tract flora. Obstet Gynecol 2003;101:516–22.
203. Kiss H, Petricevic L, Husslein P. Prospective randomised controlled trial of an infection screening programme to reduce the rate of preterm delivery. BMJ 2004;329:371–5.
204. Larsson PG, Fahraeus L, Carlsson B, et al. Late miscarriage and preterm birth after treatment with clindamycin: a randomised consent design study according to Zelen. BJOG 2006;113:629–37.
205. American College of Obstetricians and Gynecologists. Assessment of risk factors for preterm birth. ACOG Practice Bulletin number 31. Obstet Gynecol 2001;98:709–16.
206. Rouse DJ, Caritis SN, Peaceman AM, et al. A trial of 17 alpha-hydroxyprogesterone caproate to prevent prematurity in twins. N Engl J Med 2007;357:454–61.
207. Northen AT, Norman GS, Anderson K, et al. Follow-up of children exposed in utero to 17 alpha-hydroxyprogesterone caproate compared with placebo. Obstet Gynecol 2007;110:865–72.

208. Meis PJ, Society for Maternal-Fetal Medicine. 17 Hydroxyprogesterone for the prevention of preterm delivery. Obstet Gynecol 2005;105:1128–35.
209. Christian MS, Brent RL, Calda P. Embryo-fetal toxicity signals for 17alpha-hydroxyprogesterone caproate in high-risk pregnancies: a review of the non-clinical literature for embryo-fetal toxicity with progestins. J Matern Fetal Neonatal Med 2007;20:89–112.
210. Petrini JR, Callaghan WM, Klebanoff M. Estimated effect of 17 alpha hydroxy-progesterone caproate on preterm birth in the United States. Obstet Gynecol 2005;105:267–72.
211. Bailit JL, Votruba ME. Medical cost savings associated with 17 alpha-hydroxy-progesterone caproate. Am J Obstet Gynecol 2007;196:219 e1–7.
212. Armstrong J. 17 Progesterone for preterm birth prevention: a potential $2 billion opportunity. Am J Obstet Gynecol 2007;196:194–5.
213. Shapiro-Mendoza CK, Tomashek KM, Kotelchuk M, et al. Effect of late-preterm birth and maternal medical conditions on newborn morbidity risk. Pediatrics 2008;121:e223–32.
214. Sibai BM, Mabie WC, Shamsa F, et al. A comparison of no medication versus methyldopa or labetalol in chronic hypertension during pregnancy. Am J Obstet Gynecol 1990;162:960–6.
215. Redman CW. Controlled trials of antihypertensive drugs in pregnancy. Am J Kidney Dis 1991;17:149–53.
216. Chang J, Elam-Evans LD, Berg CJ, et al. Pregnancy-related mortality surveil-lance—United States, 1991–1999. MMWR Surveill Summ 2003;52:1–8.
217. US Department of Health and Human Services. Healthy people. Available at: http://www.healthypeople.gov/.
218. Antepartum fetal surveillance. ACOG Practice Bulletin number 9. American College of Obstetricians and Gynecologists 1999.
219. Reid R, Ivey KJ, Rencoret RH, et al. Fetal complications of obstetric cholestasis. BMJ 1976;1:870–2.
220. Al Inizi S, Gupta R, Gale A. Fetal tachyarrhythmia with atrial flutter in obstetric cholestasis. Int J Gynaecol Obstet 2006;93:53–4.
221. Mathews TJ, MacDorman MF. Infant mortality from the 2005 period linked birth/infant death data set. Natl Vital Stat Rep 2008;57.
222. Ananth CV, Gyamfi C, Jain L. Characterizing risk profiles of infants who are deliv-ered at late preterm gestations: does it matter? Am J Obstet Gynecol 2008;199:329–31.
223. Ananth CV, Joseph KS, Oyelese Y, et al. Trends in preterm birth and perinatal mortality among singletons: United States, 1989 through 2000. Obstet Gynecol 2005;105:1084–91.

Health Issues of the Late Preterm Infant

Ashwin Ramachandrappa, MD, MPH*, Lucky Jain, MD, MBA

KEYWORDS

• Late preterm • Near term • Early term
• Fetal lung fluid clearance

"Late preterm" birth is not such an unusual occurrence. This group of premature infants was the first group that pediatricians learned to treat. These infants were treated with such remarkable success that pediatricians no longer consider them to be at high risk. So, why the sudden interest in this group? There is now growing evidence that this population is not as healthy as previously thought; it has increased mortality when compared to term infants and is at higher risk for several complications such as transient tachypnea of newborn (TTN), respiratory distress syndrome (RDS), persistent pulmonary hypertension (PPHN), respiratory failure, temperature instability, jaundice, feeding difficulties, and prolonged neonatal intensive care unit (NICU) stay. Evidence is emerging that late preterm infants make up a majority of preterm births, take up a significant amount of healthcare resources, have increased mortality/ morbidity, and may even have long-term neurodevelopmental consequences secondary to their late prematurity.

DEFINITION

They have been called by several names: near term, moderately preterm, minimally preterm, and marginally preterm. These terms can be misleading, implying that late preterm infants are healthy, although recent research has shown that they have increased morbidity and mortality associated with preterm gestation.[1-6] The National Institute of Child Health and Human Development (NICHD) of the National Institutes of Health (NIH) convened a workshop in July 2005 that recommended that infants born between 34 0/7 weeks (239 days gestation) and 36 6/7 weeks (259 days gestation) be referred to as "late preterm" infants (**Fig. 1**).[7]

EPIDEMIOLOGY

The preterm birth rate has seen a steady increase in the last 25 years. Preterm infants comprise 12.8% of all live births (~546,000), with late preterm births making up 72%

Division of Neonatology, Department of Pediatrics, Emory University School of Medicine, 2015 Uppergate Drive NE, Atlanta, GA 30322, USA
* Corresponding author.
E-mail address: ashwin_ramachandrappa@oz.ped.emory.edu (A. Ramachandrappa).

Pediatr Clin N Am 56 (2009) 565–577
doi:10.1016/j.pcl.2009.03.009
0031-3955/09/$ – see front matter © 2009 Elsevier Inc. All rights reserved.

pediatric.theclinics.com

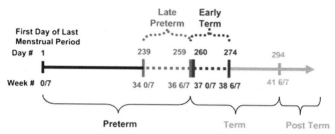

Fig. 1. Definition of "late preterm" and "early term". (*From* Engle WA, Kominiarek MA. Late preterm infants, early term infants, and timing of elective deliveries. Clinics in Perinatology 2008;35:325; with permission.)

of the overall preterm population. While preterm births less than 34 weeks have increased by a modest 10% since 1990, late preterm births have increased by nearly 25% (**Fig. 2**).[8] Most races including Hispanics, African-American and non-Hispanic whites, have seen an increase in late preterm births; emerging data suggests that late preterm births are becoming increasingly common throughout the world.

ETIOLOGY

Why have late preterm births increased in recent times? There is no one particular explanation, but a multitude of factors that have contributed to this rise. Preterm labor, preeclampsia and premature rupture of membranes are known contributors to preterm birth; however, recent spikes in inductions, cesarean sections and other obstetrical

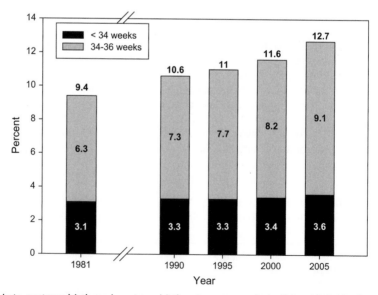

Fig. 2. Late preterm birth and preterm birth rate compared to all live births in the United States 1981–2005. (*Data from* CDC/NCHS, National Vital Statistics System; and *from* Tomashek KM, Shapiro-Mendoza CK, et al. Differences in mortality between late-preterm and term singleton infants in the United States, 1995–2002. J Pediatr 2007;151:450.)

practices, as well as a modest change in maternal demographics, have played a key role in the increase in late preterm births.[1,8-10]

Nearly one in four births today are born by induction of labor; induction rates have more than doubled since 1990 (from 9.5% to 22.5%) with late preterm and term births showing the largest increase in induction rates.[8] In addition, cesarean sections have continued to increase over the last decade and are at the highest reported level (31.1% of all live births or nearly one in three live births). If a woman has a primary cesarean section, she has a 92% probability of having a repeat cesarean section; primary cesarean sections have thus contributed to the dramatic increase in the total cesarean section rate.[8] Davidoff and colleagues[1] found a shift towards earlier gestations among births by medical intervention (cesarean sections and inductions), with the majority of the increases seen among the late preterm (34–36 weeks) and early term infants (37–39 weeks). There is also an increasing demand for cesarean sections at maternal request, spurred by the perceived safety of surgical procedures, desire for smaller families, and the fear of complications/risks associated with vaginal birth.[11] A national consensus meeting in 2006 convened by the NIH coined the term "cesarean section on maternal request" for cesarean births with no medical indication.[12] It is estimated that nearly 2.5%–18% of all live births are being delivered by cesarean section on maternal request,[7,11] although others disagree, contending that the increase in cesarean section rates is largely caused by changing maternal demographics and practice standards of medical professionals, and the ever-increasing risk of malpractice litigation.[13,14] Higher use of intrapartum fetal monitoring and prenatal ultrasound, coupled with a substantial increase in obesity and gestational diabetes (leading to fetal macrosomia) can all result in overestimation of gestational age, prompting inductions and cesarean sections at earlier than intended gestational age.[15,16] Finally, a striking rise in multiple births from use of assisted reproductive technologies has added to the rise in late preterm births.[17]

PATHOPHYSIOLOGY AND OUTCOMES

As mentioned earlier, late preterm infants can present with a multitude of clinical problems including respiratory distress, hyperbilirubinemia, temperature instability, feeding difficulties, hypoglycemia, apnea, and late onset sepsis, leading to prolonged hospital stay and readmission after discharge.[2,5,16,18-20] A few of the complications that are of relevance to the practicing pediatrician are discussed here.

Respiratory

Several studies have consistently shown that late preterm infants are at higher risk for TTN, RDS, PPHN and respiratory failure than term infants.[3-5,21-25] The lungs in the fetus are filled with fluid, which is rapidly cleared and filled with air soon after birth. Traditional explanations such as vaginal squeeze and starling forces can only account for a fraction of the fluid that is absorbed; studies show that the epithelium sodium channels (ENaC) plays an important role in the transepithelial movement of fetal lung fluid. Increased numbers and activation of the ENaC channels close to birth and after birth lead to movement of sodium from the alveolar lumen across the apical membrane into the cell, with subsequent extrusion out of the cell by Na^+/K^+-ATPase. Peak expression of the ENaC channels occurs at term gestation; late preterm infants are therefore born with lower expression of ENaC, which reduces their ability to clear lung fluid after birth (**Fig. 3**).[20]

Several studies have shown that the incidence of respiratory distress increases with decreasing gestational age.[3,5,19,21,24,26-28] Wang and colleagues[5] showed that

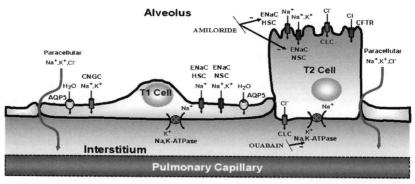

Fig. 3. Epithelial sodium (Na) absorption in the fetal lung near birth. Na enters the cell through the apical surface of both ATI and ATII cells via amiloride-sensitive epithelial Na channels (ENaC), both highly selective channels (HSC) and nonselective channels (NSC), and via cyclic nucleotide gated channels (seen only in ATI cells). Electroneutrality is conserved with chloride movement through cystic fibrosis transmembrane conductance regulator (CFTR) or through chloride channels (CLC) in ATI and ATII cells, and/or paracellularly through tight junctions. The increase in cell Na stimulates Na-K-ATPase activity on the basolateral aspect of the cell membrane, which drives out three Na ions in exchange for two K ions, a process that can be blocked by the cardiac glycoside ouabain. If the net ion movement is from the apical surface to the interstitium, an osmotic gradient would be created, which would in turn direct water transport in the same direction, either through aquaporins or by diffusion. (*From* Jain L. Respiratory morbidity in late-preterm infants: prevention is better than cure! Am J Perinatol 2008;25(2):75–8; with permission.)

late preterm infants had nine times the odds of respiratory distress than term infants (28.9% versus 4.2%; $P<0.00001$). Recent data from the British Columbia Perinatal Database Registry found that late preterm infants (33–36 weeks) had 4.4 times the relative risk of respiratory morbidity than term infants.[27] A large population-based study from California found that the incidence of RDS was 7.4% at 34 weeks, 4.5% at 35 weeks and 2.3% at 36 weeks with 6.3% infants requiring mechanical ventilation at 34 weeks, 3.6% at 35 weeks and 2.3% at 36 weeks.[26] More recent studies have shown that 23%–33% of the late preterm infants require respiratory support, and up to 3.3% of them require some form of mechanical ventilation.[25] Prematurity by itself is responsible for significant respiratory morbidity, but when coupled with cesarean section and absence of labor, it can exaggerate the incidence of respiratory distress. Several studies of term infants have shown increased odds of respiratory distress for births by cesarean section without labor; this risk increases substantially with a drop in gestational age. Morrison and colleagues[29] found that the incidence of respiratory morbidity was significantly higher for the group delivered by caesarean section before the onset of labor (35.5/1000) compared with vaginal delivery (5.3/1000) (OR 6.8; 95% CI 5.2–8.9; $P < 0.001$). A large Dutch study similarly found increasing odds of severe respiratory distress with decreasing gestational age; at 37 weeks, infants born by cesarean section without labor had five times the odds of severe respiratory morbidity than those born by vaginal delivery at 39 weeks.[30]

RDS and TTN in the late preterm infants can prolong hospital stay requiring the use of mechanical ventilation, but of even greater concern are the small number of these infants who develop PPHN and severe hypoxic respiratory failure requiring ECMO.[21,31]

Feeding Difficulties

Late preterm infants have poor suck and swallow coordination because of neuronal immaturity and decreased oromotor tone, which can lead to poor caloric intake and dehydration. Wang and colleagues[5] found that nearly 27 percent of the late preterm infants required intravenous fluids compared to 5% term infants (OR 6.5, 95% CI: 2.3–23), and 76% of the late preterm infants with poor feeding required a prolonged hospital stay with a delay in discharge. Vachharajani and colleagues found that nearly 7.3% of infants at 35 weeks gestation were admitted to the NICU for feeding difficulties. In a study of rehospitalization by Escobar and colleagues,[2] it was found that nearly 26% of the late preterm and term infants required rehospitalization for feeding difficulties and late preterm infants were more likely to get readmitted (4.4% in late preterm versus 2% in term). Dehydration from poor oral intake also exacerbates physiological jaundice and predisposes the late preterm infant to rehospitalizations.

Hyperbilirubinemia

Hyperbilirubinemia in the late preterm infant results from excess bilirubin load caused by reduced hepatic uptake or decreased conjugation of bilirubin secondary to decreased activity of hepatic uridine diphosphate glucoronyltransferase enzyme and increased enterohepatic circulation caused by immature gastrointestinal function and motility.[32] This condition puts them at risk for high serum bilirubin levels and sometimes severe, prolonged jaundice, and kernicterus. A retrospective study looking at data from 11 northern California hospitals found that infants born at 36 weeks gestation have nearly four times the odds for developing serum bilirubin levels >20 mg/dL (343 μmol/L) when compared to those born at 39–40 weeks.[33] Gestational age was a strong predictor of severe jaundice in this study, which indicates that physicians were treating late preterm infants with less aggressive treatment protocols applicable to term infants. In another retrospective study, infants at 35 to 36 weeks, 36 to 37 weeks, and 37 to 38 weeks gestation were 13.2, 7.7, and 7.2 times more likely to be readmitted to the hospital and require phototherapy for significant hyperbilirubinemia than those greater than or equal to 40 weeks gestation[34] In a prospective study by Sarici and colleagues, late preterm infants were 2.4 times more likely to develop significant hyperbilirubinemia than term infants; and nearly one in four late preterm infants required phototherapy for jaundice. In this study, they had significantly higher bilirubin levels on day 5 and day 7, indicating that these infants have a relatively delayed bilirubin peak with a tendency to persist for a longer duration. This study developed an age-specific percentile based nomogram-utilizing sensitivity, specificity, and negative and positive predictive values (fifth percentile track with greatest sensitivity and negative predictive value, and 95th percentile track with greatest specificity and positive predictive value) in the assessment of the predictive ability of the 6- and 30-hour serum bilirubin value in determining the development of significant hyperbilirubinemia (**Fig. 4**). Therefore, considering their high-risk status, late preterm infants should not be treated as term infants. They require aggressive treatment based on their risk status using percentile distribution of the serum bilirubin values on postnatal age, rather than using traditional birthweight-based thresholds; a longer follow-up is also required because of the delayed bilirubin peak and prolonged duration of jaundice.[35]

Hypothermia

Term infants can generate heat by breaking down brown adipose tissue with the help of hormones, such as norepinephrine, prolactin, triiodothyronine and cortisol, which

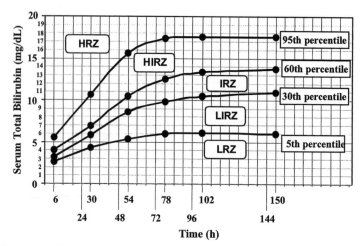

Fig. 4. Risk zones of near-term newborns according to the percentile tracks based on the hour-specific serum bilirubin values. HRZ, high-risk zone designated >95th percentile track; HIRZ, high-intermediate risk zone between the 60th and 95th percentile tracks; IRZ, inter-mediate-risk zone between the 30th and 60th percentile tracks; LIRZ, low-intermediate risk zone between the 5th and 30th percentile tracks; LRZ, low-risk zone <5th percentile track. (*From* Sarici SU, Serdar MA. Incidence, course, and prediction of hyperbilirubinemia in near-term and term newborns. Pediatrics 2004;113:775; with permission.)

peak at term gestation. Late preterm infants have decreased brown adipose tissue stores and hormones necessary for their breakdown. They also have decreased insu-lation in the form of white adipose tissue and increased body–surface area to body–weight ratio, putting them at risk for increased heat loss.[36,37] Wang and colleagues[5] found that late preterm infants were more likely to present with temperature instability (**Fig. 5**). In another study, hypothermia was cited as the primary reason for admission in 5.2% of all late preterm infants who were admitted to the NICU.[25] Cold stress can lead to poor respiratory transition in late preterm infants and exacerbate hypogly-cemia, prompting work-ups for sepsis, which require further laboratory tests and anti-biotics. Temperature regulation is important in late preterm infants and, if not properly managed, can lead to significant morbidity.

Hypoglycemia

Newborn infants produce glucose primarily by hepatic glycogenolysis and gluconeo-genesis. There is a surge of catecholamines and glucacon after birth with a drop in circulating insulin; these changes help in maintaining euglycemic control. Late preterm infants have immature hepatic enzymes for gluconeogenesis and glycogenolysis; they also have decreased hepatic glycogen stores, which normally accumulate in the third trimester. In addition, hormonal regulation and insulin secretion by pancreatic β cells is immature, resulting in unregulated insulin secretion during hypoglycemia. This quick depletion of the inadequate glycogen stores, associated conditions such as cold stress, sepsis and feeding difficulties, in the late preterm infants puts them at increased risk for hypoglycemia.[12,38] In a study by Wang and colleagues[5] hypogly-cemia (blood glucose <40 mg/dL) was three times more common in late preterm infants than term infants and nearly 27% of them required intravenous fluids when compared to 5% among term infants. It is well known that severe hypoglycemia is

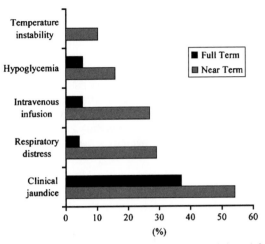

Fig. 5. Graph of clinical outcomes in near-term (35–36 6/7 weeks) and full-term infants as percentage of patients studied. (*From* Wang ML, Dorer DJ, Fleming MP, et al. Clinical outcomes of near-term infants. Pediatrics 2004;114:372; with permission.)

a risk factor for neuronal cell death and adverse neurodevelopmental outcomes,[38] but more studies of the late preterm infant are needed to identify the threshold for severe hypoglycemia.

Infection

Late preterm infants have approximately four times the odds for being screened for sepsis than term infants (36.7% versus 12.6%; OR: 3.97, $P < 0.01$); the majority of the late preterm infants who were screened for sepsis were treated with antibiotics and were likely to be treated longer (30% versus 17% in term infants).[5] The likelihood of having a sepsis screen increases with decreasing gestational age. McIntire and colleagues[28] found that 33% versus 12% of infants were screened for sepsis at 34 and 39 weeks respectively and only 0.4% of those screened had culture proven sepsis. Late preterm infants often have conditions such as mild RDS, TTN, hypoglycemia and hypothermia, which are all related to their prematurity, but these conditions may be enough to prompt the clinician to screen and treat these infants for suspected sepsis. Most of these infants have sterile blood cultures and rarely is pneumonia a cause for their respiratory distress. This situation presents a common dilemma to the practitioner, who most likely will decide to treat these infants for pneumonia and clinical sepsis per conventional practices applicable to term infants, thus prolonging hospital stay and antibiotic therapy.[5]

Morbidity and Mortality

As described above, late preterm infants are at significant risk of morbidity and are susceptible to multiple illnesses because of their relative physiological immaturity. Shapiro-Mendoza and colleagues estimated that late preterm infants are 20, 10, and 5 times more likely to experience morbidity at 34, 35, and 36 weeks respectively. A large population-based cohort of linked birth–death certificate data from the United States and Canada showed that late preterm infants were 2.9 (95% CI; 2.8–3) and 4.5 (95% CI; 4–5) times more likely to die than term infants respectively.[39] Tomashek and colleagues, using United States period-linked infant birth/death files for 1995 to 2002, found that despite significant declines in mortality from 1995, infant mortality rate was three times higher for late preterm infants than term infants (7.9 versus 2.4 deaths per 1000 live births); early, late, and postneonatal rates were six, three, and two times higher, respectively. Late preterm infants were four times more like than term infants to die of congenital malformations, newborn bacterial sepsis, and complications of placenta, cord, and membranes. Young and colleagues,[6] in a large population-based study, have shown that mortality and the relative risk of death increases with each decreasing week in gestational age (**Table 1**). The United States mortality rate for late preterm infants continues to be high when compared to term infants, with the rates in 2005 being 7.3 per 1000 live births versus 2.43 per 100 live births in term infants. It is now clear that prematurity even by a few weeks carries with it significant morbidity and mortality risks.

Long-term Outcomes

It is hard to believe that infants just a few weeks shy of term gestation can have long-term morbidity associated with it, but several studies are now beginning to show the long-term consequences of late prematurity. The cerebral volume of the late preterm brain is only 53% of the term 40-week infant and weighs one third less than the term 40-week gestation brain. The cerebral cortex has less gyri/sulci, and is smooth when compared to the term brain. Myelination and interneuronal connectivity is incomplete and any interruption or insult during this stage of development can lead to poor long-term neurodevelopmental outcomes.[40] A large population-based study from Sweden including ~900,000 children and nearly 33,000 late preterm infants born without any congenital anomalies between 1967 and 1983, who were followed until 2003, found a higher incidence of cerebral palsy (RR 2.7; $P < 0.001$), mental retardation (RR 1.6; $P < 0.001$), psychological developmental problems, behavioral and emotional disturbances, and other major disabilities, such as blindness, decreased vision, hearing loss and epilepsy.[41] Lindstorm and colleagues looking at a large Swedish cohort of ~500,000 adults in their twenties found that infants born at 33–36 weeks gestation were more likely to receive disability allowance and were less likely to attain university or post-secondary education. Chyi and colleagues[42] using the Early Childhood Longitudinal Study–Kindergarten Cohort found that late preterm infants had lower scores for reading in kindergarten and first grade (using direct child assessment tests) and scored lower for reading and math using teacher academic rating scale scores. These

Table 1
Mortality rates and risk ratios for death according to gestational age

Gestational Age, wks	Early Neonatal Mortality Rate (1–7 Days)		Infant Mortality Rate (1–365 Days)	
	Mortality Rate[a]	Risk Ratio	Mortality Rate[a]	Risk Ratio
34	7.2	25.5[b]	12.5[b]	10.5
35	4.5	16.1[b]	8.7[b]	7.2
36	2.8	9.8[b]	6.3[b]	5.3
37	0.8	2.7[b]	3.4[b]	2.8
38	0.5	1.7	2.4[b]	2.0
39	0.2	0.8	1.2	1.2
40	0.3	ref	1.4	ref

[a] Mortality rates are per 1000 live births.
[b] Risk ratios are significantly different from 40 weeks.
Data from Young PC, Glasgow TS, Li X, et al. Mortality of late-preterm (near-term) newborns in Utah. Pediatrics 2007;119:e659.

studies show that late preterm birth has a significant impact on the growing brain, but further prospective studies are needed to confirm causality.

Economic Burden

Increase in direct costs for late preterm infants is 2.9 times that of a term infant, resulting in a cost increase of $2,630 per infant (P < 0.0004).[5] In a 1996 study by Gilbert and colleagues using hospital discharge data from California, the authors show increasing hospital costs with decreasing gestational age, with costs ranging from $7,200, $4,200, $2,600, and $1,100 for 34, 35, 36, and 38 week infants respectively. The average cost for treating a premature infant at 25 weeks and 35 weeks was ~$202,000 and $4,200 respectively, but when the total costs for each gestational age group was looked at, the average cost for treating infants at 25 weeks gestation was 38.9 million dollars and for 35 weeks gestation was 41.1 million dollars.[26] Although the extremely premature infants are expensive to treat, the overall cost for treating late preterm infants is similar or higher because of their large numbers. With 72% of all preterm births being late preterm and nearly 30%–50% requiring prolonged hospital stay or NICU care, the cost of their care continue to rise.

MANAGEMENT

It should now be clear that late preterm infants are not term infants, even though they are often of good size and look healthy. It is of great importance that clinicians treat these infants with the monitoring and care which they deserve and not club them with term infants. The authors, along with other colleagues at their institution, recently developed a clinical consensus document to serve as a guide for the care of the late preterm infant. Salient points of this guide are summarized in **Box 1** and described below.[43] Similar guidelines have been published by Engle and colleagues.[18]

Admission

Infants < 35 weeks gestation and/or <2300 g should be admitted to an area where they can be monitored closely for stability. They should have a physical exam on admission and discharge with determination of accurate gestation age on admission exam. The authors recommend using the obstetrical estimate of gestational age if it is based on a first trimester ultrasound. If there is a discrepancy between the gestational ages based on the obstetrical estimate and the newborn examination, the authors then use gestational age, based on the newborn exam. Vital signs and pulse oximeter check should be performed on admission, followed by vital signs every 3–4 hours in the first 24 hours, and every shift thereafter. The authors recommend caution against the use of oxyhoods with high FiO2 and recommend transfer to high risk NICU/environment if FiO2 exceeds 0.4. A feeding plan should be developed with formal evaluation and documentation of breast-feeding by caregivers trained in breast-feeding at least twice daily after birth. Serum glucose screening should be performed per existing protocols for infants at high risk of hypoglycemia, such as SGA/LGA/IDM. They should be transferred to the mother's room or regular "term" nursery only if they demonstrate stability of temperature, vital signs, blood sugar, and oral feeding.

Discharge Criteria

Discharge should not be considered before 48 hours after birth. Vital signs should be within normal range for the 12 hours preceeding discharge (ie, respiratory rate <60/min, heart rate 100–160/bpm, axillary temperature 36.5–37.4°C in an open crib with appropriate clothing). There should be documentation of passage of at least one stool

---

Box 1
Management of late preterm infant: admission and discharge criteria

Admission Criteria

- Admit all infants <35 weeks and/or <2300 g.

  They should not to be sent to their mothers' rooms in the first 24 hours until stable, unless arrangements can be made to provide transitional care and close monitoring in the mother's room.

Hospital Management

- Physical exam on admission and discharge.
- Determination of accurate gestation age on admission exam.
- Vital signs and pulse oximeter check on admission, followed by vital signs q 3–4 hours in the first 24 hours, and q shift thereafter.
- Caution against use of oxyhoods with high FiO_2. Consider transfer to NICU/tertiary care center if FiO_2 exceeds 0.4.
- A feeding plan should be developed. Formal evaluation of breast-feeding and documentation in the record by caregivers trained in breast-feeding at least twice daily after birth.
- Serum glucose screening per existing protocols for infants at high risk of hypoglycemia.

Discharge Criteria

- Discharge should not be considered before 48 hours after birth.
- Vital signs should be within normal range for the 12 hours proceeding discharge.
- Passage of one stool spontaneously.
- Adequate urine output.
- 24 hours of successful feeding: ability to coordinate sucking, swallowing and breathing while feeding.
- If weight loss greater than 7% in 48 hours, consider further assessment before discharge.
- Risk assessment plan for jaundice for infants discharged within 72 hours of birth.
- No evidence of active bleeding at circumcision site for at least 2 hours.
- Initial hepatitis B vaccine has been given or an appointment scheduled for its administration.
- Metabolic and genetic screening tests have been performed in accordance with local or hospital requirements.
- The late preterm infant has passed a car seat safety test.
- Hearing assessment is performed and results documented in the medical records. Follow-up, if necessary, has been arranged.
- Family, environmental, and social risk factors have been assessed. When risk factors are present discharge should be delayed until a plan for future care has been generated.
- Identification of a physician with a follow-up visit arranged for 24–48 hours.
- Give the mother and caregivers training and competency in the care of the infant.

---

spontaneously, with adequate urine output, and 24 hours of successful/adequate oral feeding; there should be confirming coordination of sucking, swallowing and breathing while feeding. If weight loss is greater than 7% in 48 hrs, consider further assessment before discharge. There should be a risk assessment plan for jaundice in infants discharged within 72 hours of birth; predischarge bilirubin check (serum or transcutaneous) should be done before discharge. If transcutaneous bilirubin is >12 mg, it must be confirmed with a serum bilirubin for determination of accuracy of bilirubin. Bilirubin normograms should be used to determine the need for follow-up or treatment. There should be no evidence of active bleeding at the circumcision site for at least 2 hours. Initial hepatitis B vaccine should be given, or an appointment scheduled for its administration, and the metabolic/genetic screening tests should have been performed in accordance with local or hospital requirements. A car seat safety test and a hearing assessment must be performed; the results must be documented in the medical records. Family, environmental, and social risk factors should have been assessed, and when risk factors are present, discharge should be delayed until a plan for future care has been generated. A follow-up visit with a physician must be arranged for 24–48 hours from discharge. The mother and caregivers should receive training and demonstrate competency in the following activities: determining urine/stool frequency, umbilical cord and skin care, identification of common signs and symptoms of illness, specific instructions concerning jaundice, specific instructions regarding sleeping patterns and positions, instructions on thermometer use, and instruction regarding responses to an emergency. Much of the morbidity is preventable using low cost and low technology interventions, which should become a priority for pediatricians and neonatologists everywhere.

REFERENCES

1. Davidoff MJ, Dias T, Damus K, et al. Changes in the gestational age distribution among U.S. singleton births: impact on rates of late preterm birth, 1992 to 2002. Semin Perinatol 2006;30:8–15.
2. Escobar GJ, Greene JD, Hulac P, et al. Rehospitalisation after birth hospitalisation: patterns among infants of all gestations. Arch Dis Child 2005;90:125–31.
3. Roth-Kleiner M, Wagner BP, Bachmann D, et al. Respiratory distress syndrome in near-term babies after caesarean section. Swiss Med Wkly 2003;133:283–8.
4. Ventolini G, Neiger R, Mathews L, et al. Incidence of respiratory disorders in neonates born between 34 and 36 weeks of gestation following exposure to antenatal corticosteroids between 24 and 34 weeks of gestation. Am J Perinatol 2008; 25:79–83.
5. Wang ML, Dorer DJ, Fleming MP, et al. Clinical outcomes of near-term infants. Pediatrics 2004;114:372–6.
6. Young PC, Glasgow TS, Li X, et al. Mortality of late-preterm (near-term) newborns in Utah. Pediatrics 2007;119:e659–65.
7. Raju TN. The problem of late-preterm (near-term) births: a workshop summary. Pediatric research 2006;60:775–6.
8. Martin JA, Hamilton BE, Sutton PD, et al. Births: Final data for 2006. In: National vital statistics reports; vol 57 no 7. Hyattsville (MD): National Center for Health Statistics; 2009. p. 1–102.
9. Institute of Medicine Committee on Understanding Premature Birth and Assuring Healthy Outcomes. Preterm birth: causes, consequences, and prevention. In: Behrman RE, Butler AS, editors. Summary, 1st edition. Washington DC: National Acamedies Press; 2007. p. 1–30.
10. Bettegowda VR, Dias T, Davidoff MJ, et al. The relationship between cesarean delivery and gestational age among US singleton births. Clin Perinatol 2008;35:309–23.

11. Ramachandrappa A, Jain L. Elective cesarean section: its impact on neonatal respiratory outcome. Clin Perinatol 2008;35:373–93.
12. Raju TN, Higgins RD, Stark AR, et al. Optimizing care and outcome for late-preterm (near-term) infants: a summary of the workshop sponsored by the National Institute of Child Health and Human Development. Pediatrics 2006; 118:1207–14.
13. Declercq E, Sakala C, Corry M, et al. Listening to mothers II: the second national U.S. survey of women's childbearing experiences. In: New York: Childbirth Connection; 2006. p. 1–9.
14. McCourt C, Weaver J, Statham H, et al. Elective cesarean section and decision making: a critical review of the literature. Birth 2007;34:65–79.
15. Engle WA, Kominiarek MA. Late preterm infants, early term infants, and timing of elective deliveries. Clin Perinatol 2008;35:325–41.
16. Raju TN. Epidemiology of late preterm (near-term) births. Clin Perinatol 2006;33: 751–63.
17. Centers for Disease Control and Prevention, American Society for Reproductive Medicine, Society for Assisted Reproductive Technology. 2005 assisted reproductive technology success rates: National Summary and Fertility Clinic reports. Atlanta: Centers for Disease Control and Prevention; 2007. p. 1–574.
18. Engle WA, Tomashek KM, Wallman C. "Late-preterm" infants: a population at risk. Pediatrics 2007;120:1390–401.
19. Escobar GJ, Clark RH, Greene JD. Short-term outcomes of infants born at 35 and 36 weeks gestation: we need to ask more questions. Semin Perinatol 2006;30: 28–33.
20. Jain L, Eaton DC. Physiology of fetal lung fluid clearance and the effect of labor. Semin Perinatol 2006;30:34–43.
21. Dudell GG, Jain L. Hypoxic respiratory failure in the late preterm infant. Clin Perinatol 2006;33:803–30.
22. Heritage CK, Cunningham MD. Association of elective repeat cesarean delivery and persistent pulmonary hypertension of the newborn. Am J Obstet Gynecol 1985;152:627–9.
23. Jain L. Respiratory morbidity in late-preterm infants: prevention is better than cure! Am J Perinatol 2008;25:75–8.
24. Tita AT, Landon MB, Spong CY, et al. Timing of elective repeat cesarean delivery at term and neonatal outcomes. N Engl J Med 2009;360:111–20.
25. Vachharajani AJ, Dawson JG. Short-term outcomes of late preterms: an institutional experience. Clin Pediatr (Phila) 2009;48(4):383–8.
26. Gilbert WM, Nesbitt TS, Danielsen B. The cost of prematurity: quantification by gestational age and birth weight. Obstet Gynecol 2003;102:488–92.
27. Khashu M, Narayanan M, Bhargava S, et al. Perinatal outcomes associated with preterm birth at 33 to 36 weeks' gestation: a population-based cohort study. Pediatrics 2009;123:109–13.
28. McIntire DD, Leveno KJ. Neonatal mortality and morbidity rates in late preterm births compared with births at term. Obstet Gynecol 2008;111:35–41.
29. Morrison JJ, Rennie JM, Milton PJ. Neonatal respiratory morbidity and mode of delivery at term: influence of timing of elective caesarean section. Br J Obstet Gynaecol 1995;102:101–6.
30. Hansen AK, Wisborg K, Uldbjerg N, et al. Risk of respiratory morbidity in term infants delivered by elective caesarean section: cohort study. BMJ 2008;336: 85–7.

31. Keszler M, Carbone MT, Cox C, et al. Severe respiratory failure after elective repeat cesarean delivery: a potentially preventable condition leading to extracorporeal membrane oxygenation. Pediatrics 1992;89:670–2.
32. Bhutani VK, Johnson L. Kernicterus in late preterm infants cared for as term healthy infants. Semin Perinatol 2006;30:89–97.
33. Newman TB, Escobar GJ, Gonzales VM, et al. Frequency of neonatal bilirubin testing and hyperbilirubinemia in a large health maintenance organization. Pediatrics 1999;104:1198–203.
34. Maisels MJ, Kring E. Length of stay, jaundice, and hospital readmission. Pediatrics 1998;101:995.
35. Sarici SU, Serdar MA, Korkmaz A, et al. Incidence, course, and prediction of hyperbilirubinemia in near-term and term newborns. Pediatrics 2004;113:775–80.
36. Sedin G. The thermal environment of the newborn infant. In: Martin JA, Fanaroff AA, Walsh MC, editors. Fanaroff and Martin's neonatal-perinatal medicine: diseases of the fetus and infant, volume 1. 8th edition. Philadelphia: Mosby; 2006. p. 585–97.
37. Power GG, Blood AB, Hunter CJ. Perinatal thermal physiology. In: Polin RA, Fox WW, Abman SH, editors. Fetal and neonatal physiology, vol. 1. 3rd edition. Philadelphia: Saunders; 2003. p. 541–7.
38. Garg M, Devaskar SU. Glucose metabolism in the late preterm infant. Clin Perinatol 2006;33:853–70.
39. Kramer MS, Demissie K, Yang H, et al. The contribution of mild and moderate preterm birth to infant mortality. Fetal and Infant Health Study Group of the Canadian Perinatal Surveillance System. JAMA 2000;284:843.
40. Kinney HC. The near-term (late preterm) human brain and risk for periventricular leukomalacia: a review. Semin Perinatol 2006;30:81–8.
41. Moster D, Lie RT, Markestad T. Long-term medical and social consequences of preterm birth. N Engl J Med 2008;359:262–73.
42. Chyi LJ, Lee HC, Hintz SR, et al. School outcomes of late preterm infants: special needs and challenges for infants born at 32 to 36 weeks gestation. J Pediatr 2008;153:25–31.
43. Jain L. The late preterm infant - clinical consensus. Atlanta: Emory University; 2007. p. 1–4.

Advances in the Diagnosis and Management of Persistent Pulmonary Hypertension of the Newborn

G. Ganesh Konduri, MD*, U. Olivia Kim, MD

KEYWORDS

- Pulmonary hypertension • Respiratory failure in the newborn
- Nitric oxide • Extracorporeal membrane oxygenation
- Outcomes of persistent pulmonary hypertension of the newborn

Persistence of pulmonary hypertension leading to respiratory failure in the neonate has been recognized for 40 years since its original description by Gersony and colleagues[1] in 1969. Fox and colleagues[2] reported suprasystemic pulmonary artery pressures and systemic desaturation in a group of neonates who had perinatal aspiration syndrome and absence of congenital heart disease (CHD) documented by cardiac catheterization. The hypoxemia in these neonates was attributable to right-to-left extrapulmonary shunting of blood across a patent foramen ovale (PFO) or patent ductus arteriosus (PDA).[1,2] The term originally used to describe this syndrome was *persistent fetal circulation*,[1] which was subsequently changed to *persistent pulmonary hypertension of the newborn* (PPHN) because it describes the pathophysiology more accurately.

PPHN occurs when the pulmonary vascular resistance (PVR) fails to decrease at birth. Affected neonates fail to establish adequate oxygenation during postnatal life and may develop multiorgan dysfunction. The condition usually presents at or shortly after birth. Although high pulmonary artery pressure and an oxygen tension of 20 to 30 mm Hg are normal during fetal life, they are poorly tolerated after birth. The severity of PPHN can run the full spectrum from mild and transient respiratory distress to severe

This article was supported by grant RO1 HL57268 from the National Heart, Lung, and Blood Institute and grants from the Advancing Healthier Wisconsin Foundation and Children's Research Institute of Wisconsin.

Division of Neonatology, Department of Pediatrics, Children's Research Institute and Medical College of Wisconsin, Milwaukee, WI 53226, USA

* Corresponding author.

E-mail address: gkonduri@mcw.edu (G.G. Konduri).

hypoxemia and cardiopulmonary instability requiring intensive care support. Prompt diagnosis and management, including a timely referral to a tertiary care center, can dramatically improve the chances of survival. Although mortality for PPHN was reported as 11% to 34% during 1980s,[3–5] current mortality is lower than 10% at most tertiary care centers.[6] Most cases of PPHN are associated with lung parenchymal disease, such as meconium aspiration syndrome (MAS) and respiratory distress syndrome (RDS); however, some present without known lung disease as primary PPHN. Some infants who have PPHN have lethal causes of respiratory failure, such as alveolar-capillary dysplasia (ACD),[7] genetic defects in surfactant synthesis,[8] or severe lung hypoplasia secondary to oligohydramnios or congenital anomalies.

VASCULAR BIOLOGY OF NORMAL TRANSITION

Translational biology studies in animal models have led to rapid advances in our understanding and management of PPHN. PPHN represents a failure of the unique adaptations that occur at birth in the pulmonary circulation. The fetal lung is a fluid-filled organ that does not participate in gas exchange and offers high resistance to blood flow.[9] Fetal lungs receive only 5% to 15% of the right ventricular output, with the remainder shunted across the PDA to the descending aorta and placental circulation.[10] Low oxygen tension present during fetal life and release of the endogenous vasoconstrictors endothelin-1 and thromboxane facilitate the maintenance of high PVR.[11] Fetal pulmonary circulation becomes more responsive to the vasodilator effect of oxygen with maturation, acquiring this response after 31 weeks of gestation in the human fetus and at a comparable time point in fetal sheep.[12,13] PVR undergoes a dramatic decrease as the lungs take over gas exchange function at birth. The decrease in PVR results in a 50% decrease in pulmonary artery pressure and a nearly 10-fold increase in pulmonary blood flow during the first few minutes of this transition.[10] The increase in pulmonary blood flow facilitates gas transport across the air-blood interface in the lung. The physiologic stimuli that initiate pulmonary vasodilation include the clearance of lung liquid, distention of air spaces, increase in oxygen tension, and shear stress from increased blood flow.[13–16] Oxygen is the most important stimulus for pulmonary vasodilation, although a decrease in $Paco_2$ and increase in pH also contribute to this response.[13] Together, these physiologic stimuli promote the release of several vasodilators, including endothelium-derived mediators, nitric oxide (NO), and vasodilator prostaglandins (PGs) **(Fig. 1)**.[16–19]

Endothelial nitric oxide synthase (eNOS) plays a critical role in the transition of pulmonary circulation by releasing NO. eNOS converts l-arginine to l-citrulline and NO in the presence of oxygen. Oxygen stimulates NO release directly[18] and indirectly by an increase in oxidative phosphorylation and release of ATP from oxygenated fetal red blood cells.[20,21] A maturational increase in the eNOS protein level at term gestation occurs[22] and is critical to this adaptation, because NO is not stored in the cell and its increased synthesis at birth requires high expression of the enzyme. NO initiates rapid vasodilation by stimulating soluble guanylate cyclase in the vascular smooth muscle cell, which, in turn, converts the nucleotide guanosine triphosphate to cyclic guanosine monophosphate (cGMP) (see **Fig. 1**). An increase in intracellular cGMP levels leads to a decrease in Ca^{2+} influx and relaxation of the vascular smooth muscle cell. Type 5 phosphodiesterase (PDE-5) in the vascular smooth muscle cell breaks down cGMP and limits the duration of vasodilation. In addition to the vasodilator effect, NO plays a major role in promoting the growth of blood vessels in the pulmonary circulation in utero in response to vascular endothelial growth factor (VEGF).[23] Loss of NO and inhibition of VEGF receptors in utero cause decreased growth of

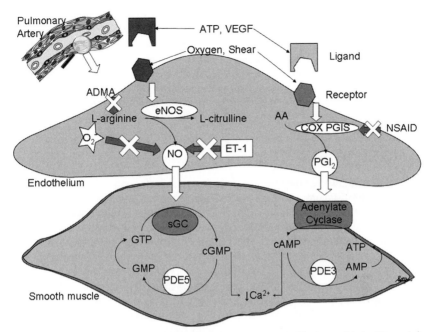

Fig. 1. Mechanism of endothelium-dependent pulmonary vasodilation at birth. NO and pros-tacyclin (PGI_2) are released in response to birth-related stimuli. NO and PGI_2 increase the cyclic guanosine monophosphate (cGMP) and cyclic adenosine monophosphate (cAMP) levels in the smooth muscle cell. Type 5 and type 3 phosphodiesterases (PDEs) degrade these cyclic nucleo-tides. A decrease in intracellular Ca^{2+} levels leads to relaxation of vascular smooth muscle. NO levels are decreased by asymmetric dimethyl arginine (ADMA), superoxide (O_2^-), and endo-thelin (ET-1). Nonsteroidal anti-inflammatory drugs (NSAIDs) inhibit cyclooxygenase (COX). AA, arachidonic acid; eNOS, endothelial nitric oxide synthase; GMP, guanosine monophos-phate; GTP, guanosine triphosphate; PGIS, PGI_2 synthase; sGC, soluble guanylate cyclase; VEGF, vascular endothelial growth factor. (*Adapted from* Berger S, Konduri GG. Pulmonary hypertension in children. Pediatr Clin North Am 2006;53:966; with permission).

pulmonary vessels and air spaces, suggesting a coordinated development of the vasculature and parenchyma during fetal life.[24] The intracellular cGMP levels in the smooth muscle can also be augmented by the natriuretic peptides, atrial natriuretic peptide (ANP) and B-type natriuretic peptide (BNP), which stimulate the particulate guanylate cyclase, an isoform of soluble guanylate cyclase. Although the role of ANP and BNP in the perinatal transition has not been delineated, they dilate pulmonary arteries in the newborn lung.[25] The natriuretic peptide-cGMP system may offer redun-dancy to the NO-cGMP system in the pulmonary circulation.

The PG system is also activated by birth-related stimuli in the fetal lung[26] and medi-ates pulmonary vasodilation in a complementary fashion to the NO-cGMP system (see **Fig. 1**). Prostacyclin (PGI_2) is the most potent of the vasodilator PGs and activates the enzyme adenylate cyclase in the vascular smooth muscle cell, which converts ATP to cyclic adenosine monophosphate (cAMP). An increase in intracellular cAMP also results in the relaxation of vascular smooth muscle cell by decreasing Ca^{2+} influx. Type 3 phosphodiesterase (PDE-3) breaks down cAMP and limits the duration of vasodilation. Therefore, pulmonary vasodilation can be achieved by increasing the levels of oxygen and arginine, which are substrates for eNOS, providing NO or PGI_2

or by inhibition of their corresponding cyclic nucleotide PDE-5 by sildenafil or PDE-3 by milrinone (see **Fig. 1**). Vascular smooth muscle cells in the pulmonary artery also show independent responses to oxygen and hypoxia by means of activation of specific potassium channels.[27,28] Despite decades of investigation, the fundamental mechanisms involved in the opposing effects of oxygen, hypoxia, and acidosis on the pulmonary and systemic vessels remain unknown. Understanding the nature of these differences in the basic physiology of pulmonary and systemic vessels may provide additional targeted therapies to decrease the pulmonary artery pressure in PPHN selectively.

ALTERED VASCULAR BIOLOGY IN PERSISTENT PULMONARY HYPERTENSION OF THE NEWBORN

Failure of postnatal vasodilation may result from inadequate oxygenation or lung expansion or from failure of NO or PG release at birth. Neonates who have MAS or RDS may present with reversible pulmonary hypertension attributable to a failure of alveolar expansion or oxygenation. Biochemical alterations in the NO-cGMP pathway reported in neonates who have PPHN include decreased expression of eNOS,[29] decreased availability of arginine,[30] and decreased NO production reflected by lower NO metabolites in the urine.[30] The fetal lamb model of PPHN shows a consistent decrease in eNOS expression in pulmonary arteries.[31,32] The naturally occurring arginine analogue asymmetric dimethyl arginine can induce competitive inhibition of eNOS and decrease NO production (see **Fig. 1**), as previously reported in animal models of PPHN[33] and in adult patients who have pulmonary hypertension.[34] An increase in endothelin-1 peptide levels in PPHN[35] can cause pulmonary hypertension by inhibition of eNOS and constriction of the vascular smooth muscle.[36] Superoxide, a free radical present in vascular cells, can scavenge NO and cause pulmonary vasoconstriction (see **Fig. 1**). Increased superoxide levels have been demonstrated in the pulmonary arteries obtained from fetal lambs that have PPHN.[37,38] A decrease in the expression of soluble guanylate cyclase, which leads to decreased availability of cGMP in the pulmonary artery smooth muscle, also occurs in this model.[39] In summary, one or several of the steps in NO-cGMP signaling may be altered and contribute to impaired pulmonary vasodilation in PPHN.

Inhibition of PG synthesis by prenatal exposure to nonsteroidal anti-inflammatory drugs (NSAIDs) that inhibit cyclooxygenase also increases the risk for PPHN.[40,41] PPHN occurs in these babies as a result of prenatal constriction of the PDA from maternal intake of NSAIDs.[42] Prenatal ductal constriction consistently reproduces the clinical and structural features of PPHN in fetal lambs.[43,44] Constriction of the PDA leads to sustained elevation of pulmonary artery pressure in utero[45] and persistence of right-to-left shunts after birth. Studies in this animal model have led to major advances in the understanding of altered vascular biology in PPHN. Pulmonary arteries in this PPHN model show decreased NO release and increased levels of the reactive oxygen species superoxide, hydrogen peroxide, and peroxynitrite.[31,32,37,38] Scavengers of superoxide improve the vasodilation and oxygenation in lambs that have PPHN.[46] Recent studies demonstrated that in utero pulmonary hypertension from ductal constriction leads to impaired development of pulmonary vasculature and alveoli.[47] These data suggest that pressure elevation at a critical phase in lung development leads to structural alterations in the fetal lung.

INCIDENCE

PPHN primarily affects full-term and near-term neonates, although some premature neonates at less than 32 weeks of gestation show echocardiographic evidence of

PPHN.[48] The incidence of PPHN in term and near-term newborns is estimated to be 2 per 1000 live births, based on an observational study by Walsh Sukys and colleagues[49] that included neonatal intensive care units (NICUs) at 12 large academic centers from 1993 to 1994. This study and subsequent large multicenter trials of inhaled nitric oxide (iNO) have demonstrated that MAS is the most common underlying diagnosis of PPHN, followed by primary PPHN (**Fig. 2**). Other diagnoses include RDS, pneumonia or sepsis, pulmonary vasoconstriction from asphyxia, and pulmonary hypoplasia secondary to congenital diaphragmatic hernia (CDH) or oligohydramnios. The incidence of lung diseases associated with PPHN has changed over the past 8 years. The overall incidence of MAS has declined, coinciding with a decrease in the number of postterm pregnancies.[50] In contrast, RDS in preterm neonates delivered by elective or indicated Cesarean section at 34 to 37 weeks of gestation has become a more frequent cause of PPHN. Yoder and colleagues[50] compared the incidence of MAS over two periods: 1990 to 1992 and 1997 to 1998. The incidence of MAS declined by fourfold from 5.8% to 1.5% of all the meconium-stained infants in the second period. These researchers attribute this to a 33% reduction in the number of deliveries at greater than 41 weeks of gestation. They observed a reciprocal 33% increase in deliveries at 38 to 39 weeks of gestation and an increase in deliveries at 34 to 36 weeks of gestation over the same period.[51] The median age at delivery decreased from 40 to 39 weeks of gestation.[51] These recent secular trends should be factored into the changing demographics of neonates who have PPHN, with important implications for their management and long-term outcome. The incidence of lung diseases associated with PPHN from a multicenter trial of early iNO therapy[6] is shown in **Fig. 2**.

MECONIUM ASPIRATION SYNDROME

Although meconium staining of amniotic fluid occurs in 10% to 15% of pregnancies, MAS occurs infrequently, in up to 5% of neonates born through meconium-stained fluid. As noted previously, the incidence of MAS among meconium-stained neonates has declined in recent years[50] with the decline in postterm pregnancies. This observation suggests that MAS is often a result of in utero stress with aspiration of meconium

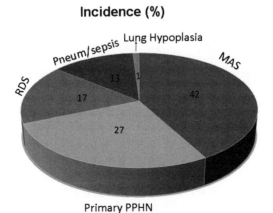

Fig. 2. Lung diseases associated with PPHN in 299 neonates enrolled in the early iNO study in term and near-term neonates.[6] MAS was the most frequent diagnosis, followed by primary PPHN, RDS, and pneumonia (Pneum) or sepsis. Infants who had congenital diaphragmatic hernia were excluded from this study.

by a compromised fetus. Meconium can cause respiratory failure from several mechanisms. Meconium causes mechanical obstruction to the airways, particularly during exhalation, resulting in air trapping, hyperinflation, and increased risk for pneumothorax. Meconium components also inactivate surfactant,[52] incite an inflammatory response with release of cytokines, and increase the production of the vasoconstrictors endothelin and thromboxane.[53] MAS can result in PPHN by the same mechanisms that were described previously. Recent advances in the management of PPHN has resulted in an excellent outcome for neonates who have MAS.[54]

PRIMARY PERSISTENT PULMONARY HYPERTENSION OF THE NEWBORN

Neonates with primary PPHN usually have hypoxemia in the absence of a recognizable parenchymal lung disease. The cause of primary PPHN remains elusive; however, prenatal constriction of the ductus arteriosus has been identified as an important contributor. Association of PPHN with maternal intake of NSAIDs has been recognized in case reports since 1970s.[40,41] In a controlled prospective study, NSAIDs were detected by meconium drug analysis in 88% of babies who had PPHN and were delivered in an urban population, indicating prenatal exposure.[42] The concentration of NSAIDs in the meconium correlated with the incidence and severity of PPHN in this study. A strong causal association is also suggested by the consistent reproduction of hemodynamic and structural features of PPHN by fetal ductal constriction.[43,44] Recently, an epidemiologic study suggested an increased incidence of PPHN with prenatal exposure to selective serotonin reuptake inhibitors (SSRIs) during the third trimester of pregnancy.[55] Another study[56] that compared the incidence of PPHN among mothers exposed to SSRIs during the third trimester and control mothers without exposure found no such association (incidence among SSRI-exposed mothers of 2.14 per 1000 and incidence among control mothers of 2.72 per 1000), however. There are methodologic differences between the two studies that may account for these different study findings. Larger population-based studies are needed to define the risk for SSRI exposure in causing PPHN. The potential mechanism of the effect of SSRIs on the fetal pulmonary circulation also requires further investigation. For NSAID and SSRIs, some control babies with prenatal exposure did not develop PPHN, suggesting that a biologic susceptibility to these drugs plays a role in the pathogenesis. Some neonates delivered through meconium-stained amniotic fluid develop PPHN without radiographic evidence of MAS. This observation suggests that the intrauterine stress leading to meconium passage in utero also may result in PPHN; however, the nature of this stress is unknown.

PNEUMONIA AND SEPSIS

PPHN can be a complication of pneumonia or sepsis secondary to common neonatal pathogens, group B *Streptococcus*, and gram-negative organisms.[57] Bacterial endotoxin causes pulmonary hypertension from several mechanisms, including the release of thromboxane, endothelin, and several cytokines (eg, tumor necrosis factor-α).[58,59] Sepsis also leads to systemic hypotension from activation of inducible NOS with excess NO release in the systemic vascular beds, impaired myocardial function, and multiorgan failure. Addressing pulmonary hypertension should be a component of the overall management of septic shock and prevention of multiorgan failure in the affected neonates.

RESPIRATORY DISTRESS SYNDROME

PPHN can occur as a complication of RDS in near-term premature neonates, often in those delivered by elective or indicated Cesarean section at 34 to 37 weeks of gestation.[60] The increasing reactivity of pulmonary arteries at this gestation period predisposes these neonates to pulmonary hypertension when gas exchange is impaired because of surfactant deficiency.

PULMONARY HYPOPLASIA

CDH and oligohydramnios secondary to renal anomalies or premature rupture of membranes leads to pulmonary hypoplasia. Pulmonary hypertension often occurs as a complication because of the decreased number of blood vessels and increased reactivity of the vessels in the hypoplastic lungs. PPHN is usually more chronic and less responsive to vasodilator therapy in these babies. The outcome of these babies is related to the degree of lung hypoplasia, associated anomalies, and duration of pulmonary hypertension.[61] The outcome for neonates who have CDH has improved since gentle ventilation and permissive hypercapnia have been incorporated into the management, with many centers reporting 75% survival in recent years.[61,62]

LETHAL CAUSES OF PERSISTENT PULMONARY HYPERTENSION OF THE NEWBORN

ACD can present at birth or several days after birth with progressive cyanosis and severe pulmonary hypertension.[7,63] The diagnosis is made by lung biopsy or postmortem lung sections that show characteristic features of an abnormal air-blood interface with increased distance between the alveolar epithelium and capillaries.[64] Misalignment of pulmonary veins also occurs because they appear next to the bronchus and pulmonary artery in a bronchovascular bundle instead of in their usual location in the interlobular septum. Recurrence of ACD in some families, sometimes by autosomal recessive inheritance, has been reported.[7,63] In some case series, 50% of neonates who have ACD have associated renal, gastrointestinal, and cardiac anomalies.[63]

PPHN was also reported in association with respiratory failure in term neonates caused by inherited defects in surfactant components. Mutations in the surfactant protein B (SP-B) gene that lead to defective synthesis or processing can cause severe respiratory failure and PPHN.[65] Originally referred to as congenital alveolar proteinosis, the most common defect in SP-B synthesis is attributable to a mutation in codon 121 of the SP-B gene.[65] These neonates present with signs of hyaline membrane disease that shows only short-term improvement with surfactant replacement therapy. The outcome is poor despite support with surfactant, iNO, and extracorporeal membrane oxygenation (ECMO). Lung transplantation is offered by some centers for the affected infants. Diagnosis is usually made in suspected infants by blood DNA analysis for the common mutations.[65] A related series of neonates with fatal respiratory failure attributable to ATP-binding cassette protein member A3 deficiency, an inborn error in surfactant synthesis, has also been reported.[66] The affected neonates can develop severe PPHN unresponsive to iNO.[8]

DIAGNOSIS OF PERSISTENT PULMONARY HYPERTENSION OF THE NEWBORN

A term or late-preterm newborn with symptoms of respiratory distress shortly after delivery may have a variety of pulmonary diseases as described previously or simply a delayed transition to extrauterine life. If the newborn has respiratory distress complicated by labile oxygenation and hypoxemia out of proportion to the degree of lung disease, however, PPHN should be suspected. Physical examination of a neonates who has PPHN usually reveals tachypnea, retractions, grunting, and cyanosis. Abnormal cardiac sounds, such as a systolic murmur of tricuspid regurgitation or a prominent S_2, may be heard; however, these are not diagnostic for PPHN. Many of these clinical signs are also found in neonates with cyanotic CHD, and differentiation between lung disease, PPHN, and cyanotic CHD can be difficult.

A systematic approach to the hypoxemic neonates with serial interventions and tests is needed for a timely and accurate diagnosis of PPHN. The initial studies obtained in symptomatic neonates are a chest radiograph (CXR) and arterial blood gas analysis. The CXR can be normal in primary PPHN, because most affected neonates have minimal or no parenchymal lung disease (**Fig. 3**A). It is more common for PPHN to be secondary to parenchymal lung disease that is evident on the CXR, however. Apparent lung disease on the CXR does not rule out a cardiac defect, as shown in the example in **Fig. 3**B. The CXR in **Fig. 3**B was obtained in a preterm neonate (36 weeks of gestation) who presented with signs of RDS and had a poor response to surfactant therapy and a transient improvement in Po_2 with iNO therapy. After the neonate was transferred to the authors' center for evaluation of severe PPHN, an echocardiogram revealed total anomalous infradiaphragmatic pulmonary venous return to inferior vena cava. An atypical course with a poor response to surfactant therapy and hypoxemia that is out of proportion to a ventilation problem should lead the clinician to suspect cyanotic heart disease or severe PPHN. Response to supplemental oxygen has been used traditionally to differentiate lung disease from CHD. Oxygen is a potent and selective pulmonary vasodilator. A Pao_2 increase greater than 20 mm Hg or a saturation increase greater than 10% in response to oxygen suggests that hypoxemia is secondary to lung disease or mild PPHN. Higher preductal Pao_2 and oxygen saturation compared with postductal location indicates the presence of a right-to-left shunt at the PDA, which occurs in approximately half of the babies who have PPHN.[67] Ductal-dependent left-sided cardiac defects are also associated with a right-to-left shunt at the PDA and lower postductal oxygen saturation, however. The response to iNO may help to differentiate PPHN from cyanotic CHD. Most neonates who have PPHN respond rapidly to iNO, with an increase in Pao_2 and oxygen saturations. Some neonates who have severe PPHN and infants who have cyanotic

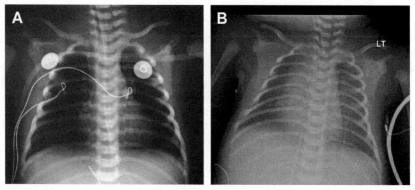

Fig. 3. (*A*) CXR on the left obtained in a neonate who had primary PPHN shows absence of parenchymal lung disease. (*B*) CXR on the right was obtained in a neonate who was suspected of having RDS and did not improve with surfactant therapy. Echocardiography demonstrated total anomalous pulmonary venous return to the inferior vena cava.

CHD may experience a small or no increase in oxygenation with iNO, however. It is important to recognize that the use of high oxygen concentrations or pulmonary vaso-dilator therapy can adversely affect systemic perfusion in a neonate who has ductal-dependent left-sided CHD, such as coarctation of the aorta or hypoplastic left heart syndrome. An echocardiogram is therefore needed to make an accurate diagnosis and initiate PG therapy for ductal-dependent CHD. Echocardiography can also document the presence of right-to-left or bidirectional shunts at the level of the PDA or PFO and estimate the pulmonary artery pressure from Doppler velocity measurement of the tricuspid regurgitation jet.

MANAGEMENT OF PERSISTENT PULMONARY HYPERTENSION OF THE NEWBORN

Neonates who have PPHN require supportive care tailored to the degree of hypoxemia and physiologic instability. The overall approach should focus on restoring the cardio-pulmonary adaptation while avoiding lung injury and adverse effects on systemic perfusion. Prolonged exposure to 100% oxygen and aggressive ventilation can be avoided by judicious application of newer therapies, such as iNO, surfactant replacement, and inotropic support. The traditional practice of targeting a high Po_2 (>100 mm Hg) and low Pco_2 to achieve pulmonary vasodilation has not been shown to improve outcome and is potentially harmful to the developing lung and cerebral perfusion. Although achieving a normal Pao_2 of 60 to 90 mm Hg is important for the postnatal adaptation, there is no evidence that a Pao_2 greater than 100 mm Hg causes a greater reduction in PVR.

Because PPHN is often associated with parenchymal lung disease or systemic illness, therapy should target the underlying disease. Neonates with mild and transient respiratory distress may respond well to supplemental oxygen alone or the use of nasal continuous positive airway pressure. Neonates with moderate respiratory distress and hypoxemia may need ventilator support and monitoring of blood gases. Management of moderate to severe PPHN requires a comprehensive approach to optimize cardiac function and achieve uniform lung expansion and pulmonary vasodi-lation. It is important to recognize that the heart and lungs are connected, are interdependent, and function as an integrated system while undergoing critical adaptation at birth. Reversal of right-to-left extrapulmonary shunts requires a reduction in pulmonary artery pressure and maintaining the systemic blood pressure. Sedation may be necessary to provide comfort and decrease oxygen consumption from agitation in hypoxemic neonates. Finally, neonates who fail to respond to optimum medical management may require ECMO. These supportive measures are discussed in sequence with the evidence presented when available to favor each approach for a critically ill neonate who has PPHN.

OPTIMUM LUNG EXPANSION

Mechanical ventilation facilitates alveolar recruitment and lung expansion, potentially improving the ventilation/perfusion (VQ) match. The ventilator strategy should target recruitment of the atelectatic segments while avoiding overdistention, which leads to lung injury and increased resistance to pulmonary blood flow. The application of surfactant therapy facilitates alveolar expansion in parenchymal lung disease. Surfactant therapy has been shown to decrease the need for ECMO in full-term neonates with severe respiratory failure.[68] The beneficial effect of surfactant was seen particularly in babies who had MAS and sepsis.[68] The use of surfactant in PPHN has increased over recent years, with nearly 80% of neonates with moderate to severe respiratory failure currently receiving this therapy.[6,69] High-frequency oscillation (HFO) may help to optimize lung expansion in neonates who have PPHN secondary to lung disease. Kinsella and colleagues[70] reported that HFO improves the oxygenation response to iNO when used in babies who have MAS and RDS.

USE OF SEDATIVES AND SKELETAL MUSCLE RELAXATION

Although widely used to minimize fluctuations in oxygenation and facilitate ventilation, these approaches have not been tested in randomized trials. These drugs have significant adverse effects and commonly induce hypotension, generalized edema, and deterioration of lung function with prolonged use. Hypotension is more common when a combination of sedatives and muscle relaxants is used. The use of skeletal muscle relaxation has been linked to an increased incidence of hearing impairment in survivors of PPHN; however, the mechanism of this association is unclear.[71] Diuretics, often used to treat edema secondary to skeletal muscle relaxation, also increase the risk for hearing loss.[72] Although sedation may be needed for comfort in ventilated neonates, the authors do not recommend the routine use of skeletal muscle relaxation and limit its use when necessary to less than 48 hours. Pulmonary vasodilation with iNO can ameliorate the fluctuations in pulmonary artery pressure and oxygenation, and its safety has been demonstrated in randomized trials as described elsewhere in this article.

HYPERVENTILATION AND ALKALOSIS

These therapies were widely used in the management of PPHN before the introduction of iNO. Studies in animal models and limited studies in babies who had PPHN demonstrated that low $Paco_2$ and an increase in pH cause pulmonary vasodilation.[73–75] These studies demonstrated only short-term improvements in pulmonary hypertension and oxygenation, however. The effect of hyperventilation on the pulmonary circulation seems to be primarily related to its effect on increasing pH.[75] Hypocarbia and alkalosis decrease cerebral perfusion and have been associated with hearing loss and neurologic injury in the follow-up studies of infants who survived PPHN.[76,77] They induce hypocalcemia, myocardial dysfunction, and systemic hypotension. Alkalosis also decreases the unloading of oxygen from hemoglobin (Hb), which can potentially decrease oxygen delivery to the tissues. Use of high tidal volumes to induce hypocarbia also leads to lung injury and can prolong the hospital stay for these neonates. The development of new and specific pulmonary vasodilators has led to the decreased use of these therapies. Although correction of respiratory and metabolic acidosis facilitates pulmonary vasodilation, the authors do not advocate the use of hypocarbia and metabolic alkalosis in neonates who have PPHN.

CARDIOTONIC THERAPY

Dopamine, dobutamine, and epinephrine have been widely used in the management of PPHN, primarily to optimize cardiac function, stabilize systemic blood pressure, and reduce right-to-left shunting. Recently, norepinephrine has been shown to increase systemic pressure and oxygenation in neonates who have PPHN.[78] An increase in systemic pressure, however, may not reflect an improvement in cardiac output. The use of vasopressor support should be considered one component of an overall approach to PPHN.

INHALED NITRIC OXIDE THERAPY

The introduction of iNO therapy has been the most significant milestone in the era of vasodilator therapy for PPHN. Development of this approach for PPHN is a remarkable example of the bench-to-bedside translational biology research done by several investigators. A short time after the discovery of NO as the endogenous vasodilator released by blood vessels, iNO was shown to cause selective pulmonary vasodilation at doses less than 100 ppm in a sheep model of pulmonary hypertension.[79] NO gas given by inhalation reaches the alveolar space and diffuses to the vascular smooth muscle of the adjacent pulmonary artery from the abluminal side (**Fig. 4**). iNO causes vasodilation by increasing the intracellular cGMP levels in the smooth muscle. As NO continues to diffuse into the lumen of the pulmonary artery, it is rapidly bound and inactivated by Hb, limiting its effect to the pulmonary circulation. iNO is also preferentially distributed to the ventilated segments of the lung, resulting in increased perfusion of the ventilated segments, optimizing VQ match (see **Fig. 4**). The effect of iNO on pulmonary circulation is not limited by the presence of extrapulmonary right-to-left shunts, which often result in hypotension with intravenously given vasodilators. These properties make iNO the ideal pulmonary vasodilator in neonatal respiratory failure. Recent studies have demonstrated that NO levels in the nasal cavity of premature infants can reach 50 to 100 parts per billion.[80,81] Significant exhaled NO concentrations are measured in these neonates, suggesting that inhalation of NO occurs physiologically during tidal respiration.[80] Pilot studies in neonates who had PPHN reported a rapid and sustained improvement in oxygenation with iNO.[82,83] The improvement in oxygenation is usually evident within a few minutes of starting iNO, which facilitates the rapid stabilization of a severely hypoxic and compromised neonate. Several large randomized clinical trials demonstrated that iNO therapy decreases the need for ECMO in addition to mortality in full-term and near-term neonates with hypoxic respiratory failure and pulmonary hypertension.[67,84–87] iNO improves oxygenation in 70% or more of neonates who have PPHN, with the best responses observed in idiopathic PPHN.[6,67,86] iNO therapy has been approved for clinical use in term and near-term newborns (>34 weeks of gestation) with hypoxic respiratory failure since 2000 by the US Food and Drug Administration (FDA).[88]

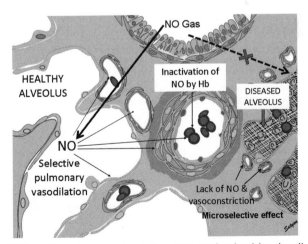

Fig. 4. Effect of iNO on the pulmonary circulation. iNO reaches healthy alveoli, shown on the left, and diffuses to the adjacent pulmonary arteries to cause vasodilation. As NO reaches the lumen of the pulmonary artery, it is inactivated by Hb, limiting its effect to the pulmonary circulation. NO does not reach the atelectatic alveoli, shown on the right, maintaining constriction of the adjacent pulmonary arteries. Increased perfusion of the ventilated segments of the lung improves the VQ match and oxygenation in parenchymal lung disease.

Previous clinical trials suggested that the ideal starting dose for iNO is 20 ppm, with the effective dose being between 5 and 20 ppm.[6] Doses greater than 20 ppm did not increase efficacy and were associated with more adverse effects in these neonates.[67,89] The timing of initiation of iNO therapy is an important consideration in the management of PPHN. Based on a review of the previous clinical trials (**Fig. 5**), the authors recommend initiation of iNO therapy when the respiratory failure progresses and oxygenation index (OI) reaches 20 on at least two blood gases. The severity of respiratory failure, as assessed by the OI, differed widely at the time of initiation of iNO in these six trials. The ECMO rates observed for iNO-treated neonates in these trials correlate well with the OI at the time of initiation of iNO and range from 40%[84] to 11%.[6] The optimum time for initiation of iNO is before the neonate develops severe respiratory failure secondary to progression of lung disease or lung injury. The randomized controlled studies of iNO also demonstrated the short-term and long-term safety of this therapy in infants who have PPHN. iNO therapy can lead to three potential adverse events: methemoglobinemia generated by oxidation of Hb by NO, exposure to nitrogen dioxide generated by reaction of NO and oxygen, and inhibition of platelet aggregation by NO. Previous iNO trials reported low methemoglobin levels and no significant exposure to nitrogen dioxide when doses less than 20 ppm were used. Davidson and colleagues[89] reported that at doses of 80 ppm, the average methemoglobin levels peak at greater than 5%, with up to a third of neonates having levels greater than 7%. Significant levels of nitrogen dioxide were also measured at the 80-ppm dose.[89] Although altered platelet function is a potential complication, Christou and colleagues[90] found no difference in platelet activation by ADP in neonates receiving 40 ppm of iNO and a placebo group.

Exposure to iNO even for a brief period can sensitize the pulmonary circulation to rebound vasoconstriction during discontinuation of iNO therapy. A significant decrease in Pao_2 during withdrawal of iNO can be avoided by weaning the dose gradually in steps from 20 ppm to the lowest dose possible (0.5–1 ppm) for a period before its discontinuation.[91] Even in babies who show no response to iNO, sudden discontinuation can precipitate pulmonary vasoconstriction and rapid deterioration.[92] When iNO therapy is used in centers that do not provide ECMO, it should be continued during transport of the neonate to a center that does provide ECMO.[88] Centers that do not provide ECMO should establish treatment failure criteria for iNO in

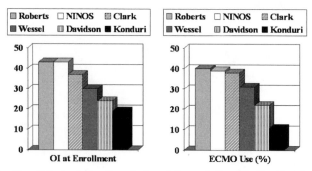

Fig. 5. Relationship of the severity of respiratory failure, defined by the OI at the time of initiation of iNO therapy, to the ECMO rates observed in these neonates. Data are from six randomized trials in term or near-term neonates for babies assigned to the iNO arm in these trials.[6,67,84,86,87,89] The trials are labeled by the name of the first investigator and are shown in the order of highest to lowest OI. NINOS, Neonatal Inhaled Nitric Oxide Study Group. The ECMO rate correlates with the severity of respiratory failure at the time of iNO initiation.

collaboration with the nearest center that does provide ECMO so that transfer of an ill infant is not delayed while waiting for a response to iNO.

Based on the efficacy and safety of iNO from controlled clinical trials, the authors recommend using this therapy before prolonged exposure to a high fraction of inspired oxygen (FIO_2) or to maximal ventilator support. Exposure to 100% oxygen even for a brief period can induce vascular dysfunction, increase oxidative stress, and impair the subsequent response to iNO.[93] iNO facilitates rapid weaning of FIO_2 and decreases oxidative stress from oxygen in an animal model of PPHN.[46]

ALTERNATIVES TO INHALED NITRIC OXIDE THERAPY IN PERSISTENT PULMONARY HYPERTENSION OF THE NEWBORN

iNO therapy has not been as effective in babies who have CDH, despite clinical and echocardiographic evidence of PPHN in most of these neonates.[94] iNO does not reduce the mortality or the ECMO rate in babies who have CDH.[94] In addition, nearly 30% of neonates who have PPHN did not show an improvement in oxygenation in randomized trials of iNO.[6,67] As shown in **Fig. 1**, inhibition of PDE-5 by sildenafil to preserve cGMP, activation of cAMP by PGI_2, and PDE-3 inhibition by milrinone offer additional tools to achieve pulmonary vasodilation. To date, these therapies have been tested in limited clinical trials in patients who did not respond to iNO or when iNO was not available. After the introduction of sildenafil for erectile dysfunction, it was tested in adults with pulmonary hypertension, because the pulmonary circulation has a high expression of PDE-5. The initial promising results led to randomized clinical trials that demonstrated the efficacy and relative safety of oral sildenafil in adult primary pulmonary hypertension. Studies in the fetal lamb model of PPHN demonstrated increased expression of PDE-5 in pulmonary arteries, which contributes to impaired vasodilation.[95] Sildenafil has been shown to decrease pulmonary artery pressure and prevent rebound pulmonary hypertension after iNO withdrawal during the postoperative period, after repair of congenital heart defects.[96] A randomized placebo-controlled trial of oral sildenafil in PPHN was halted early after five of six neonates in the placebo group died compared with one of seven neonates in the sildenafil group.[97] A significant improvement in oxygenation occurred in the sildenafil-treated neonates 6 to 12 hours after the first dose. Systemic hypotension was not observed in these studies with oral sildenafil. These data suggest a beneficial effect of oral sildenafil used as primary therapy for PPHN when iNO is not available. Intravenous sildenafil, which is currently not available for clinical use, has been reported to cause systemic hypotension.[98] The authors currently use oral sildenafil for PPHN in iNO nonresponders. An alternative to sildenafil is inhaled PGI_2, which can be used in conjunction with iNO therapy. The effects of inhaled PGI_2 can be complementary to those of iNO because they stimulate different cyclic nucleotides. Kelly and colleagues[99] demonstrated an additive effect of inhaled PGI_2 given with iNO in four neonates who had severe PPHN unresponsive to iNO therapy alone. Although inhaled PGI_2 requires continuous administration because of its short half-life, a more stable analogue, iloprost, can be given by intermittent nebulization. Although no clinical trials have been reported with inhaled iloprost in neonates, the authors' preliminary experience suggests an effect similar to that of inhaled PGI_2 in neonates who have CDH. The PDE-3 inhibitor milrinone ameliorates postoperative pulmonary hypertension and improves cardiac function after surgical repair of CHD.[100] Milrinone infusion has been tested as a pulmonary vasodilator in PPHN in uncontrolled studies. Bassler and colleagues[101] and McNamara and colleagues[102] reported an increase in PaO_2 and decrease in OI in response to milrinone infusion in neonates who have PPHN and are unresponsive to iNO. Whether the improvement is related to milrinone or to gradual resolution of underlying disease can only be determined by a randomized trial. The effect of milrinone on cAMP may be additive to inhaled PGI_2 and complementary to iNO therapy to amplify the vasodilation.

EXTRACORPOREAL MEMBRANE OXYGENATION

ECMO was introduced as a rescue therapy to support neonates in severe respiratory failure with greater than 80% predicted mortality during the 1970s by Bartlett and colleagues.[103] ECMO has significantly improved the survival of neonates with severe but reversible lung disease.[104,105] ECMO provides respiratory and cardiac support to facilitate the occurrence of postnatal adaptation while allowing the lungs to recover from barotrauma and oxygen toxicity. ECMO requires cannulation of the right carotid artery and jugular vein for venoarterial bypass or cannulation of the jugular vein alone for venovenous bypass, however. The infants on ECMO support also require anticoagulation with heparin to prevent clotting in the bypass circuit. In view of their vulnerability to intraventricular hemorrhage, ECMO is generally not used in premature neonates aged less than 34 weeks of gestation in most centers. Despite the obvious concerns about ligation of the carotid artery or jugular vein during cannulation, ECMO support did not have an adverse impact on the outcome of neonates who had PPHN. The 1-year outcomes for babies in severe respiratory failure treated with ECMO are comparable to those of infants who survived without ECMO support.[104] The increasing application of newer therapies, such as iNO, HFO, and surfactant, over the past 10 years has greatly reduced the need for ECMO in babies who have PPHN secondary to parenchymal lung disease or primary PPHN.[69,106] Currently, fewer than 5% of neonates who have PPHN at the authors' center receive ECMO. Most of the neonates who require ECMO support at the authors' center for PPHN have CDH with pulmonary hypoplasia as the underlying diagnosis.

PULMONARY HYPERTENSION IN PREMATURE INFANTS

PPHN has been demonstrated by echocardiography in some premature newborns aged less than 30 weeks of gestation with hypoxemia unresponsive to surfactant therapy.[48] Prolonged rupture of membranes, pulmonary hypoplasia, and intrauterine growth retardation have been identified as risk factors for hypoxemia secondary to PPHN in premature infants.[48] Although iNO has been shown to improve oxygenation in premature infants who have RDS, its efficacy in improving long-term outcome has not been demonstrated.[107] Pulmonary hypertension is also being increasingly recognized as a component of chronic lung disease (CLD) in survivors of extreme prematurity.[108] A decrease in the number of pulmonary vessels, altered lung architecture, and episodes of hypoxemia and hypercarbia together may contribute to the development of pulmonary hypertension in CLD. A retrospective observational study of 42 infants who had CLD and pulmonary hypertension by Khemani and colleagues[108] demonstrated severe pulmonary hypertension, defined as systemic or suprasystemic right ventricular pressure, in 43% of these babies. Pulmonary hypertension was diagnosed at a median postnatal age of 4.8 months. Survival for this cohort was 64% at 6 months after the diagnosis of pulmonary hypertension, and severe pulmonary hypertension was a significant risk factor for mortality. The overall prevalence of pulmonary hypertension in survivors of extreme prematurity who have CLD remains unknown, however. It is important to recognize that pulmonary hypertension can develop as a complication of CLD in extremely low birth weight infants after their discharge from the NICU. iNO and sildenafil have been reported to be beneficial in these infants in decreasing the pulmonary artery pressure. Although the long-term safety of sildenafil is unclear, it has been used for as long as 1 to 2 years without adverse effects in isolated case reports and uncontrolled trials.[109] A case report of severe retinopathy of prematurity (ROP) that developed in a premature neonate treated at 29 weeks of gestational age with sildenafil raises concerns about the safety of this drug during the window of vulnerability for ROP.[110] Whether iNO or sildenafil improves survival and stimulates angiogenesis and lung growth in infants who have CLD remains unknown, although these beneficial effects were suggested in animal models.[107]

LONG-TERM OUTCOMES FOR SURVIVORS OF PERSISTENT PULMONARY HYPERTENSION OF THE NEWBORN

Several randomized trials of iNO evaluated the neurodevelopmental status of survivors of PPHN at 18 to 24 months of age. These studies identified a significant risk for hearing loss and neurodevelopmental impairments among survivors of PPHN.[111–114] Late-onset hearing loss has been identified in infants who initially pass their hearing screen before discharge from the NICU.[113] This observation highlights the need for close follow-up of these infants after discharge from the NICU. Two recent follow-up trials at 18 to 24 months of age reported on the outcome for babies with moderate and severe PPHN, respectively.[111,112] The 299 babies enrolled in the early iNO therapy trial presented with a moderate degree of respiratory failure. Among the 234 survivors seen at follow-up, 24% had hearing impairment and 26% had neurodevelopmental impairment, defined as moderate to severe cerebral palsy (CP), permanent hearing loss requiring amplification or vision loss, or Bayley mental developmental index or psychomotor developmental index less than 70. CP occurred in 7%, and an abnormal neurologic examination was documented in 13% of the infants in this cohort. These data demonstrate a need for close follow-up of survivors of PPHN because they remain at a high risk for adverse outcomes, despite survival rates that exceed 90%. The authors currently follow all neonates admitted with PPHN severe enough to need iNO therapy at 6-month intervals until 2 years of age to identify these long-term deficits. Future therapies to be tested in neonates with PPHN should focus on improving their long-term outcomes, in addition to survival.

FUTURE THERAPIES FOR PERSISTENT PULMONARY HYPERTENSION OF THE NEWBORN

Recent investigations in a fetal lamb model of PPHN demonstrated an increase in oxidative stress in the pulmonary arteries.[37,38] The oxidative stress contributes to impaired pulmonary vasodilation and lack of response to iNO.[46] The free radical superoxide is a vasoconstrictor and reacts with NO to reduce its bioavailability for vasodilation. Superoxide scavengers, such as recombinant human superoxide dismutase, decrease the pulmonary artery pressure and improve the oxygenation response to iNO in this model.[46] Antenatal administration of betamethasone also reduces the oxidative stress and improves the vasodilator response to NO in fetal lambs that have PPHN.[115] Prenatal correction of vascular dysfunction may facilitate normal birth-related adaptation and prevent periods of hypoxemia during postnatal life. Antenatal betamethasone is currently being investigated by the Maternal and Fetal Medicine Units network of the National Institutes of Child Health and Human Development (NICHD) in a randomized controlled trial to reduce respiratory morbidity for late preterm deliveries at 34 to 37 weeks of gestation. Future studies should determine the potential role of these new approaches for the prevention and management of PPHN.

In summary, rapid advances in our understanding of the postnatal adaptation of pulmonary circulation have led to newer therapeutic approaches for PPHN. Many of these advances resulted from the translational biology investigations in animal models of PPHN. Our enthusiasm over the dramatic decrease in mortality over the past 20 years should be tempered by recognition of the long-term complications among survivors of PPHN. Promising new therapies that are targeted to correct the vascular dysfunction in PPHN may help to prevent the periods of cardiopulmonary instability inherent to these babies. The impact of these new approaches on the long-term neurodevelopmental outcome for neonates who have PPHN requires further investigation.

ACKNOWLEDGMENTS

The authors acknowledge the drawings for **Figs. 1** and **4** by Dr. Satyan Lakshminrusimha, Assistant Professor of Pediatrics, State University of New York, Buffalo, New York.

REFERENCES

1. Gersony WM, Duc GV, Sinclair JC. "PFC syndrome" (persistence of the fetal circulation). Circulation 1969;40(Suppl 3):87.
2. Fox WW, Gewitz MH, Dinwiddie R, et al. Pulmonary hypertension in the perinatal aspiration syndromes. Pediatrics 1977;59(2):205–11.
3. Hageman JR, Adams MA, Gardner TH. Persistent pulmonary hypertension of the newborn. Trends in incidence, diagnosis, and management. Am J Dis Child 1984;138(6):592–5.
4. John E, Roberts V, Burnard ED. Persistent pulmonary hypertension of the newborn treated with hyperventilation: clinical features and outcome. Aust Paediatr J 1988;24(6):357–61.
5. Davis JM, Spitzer AR, Cox C, et al. Predicting survival in infants with persistent pulmonary hypertension of the newborn. Pediatr Pulmonol 1988;5(1):6–9.
6. Konduri GG, Solimano A, Sokol GM, et al. A randomized trial of early versus standard inhaled nitric oxide therapy in term and near-term newborn infants with hypoxic respiratory failure. Pediatrics 2004;113(3 Pt 1):559–64.
7. Alameh J, Bachiri A, Devisme L, et al. Alveolar capillary dysplasia: a cause of persistent pulmonary hypertension of the newborn. Eur J Pediatr 2002;161(5):262–6.
8. Kunig AM, Parker TA, Nogee LM, et al. ABCA3 deficiency presenting as persistent pulmonary hypertension of the newborn. J Pediatr 2007;151(3):322–4.
9. Dawes GS, Mott JC, Widdicomb JG, et al. Changes in the lungs of the newborn lamb. J Physiol 1953;121:141–62.
10. Cassin S, Dawes GS, Mott JC, et al. The vascular resistance of the foetal and newly ventilated lung of the lamb. J Physiol 1964;171:61–79.
11. Lakshminrusimha S, Steinhorn RH. Pulmonary vascular biology during neonatal transition. Clin Perinatol 1999;26(3):601–19.
12. Rasanen J, Wood DC, Debbs RH, et al. Reactivity of the human fetal pulmonary circulation to maternal hyperoxygenation increases during the second half of pregnancy: a randomized study. Circulation 1998;97(3):257–62.
13. Morin FC, Egan EA, Ferguson W, et al. Development of pulmonary vascular response to oxygen. Am J Physiol 1988;254:H542–6.
14. Velvis H, Moore P, Heymann MA. Prostaglandin inhibition prevents the fall in pulmonary vascular resistance as a result of rhythmic distension of the lungs in fetal lambs. Pediatr Res 1991;30:62–8.

15. Walker AM, Ritchie BC, Adamson TM, et al. Effect of changing lung liquid volume on the pulmonary circulation of fetal lambs. J Appl Physiol 1988;64(1): 61–7.

16. Abman SH, Chatfield BA, Hall SL, et al. Role of endothelium-derived relaxing factor during transition of pulmonary circulation at birth. Am J Physiol 1990; 259:H1921–7.

17. Tiktinsky MH, Morin FC III. Increasing oxygen tension dilates fetal pulmonary circulation via endothelium-derived relaxing factor. Am J Physiol 1993;265(1 Pt 2):H376–80.

18. Shaul PW, Wells LB. Oxygen modulates nitric oxide production selectively in fetal pulmonary endothelial cells. Am J Respir Cell Mol Biol 1994;11(4):432–8.

19. Shaul PW, Campbell WB, Farrar MA, et al. Oxygen modulates prostacyclin synthesis in ovine fetal pulmonary arteries by an effect on cyclooxygenase. J Clin Invest 1992;90(6):2147–55.

20. Konduri GG, Mattei J. Role of oxidative phosphorylation and ATP release in birth related pulmonary vasodilation in fetal lambs. Am J Physiol Heart Circ Physiol 2002;283(4):H1600–8.

21. Konduri GG, Mital S, Gervasio CT, et al. Purine nucleotides contribute to pulmonary vasodilation caused by birth related stimuli in the ovine fetus. (Heart Circ Physiol 41). Am J Physiol 1997;272:H2377–84.

22. Shaul PW, Farrar MA, Magness RR. Pulmonary endothelial nitric oxide production is developmentally regulated in the fetus and newborn. Am J Physiol 1993;265(Heart Circ Physiol 34):H1056–63.

23. Gien J, Seedorf GJ, Balasubramaniam V, et al. Intrauterine pulmonary hypertension impairs angiogenesis in vitro: role of vascular endothelial growth factor nitric oxide signaling. Am J Respir Crit Care Med 2007;176(11):1146–53.

24. Grover TR, Parker TA, Markham NE, et al. rhVEGF treatment preserves pulmonary vascular reactivity and structure in an experimental model of pulmonary hypertension in fetal sheep. Am J Physiol Lung Cell Mol Physiol 2005;289(2): L315–21.

25. Matsushita T, Hislop AA, Boels PJ, et al. Changes in ANP responsiveness of normal and hypertensive porcine intrapulmonary arteries during maturation. Pediatr Res 1999;46(4):411–8.

26. Leffler CW, Hessler JR, Green RS. The onset of breathing at birth stimulates pulmonary vascular prostacyclin synthesis. Pediatr Res 1984;18(10):938–42.

27. Cornfield DN, Reeve HL, Tolarova S, et al. Oxygen causes fetal pulmonary vasodilation through activation of a calcium-dependent potassium channel. Proc Natl Acad Sci U S A 1996;93:8089–94.

28. Archer SL, Souil E, Dinh-Xuan AT, et al. Molecular identification of the role of voltage-gated K+ channels, Kv1.5 and Kv2.1, in hypoxic pulmonary vasoconstriction and control of resting membrane potential in rat pulmonary artery myocytes. J Clin Invest 1998;101(11):2319–30.

29. Villanueva ME, Zaher FM, Svinarich DM, et al. Decreased gene expression of endothelial nitric oxide synthase in newborns with persistent pulmonary hypertension. Pediatr Res 1998;44:338–43.

30. Pearson DL, Dawling S, Walsh W, et al. Neonatal pulmonary hypertension: urea-cycle intermediates, nitric oxide production and carbamoylphosphate synthetase function. N Engl J Med 2001;344(24):1832–8.

31. Shaul PW, Yuhanna IS, German Z, et al. Pulmonary endothelial NO synthase gene expression is decreased in fetal lambs with pulmonary hypertension. Am J Physiol 1997;272 (Lung Cell Mol Physiol):L1005–12.

32. Villamor E, Le Cras TD, Horan MP, et al. Chronic intrauterine pulmonary hypertension impairs endothelial nitric oxide synthase in the ovine fetus. Am J Physiol 1997;272(Lung Cell Mol Physiol 16):L1013–20.

33. Arrigoni FI, Vallance P, Haworth SG, et al. Metabolism of asymmetric dimethylarginines is regulated in the lung developmentally and with pulmonary hypertension induced by hypobaric hypoxia. Circulation 2003;107(8):1195–201.

34. Pullamsetti S, Kiss L, Ghofrani HA, et al. Increased levels and reduced catabolism of asymmetric and symmetric dimethylarginines in pulmonary hypertension. FASEB J 2005;19(9):1175–7.

35. Rosenberg AA, Kennaugh J, Koppenhafer SL, et al. Elevated immunoreactive endothelin-1 levels in newborn infants with persistent pulmonary hypertension. J Pediatr 1993;123(1):109–14.

36. Wedgwood S, Black SM. Endothelin-1 decreases endothelial NOS expression and activity through ETA receptor-mediated generation of hydrogen peroxide. Am J Physiol Lung Cell Mol Physiol 2005;288(3):L480–7.

37. Brennan LA, Steinhorn RH, Wedgwood S, et al. Increased superoxide generation is associated with pulmonary hypertension in fetal lambs: a role for NADPH oxidase. Circ Res 2003;92(6):683–91.

38. Konduri GG, Bakhutashvili I, Eis A, et al. Oxidant stress from uncoupled nitric oxide synthase impairs vasodilation in fetal lambs with persistent pulmonary hypertension. Am J Physiol Heart Circ Physiol 2007;292(4):H1812–20.

39. Tzao C, Nickerson PA, Russell JA, et al. Pulmonary hypertension alters soluble guanylate cyclase activity and expression in pulmonary arteries isolated from fetal lambs. Pediatr Pulmonol 2001;31(2):97–105.

40. Csaba IF, Sulyok E, Ertl T. Relationship of maternal treatment with indomethacin to persistence of fetal circulation syndrome. J Pediatr 1978;92(3):484.

41. Rubaltelli FF, Chiozza ML, Zanardo V, et al. Effect on neonate of maternal treatment with indomethacin. J Pediatr 1979;94(1):161.

42. Alano MA, Ngougmna E, Ostrea EM, et al. Analysis of nonsteroidal antiinflammatory drugs in meconium and its relation to persistent pulmonary hypertension of the newborn. Pediatrics 2001;107:519–23.

43. Abman SH, Shanley PF, Accurso FJ. Failure of postnatal adaptation of the pulmonary circulation after chronic intrauterine pulmonary hypertension in fetal lambs. J Clin Invest 1989;83:1849–58.

44. Morin FC. Ligating the ductus arteriosus before birth causes persistent pulmonary hypertension in newborn lamb. Pediatr Res 1989;25:245–50.

45. Konduri GG, Ou J, Shi Y, et al. Decreased association of HSP90 impairs endothelial nitric oxide synthase in fetal lambs with persistent pulmonary hypertension. Am J Physiol Heart Circ Physiol 2003;285(1):H204–11.

46. Lakshminrusimha S, Russell JA, Wedgwood S, et al. Superoxide dismutase improves oxygenation and reduces oxidation in neonatal pulmonary hypertension. Am J Respir Crit Care Med 2006;174(12):1370–7.

47. Grover TR, Parker TA, Balasubramaniam V, et al. Pulmonary hypertension impairs alveolarization and reduces lung growth in the ovine fetus. Am J Physiol Lung Cell Mol Physiol 2005;288(4):L648–54.

48. Danhaive O, Margossian R, Geva T, et al. Pulmonary hypertension and right ventricular dysfunction in growth-restricted, extremely low birth weight neonates. J Perinatol 2005;25(7):495–9.

49. Walsh-Sukys MC, Tyson JE, Wright LL, et al. Persistent pulmonary hypertension of the newborn in the era before nitric oxide: practice variation and outcomes. Pediatrics 2000;105(1 Pt 1):14–20.

50. Yoder BA, Kirsch EA, Barth WH, et al. Changing obstetric practices associated with decreasing incidence of meconium aspiration syndrome. Obstet Gynecol 2002;99(5 Pt 1):731–9.
51. Yoder BA, Gordon MC, Barth WH Jr. Late-preterm birth: does the changing obstetric paradigm alter the epidemiology of respiratory complications? Obstet Gynecol 2008;111(4):814–22.
52. Dargaville PA, South M, McDougall PN. Surfactant and surfactant inhibitors in meconium aspiration syndrome. J Pediatr 2001;138(1):113–5.
53. Soukka H, Jalonen J, Kero P, et al. Endothelin-1, atrial natriuretic peptide and pathophysiology of pulmonary hypertension in porcine meconium aspiration. Acta Paediatr 1998;87(4):424–8.
54. Radhakrishnan RS, Lally PA, Lally KP, et al. ECMO for meconium aspiration syndrome: support for relaxed entry criteria. ASAIO J 2007;53(4):489–91.
55. Chambers CD, Hernandez-Diaz S, Van Marter LJ, et al. Selective serotonin-re-uptake inhibitors and risk of persistent pulmonary hypertension of the newborn. N Engl J Med 2006;354(6):579–87.
56. Andrade SE, McPhillips H, Loren D, et al. Antidepressant medication use and risk of persistent pulmonary hypertension of the newborn. Pharmacoepidemiol Drug Saf 2009;18(3):246–52.
57. Shankaran S, Farooki ZQ, Desai R. Beta-hemolytic streptococcal infection appearing as persistent fetal circulation. Am J Dis Child 1982;136(8):725–7.
58. Shook LA, Pauly TH, Marple SL. Group B Streptococcus promotes oxygen radical-dependent thromboxane accumulation in young piglets. Pediatr Res 1990;27(4 Pt 1):349–52.
59. Navarrete CT, Devia C, Lessa AC, et al. The role of endothelin converting enzyme inhibition during group B Streptococcus-induced pulmonary hypertension in newborn piglets. Pediatr Res 2003;54(3):387–92.
60. Heritage CK, Cunningham MD. Association of elective repeat cesarian delivery and persistent pulmonary hypertension of the newborn. Am J Obstet Gynecol 1985;152:627–9.
61. Bohn D. Congenital diaphragmatic hernia. Am J Respir Crit Care Med 2002;166:911–5.
62. Boloker J, Bateman DA, Wung JT, et al. Congenital diaphragmatic hernia in 120 infants treated consecutively with permissive hypercapnea/spontaneous respiration/elective repair. J Pediatr Surg 2002;37(3):357–66.
63. Singh SA, Ibrahim T, Clark DJ, et al. Persistent pulmonary hypertension of newborn due to congenital capillary alveolar dysplasia. Pediatr Pulmonol 2005;40(4):349–53.
64. Eulmesekian P, Cutz E, Parvez B, et al. Alveolar capillary dysplasia: a six-year single center experience. J Perinat Med 2005;33(4):347–52.
65. Hamvas A, Cole FS, Nogee LM. Genetic disorders of surfactant proteins. Neonatology 2007;91(4):311–7.
66. Shulenin S, Nogee LM, Annilo T, et al. ABCA3 gene mutations in newborns with fatal surfactant deficiency. N Engl J Med 2004;350(13):1296–303.
67. The Neonatal Inhaled Nitric Oxide Study Group. Inhaled nitric oxide in full-term and nearly full-term infants with hypoxic respiratory failure. N Engl J Med 1997;336:597–604.
68. Lotze A, Mitchell BR, Bulas DI, et al. Multicenter study of surfactant (beractant) use in the treatment of term infants with severe respiratory failure. J Pediatr 1998;132:40–7.

69. Hintz SR, Suttner DM, Sheehan AM, et al. Decreased use of neonatal extracorporeal membrane oxygenation (ECMO): how new treatment modalities have affected ECMO utilization. Pediatrics 2000;106(6):1339–43.

70. Kinsella JP, Truog WE, Walsh WF, et al. Randomized, multicenter trial of inhaled nitric oxide and high-frequency oscillatory ventilation in severe, persistent pulmonary hypertension of the newborn. J Pediatr 1997;131:55–62.

71. Cheung PY, Tyebkhan JM, Peliowski A, et al. Prolonged use of pancuronium bromide and sensorineural hearing loss in childhood survivors of congenital diaphragmatic hernia. J Pediatr 1999;135:233–9.

72. Robertson C, Tyberkhan JM, Peliowski A. Ototoxic drugs and sensorineural hearing loss following severe neonatal respiratory failure. Acta Pædiatr 2006; 95:214–23.

73. Drummond WH, Gregory GA, Heymann MA, et al. The independent effects of hyperventilation, tolazoline, and dopamine on infants with persistent pulmonary hypertension. J Pediatr 1981;98(4):603–11.

74. Schreiber MD, Soifer SJ. Respiratory alkalosis attenuates thromboxane-induced pulmonary hypertension. Crit Care Med 1988;16(12):1225–8.

75. Schreiber MD, Heymann MA, Soifer SJ. Increased arterial pH, not decreased $PaCO_2$, attenuates hypoxia-induced pulmonary vasoconstriction in newborn lambs. Pediatr Res 1986;20(2):113–7.

76. Hendricks-Munoz KD, Walton JP. Hearing loss in infants with persistent fetal circulation. Pediatrics 1988;81(5):650–6.

77. Marron MJ, Crisafi MA, Driscoll JM Jr, et al. Hearing and neurodevelopmental outcome in survivors of persistent pulmonary hypertension of the newborn. Pediatrics 1992;90(3):392–6.

78. Tourneux P, Rakza T, Bouissou A, et al. Pulmonary circulatory effects of norepinephrine in newborn infants with persistent pulmonary hypertension. J Pediatr 2008;153(3):345–9.

79. Frostell C, Fratacci MD, Wain JC, et al. Inhaled nitric oxide. A selective pulmonary vasodilator reversing hypoxic pulmonary vasoconstriction. Circulation 1991;83(6):2038–47 [erratum in: Circulation 1991;84(5):2212].

80. Williams O, Rafferty GF, Hannam S, et al. Nasal and lower airway levels of nitric oxide in prematurely born infants. Early Hum Dev 2003;72(1):67–73.

81. Leipala JA, Williams O, Sreekumar S, et al. Exhaled nitric oxide levels in infants with chronic lung disease. Eur J Pediatr 2004;163:555–8.

82. Roberts JD, Polaner DM, Lang P, et al. Inhaled nitric oxide in persistent pulmonary hypertension of the newborn. Lancet 1992;340(8823):818–9.

83. Kinsella JP, Neish SR, Shaffer E, et al. Low-dose inhalation nitric oxide in persistent pulmonary hypertension of the newborn. Lancet 1992;340(8823):819–20.

84. Roberts JD, Fineman JR, Morin FC, et al. Inhaled nitric oxide and persistent pulmonary hypertension of the newborn. N Engl J Med 1997;336:605–10.

85. Christou H, Van Marter LJ, Wessel DL, et al. Inhaled nitric oxide reduces the need for extracorporeal membrane oxygenation in infants with persistent pulmonary hypertension of the newborn. Crit Care Med 2000;28(11):3722–7.

86. Clark RH, Kueser TJ, Walker MW, et al. Low-dose nitric oxide therapy for persistent pulmonary hypertension of the newborn. N Engl J Med 2000;342:469–74.

87. Wessel DL, Adatia I, Van Marter LJ, et al. Improved oxygenation in a randomized trial of inhaled nitric oxide for persistent pulmonary hypertension of the newborn. Pediatrics 1997;100(5):E7.

88. American Academy of Pediatrics Committee on Fetus and Newborn. Use of inhaled nitric oxide. Pediatrics 2000;106:344–5.

89. Davidson D, Barefield ES, Kattwinkel J, et al. Inhaled nitric oxide for the early treatment of persistent pulmonary hypertension of the term newborn: a randomized, double masked, placebo controlled, dose-response, multicenter study. Pediatrics 1998;101:325–34.

90. Christou H, Magnani B, Morse DS, et al. Inhaled nitric oxide does not affect adenosine 5'-diphosphate-dependent platelet activation in infants with persistent pulmonary hypertension of the newborn. Pediatrics 1998;102:1390–3.

91. Sokol GM, Fineberg NS, Wright LL. Changes in arterial oxygen tension when weaning neonates from inhaled nitric oxide. Pediatr Pulmonol 2001;32(1):14–9.

92. Davidson D, Barefield ES, Kattwinkel J. Safety of withdrawing inhaled nitric oxide therapy in persistent pulmonary hypertension of the newborn. Pediatrics 1999; 104(2 Pt 1):231–6.

93. Lakshminrusimha S, Russell JA, Steinhorn RH, et al. Pulmonary hemodynamics in neonatal lambs resuscitated with 21%, 50%, and 100% oxygen. Pediatr Res 2007;62(3):313–8.

94. Neonatal Inhaled Nitric Oxide Study Group (NINOS). Inhaled nitric oxide and hypoxic respiratory failure in infants with congenital diaphragmatic hernia. Pediatrics 1997;99:838–45.

95. Hanson KA, Ziegler JW, Rybalkin SD, et al. Chronic pulmonary hypertension increases fetal lung cGMP phosphodiesterase activity. Am J Physiol 1998; 275(5 Pt 1):L931–41.

96. Atz AM, Wessel DL. Sildenafil ameliorates effects of inhaled nitric oxide withdrawal. Anesthesiology 1999;91:307–10.

97. Baquero H, Soliz A, Neira F, et al. Oral sildenafil in infants with persistent pulmonary hypertension of the newborn: a pilot randomized blinded study. Pediatrics 2006;117(4):1077–83.

98. Travadi JN, Patole SK. Phosphodiesterase inhibitors for persistent pulmonary hypertension of the newborn: a review. Pediatr Pulmonol 2003;36(6):529–35.

99. Kelly LK, Porta NF, Goodman DM, et al. Inhaled prostacyclin for term infants with persistent pulmonary hypertension refractory to inhaled nitric oxide. J Pediatr 2002;141(6):830–2.

100. Chang AC, Atz AM, Wernovsky G, et al. Milrinone: systemic and pulmonary hemodynamic effects in neonates after cardiac surgery. Crit Care Med 1995; 23(11):1907–14.

101. Bassler D, Choong K, McNamara P, et al. Neonatal persistent pulmonary hypertension treated with milrinone: four case reports. Biol Neonate 2006;89(1):1–5.

102. McNamara PJ, Laique F, Muang-In S, et al. Milrinone improves oxygenation in neonates with severe persistent pulmonary hypertension of the newborn. J Crit Care 2006;21(2):217–22.

103. Bartlett RH, Gazzaniga AB, Huxtable RF, et al. Extracorporeal circulation (ECMO) in neonatal respiratory failure. J Thorac Cardiovasc Surg 1977;74(6): 826–33.

104. UK Collaborative ECMO Trial Group. UK collaborative randomised trial of neonatal extracorporeal membrane oxygenation. Lancet 1996;348(9020):75–82.

105. Mugford M, Elbourne D, Field D. Extracorporeal membrane oxygenation for severe respiratory failure in newborn infants. Cochrane Database Syst Rev 2008;(3):CD001340.

106. Farrow KN, Fliman P, Steinhorn RH. The disease treated with ECMO: focus on PPHN. Semin Perinatol 2005;29:8–14.

107. Arul N, Konduri GG. Inhaled nitric oxide for preterm neonates. Clin Perinatol 2009;36(1):43–61.

108. Khemani E, McElhinney DB, Rhein L, et al. Pulmonary artery hypertension in formerly premature infants with bronchopulmonary dysplasia: clinical features and outcomes in the surfactant era. Pediatrics 2007;120(6):1260–9.

109. Mourani PM, Sontag MK, Ivy DD, et al. Effects of long-term sildenafil treatment for pulmonary hypertension in infants with chronic lung disease. J Pediatr 2009; 154:379–84.

110. Marsh CS, Marden B, Newsom R. Severe retinopathy of prematurity (ROP) in a premature baby treated with sildenafil acetate (Viagra) for pulmonary hypertension. Br J Ophthalmol 2004;88(2):306–7.

111. Konduri GG, Vohr B, Robertson C. Early inhaled nitric oxide therapy for term and near-term newborn infants with hypoxic respiratory failure: neurodevelopmental follow-up. J Pediatr 2007;150(3):235–40.

112. The Neonatal Inhaled Nitric Oxide Study Group. Inhaled nitric oxide in term and near term infants: neurodevelopmental follow-up of the Neonatal Inhaled Nitric Oxide Study Group (NINOS). J Pediatr 2000;136:611–7.

113. Robertson CM, Tyebkhan JM, Hagler ME, et al. Late-onset, progressive sensorineural hearing loss after severe neonatal respiratory failure. Otol Neurotol 2002;23(3):353–6.

114. Lipkin PH, Davidson D, Spivak L, et al. Neurodevelopmental and medical outcomes of persistent pulmonary hypertension in term newborns treated with nitric oxide. J Pediatr 2002;140(3):306–10.

115. Chandrasekar I, Eis A, Konduri GG. Betamethasone attenuates oxidant stress in endothelial cells from fetal lambs with persistent pulmonary hypertension. Pediatr Res 2008;63(1):67–72.

Use of Therapeutic Hypothermia for Term Infants with Hypoxic-Ischemic Encephalopathy

Abbot R. Laptook, MD

KEYWORDS

- Hypoxia-ischemia • Encephalopathy • Hypothermia
- Asphyxia • Neonatal

Maintenance of body temperature has long been recognized as a fundamental concept of neonatal care.[1] All care providers involved with newborn infants are taught the importance of the neutral thermal environment. The importance of thermal regulation was established through high-quality randomized controlled trials dating back to the 1950s and 1960s. Silverman and colleagues[2] randomized low birth weight infants to different incubator temperatures (28.3–29.4°C versus 31.1–32.1°C) for the first 5 days following birth. Infants cared for in a warmer incubator had higher axillary temperatures in all birth weight strata of enrolled infants (<1kg, 1–1.5kg, and 1.5–2kg) and was associated with a reduction in mortality. The difference in mortality persisted at 28 days (22% versus 45.1% for warmer versus cooler infants, respectively). Other randomized trials followed and confirmed these observations in addition to determining the optimal thermal environment for care of the low birth weight infant.[3–5] Coincident with these trials was delineation of the relationship between oxygen consumption and environmental or body temperature[6,7] and the goals of maintaining infants within a neutral thermal environment. The principles of thermal regulation in the premature infant have largely been extrapolated to the late preterm and term infant without specific studies in this age group. It is therefore somewhat paradoxical to be considering hypothermia as a treatment strategy given the importance of thermal regulation for neonatal care. The following provides an overview of the biologic plausibility of therapeutic hypothermia and the investigations from animal and clinical trials for its application in neonatal intensive care.

Neonatal Intensive Care Unit, Women and Infants' Hospital of Rhode Island, Warren Alpert Medical School at Brown University, 101 Dudley Street, Suite 1100, Providence, RI 02905, USA
E-mail address: alaptook@wihri.org

Pediatr Clin N Am 56 (2009) 601–616
doi:10.1016/j.pcl.2009.03.007
0031-3955/09/$ – see front matter © 2009 Elsevier Inc. All rights reserved.

pediatric.theclinics.com

BIOLOGIC PLAUSIBILITY

Although deep hypothermia (core body temperature <20°C) during circulatory arrest to repair congenital heart disease provides neuroprotection in infants and children,[8] prolonged exposure to such low body temperatures is associated with morbidity. Therapeutic hypothermia is focused on more modest temperature reductions (2–5°C) that are compatible with ongoing bedside management and can be sustained over time with minimal adverse effects.

The majority of investigations of hypothermia as a therapeutic regimen have been focused on its application during and after hypoxia-ischemia. An important observation suggesting that interventions may be possible for perinatal hypoxia-ischemia was provided by the use of P^{31} magnetic resonance spectroscopy. Serial spectra over the first 48 hours for newborn infants born after hypoxia-ischemia indicated that there was an interval of time following birth before observing spectroscopic changes compatible with prior hypoxia-ischemia.[9] Newborn swine were used to determine the temporal changes in brain high-energy phosphorylated metabolites and intracellular pH during and following hypoxia and ischemia.[10] Brain injury could be characterized by a biphasic process (**Fig. 1**). The initial phase is the initiating hypoxic-ischemic interval, which results in brain energy failure (reductions in high-energy phosphorylated metabolites and brain acidosis). Primary energy failure can be so severe that brain injury will result; alternatively, it can be resolved (re-establishment of the brain energy state) without progression to injury depending upon the timing and effectiveness of resuscitation. At a time remote from primary energy failure (approximately 6–12 hours), a second interval of brain energy failure may occur (secondary energy failure) but without brain acidosis.[11,12] Secondary energy failure serves as a trigger or is a marker for the initiation of multiple pathways that invariably evolve to brain injury. Secondary energy failure may occur in the absence of alterations in blood pressure, oxygen tension, and substrate concentration. The observation that the cerebral energy state is restored after primary energy failure suggests that there may be a therapeutic window of time when provision of brain-specific therapies may prevent or attenuate the progression to secondary energy failure with resultant brain injury.

The biologic processes (see **Fig. 1**) associated with primary energy failure include (1) release and decreased uptake of excitatory amino acids (eg, glutamate) from the extracellular fluid, (2) loss of ionic homeostasis across membranes and organelles,

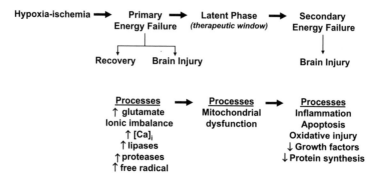

Fig. 1. A flow diagram of the sequence of pathologic events triggered by hypoxia-ischemia and culminating in brain injury. The biologic processes intimately involved with each phase of the sequence are listed below.

and resultant increases in intracellular calcium concentration, (3) liberation of lipases and proteases, (4) and generation of reactive oxygen species.[13,14] Processes involved in secondary energy failure are not completely understood but include activation of microglia with an inflammatory response, activation of specific caspase proteins that trigger apoptosis, reductions in growth factors, and protein synthesis and further accumulation of excitotoxic neurotransmitters.[15–19] Hypothermia is an attractive potential therapy because reductions in brain temperature of 2–6°C inhibit many of the processes involved in primary and secondary energy failure. Hypothermia reduces brain energy use rate and helps preserve brain energy state, attenuates the release of excitotoxic neurotransmitters and nitric oxide, decreases apoptosis, inhibits the release of platelet activating factor with a reduction in the inflammatory cascade, reduces the extent of protein and ubiquitin suppression, and decreases the extent of protein SUMOylation.[20–26] All of these processes contribute to the ability of hypothermia to attenuate the extent of secondary energy failure following prior hypoxia-ischemia and reduce the extent of brain injury.[27]

HISTORY OF THERAPEUTIC HYPOTHERMIA IN NEWBORN MEDICINE

More than 50 years ago it was established that newborn animals of different species have a longer survival time during anoxia when body temperature was hypothermic compared with normothermic.[28] It was further demonstrated that hypothermia initiated following asphyxia in newborn animals improved survival compared with normothermic body temperature.[29] These observations provided the rationale for the clinical application of body cooling when newborn infants did not respond to resuscitation at birth. Therapeutic hypothermia was used for full-term infants with 5-minute Apgar scores less than 5 who did not respond to endotracheal oxygen, bicarbonate and glucose via an umbilical vein, and cardiac massage if indicated.[30] Hypothermia was induced by immersion of the infant except for the nose and mouth in a bath of cold water with temperatures ranging from 10 to 15°C. Outcome at an average of 42 months (range 18.5–105 months) for 35 infants cooled from 1961 to 1971 was excellent with 94% survival and 3% with neurologic sequelae. However, this was an uncontrolled clinical experience and was compared with historical controls.

Interest in the use of cooling for infants at birth essentially vanished during the 1970s because of multiple factors. The randomized controlled trials referenced earlier[2–5] and an understanding of the neutral thermal environment established the critical importance of thermal regulation in the care of the low birth weight or premature infant. Specific adverse effects of cold exposure and the recognition of a cold-stress syndrome further solidified thermal regulation as a fundamental component of newborn care.[31,32] Principles of thermal regulation were extrapolated to the term infant and extended to stabilization and resuscitation at birth. Thus, the first principle in newborn care in the delivery room setting is to prevent excessive heat loss and thereby facilitate transitional physiologic events such as the fall in pulmonary vascular resistance.[33] Therapeutic hypothermia quickly fell out of favor with these developments.

RE-EMERGENCE OF HYPOTHERMIA AS A POTENTIAL THERAPY: ANIMAL INVESTIGATIONS

Research on anything but deep hypothermia remained dormant until investigators at the University of Miami published a series of astute observations.[34] This laboratory used a global ischemia model in adult rodents and examined the variability in brain histologic injury following a consistent insult. They had noted that different histopathologic injury could be obtained depending on the use of a heat lamp over the head or body. A series of experiments were conducted in which the intra-ischemic brain temperature was varied by 2 to 3 degree increments from 33 to 39°C, while maintaining a constant brain temperature before and after ischemia. Results indicated that differences in intra-ischemic temperature as little as 2°C critically determine the extent of neuronal injury in the striatum, hippocampus, thalamus, and cerebral cortex. These observations triggered the next decade of investigations on the neuroprotective effects and mechanisms of modest reductions in temperature (2–6°C) of animals and provided the basis for human clinical investigation.

Design of a hypothermia regimen for animal investigation and ultimately clinical application needs to address a number of characteristics as detailed in **Box 1**.

Time of Initiation

The parameter that has been best characterized in the perinatal period is the time of initiation of therapeutic hypothermia. Gunn and colleagues[35–37] performed a series of elegant studies in the late-gestation fetal sheep in which 30 minutes of brain ischemia was followed by 72 hours of hypothermia achieved by circulating water (8–10°C) through a cooling cap affixed to the head. Cooling was initiated at 1.5, 5.5, or 8.5 hours following brain ischemia and the extent of neuronal injury assessed at 5 days postischemia was reduced with initiation of cooling before 6 hours compared with sham controls (**Fig. 2**). No reduction in neuronal injury was observed when cooling was initiated 8.5 hours following ischemia and represents a time in this model when postischemic seizures occur. Thus, the therapeutic window is approximately 6 hours in the late-gestation sheep fetus. Data from other animals indicate that 6 hours may not be a universal value. The therapeutic window defined by the interval between re-establishment of brain-phosphorylated metabolites following hypoxia-ischemia and the start of secondary energy failure in newborn piglets is an average of 17.5 hours. Furthermore, this value is shortened with increasing severity of the initial hypoxia-ischemia.[38] In 14-day-old rats, initiation of hypothermia more than 6 hours following hypoxia-ischemia is more effective than earlier start times.[39] It is therefore difficult to extrapolate to human newborns.

Duration

The duration of hypothermia for fetal or neonatal animals has not been studied as systematically as the time of initiation. A short duration of hypothermia (temperature reduction of 2–3°C for 1 hour) initiated immediately following ischemia was associated with reduced neuronal injury and improved neurologic assessments in neonatal

---

Box 1
Components of a hypothermia regimen

Time of initiation

Duration of cooling

Temperature depth

Rate of rewarming

Mode of cooling

    Body cooling

    Head cooling

    Head and body cooling

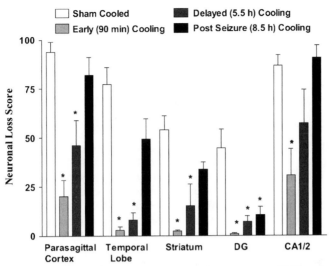

Fig. 2. The results of three studies performed by Gunn and colleagues[35–37] to determine the effect of time of initiation of cooling on neuronal loss. Fetal sheep underwent brain ischemia and were then subjected to head cooling initiated at different times following ischemia: early (90 minutes), delayed (5.5 hours), or after seizures occurred (8.5 hours). Cooling was continued for 72 hours and the extent of neuronal loss was determined 5 days following ischemia. Asterisks indicate differences ($P<.005$) compared with sham-cooled animals. (*From* Gunn AJ, Thoresen M. Hypothermic neuroprotection. NeuroRx 2006;3: 154–69; with permission.)

mini-swine.[40] Similar observations have been reported for newborn piglets subjected to 3 hours of hypothermia (temperature reduction of 4°C) initiated immediately after resolution of hypoxia.[41] However a delay of as little as 30 minutes between ischemia and 1 hour of hypothermia did not provide evidence of neuroprotection.[42] Identifying efficacy of hypothermia regimens initiated at a time remote from the hypoxia-ischemia is critical for clinical relevance in a neonatal intensive care unit. In adult rats and gerbils, increasing the duration of the hypothermia exposure allowed commencement of hypothermia at longer intervals following brain ischemia.[43–45] The use of 72 hours of hypothermia by Gunn and colleagues[35–37] provides a regimen in which it is unlikely that the duration of cooling will limit the extent of neuroprotection.

Target Temperature

The optimal target temperature for hypothermia regimens remains unclear and has received sparse attention. Newborn piglets subjected to brain hypoxia-ischemia were managed with three temperature regimens (based on rectal temperature) between 2 and 26 hours after resuscitation. Piglets were maintained normothermic at 38.5 to 39°C or were cooled to 35 or 33°C.[46] The depth of cooling altered the pattern of neuroprotection; normothermic animals had the lowest number of viable neurons in all regions surveyed while cooling to 35°C had the most viable neurons in the deep gray matter (putamen, globus pallidus, thalamus) and cooling to 33°C had more viable neurons in regions of the cortex and hippocampus. The same investigators demonstrated that cooling to 35 or 33°C between 2 and 26 hours following hypoxia-ischemia did not change the therapeutic window (biochemical assessment) and did not alter the extent of secondary energy failure during 48 hours following hypoxia-ischemia.[47]

It remains unclear whether the observed histologic differences would influence functional outcomes but raises the possibility that optimal neuroprotection may occur at different temperatures.

Rewarming

The rate of rewarming is the component of a hypothermia regimen that has received the least investigation. No systematic data exists in perinatal animals.

Mode of Cooling

Brain hypothermia may be achieved by way of different techniques that are compatible with ongoing intensive care at the bedside. The brain can be selectively cooled by cooling the head; or the brain can be cooled by cooling the body; or head and body cooling can be combined. Whether greater protection occurs with one mode of cooling compared with another is unknown but each mode of cooling is associated with unique thermal characteristics. Head cooling with a constant rectal temperature (true selective cooling) in neonatal mini-swine resulted in an increase in the temperature gradient across the brain from the warmer central structures to the cooler periphery.[48] Specifically the temperature difference between the brain at a 2 cm depth and the dura was 1.3°C, ±1.1, at baseline and 7.5°C, ±3.5, during cooling. In contrast, body cooling was associated with more homogenous cooling and an unchanged temperature gradient between brain at a 2 cm depth and the dura (1.5°C, ±1.2, at baseline and 1.1°C, ±.9, during cooling). Combining head and body cooling provides greater temperature reductions in the central regions of the brain compared with selective head cooling, and higher core-body temperatures compared with body cooling.[49] Body and head cooling may be more effective (ie, greater reduction in temperatures) in smaller compared with larger subjects because of a higher head surface-area-to-volume ratio.[46]

Duration of Neuroprotection

Demonstration of reduction in neuronal injury or other markers of neuroprotection have been assessed in most studies within 2 to 5 days of hypoxia-ischemia. There has been concern that neuroprotection may not persist over extended time intervals as demonstrated in 7-day-old rat pups[50] and adult rats.[51] However, long-lasting evidence of neuroprotection has been demonstrated in 7-day-old rat pups undergoing 26 hours of hypothermia initiated 2 hours following resolution of hypoxia-ischemia.[52] At 5 weeks of recovery, hypothermia was associated with less spatial memory deficits and reduced tissue loss on MRI compared with animals maintained normothermic. Similar long-lasting neuroprotection has been demonstrated in adult gerbils.[53]

CHALLENGES FOR CLINICAL TRIALS OF THERAPEUTIC HYPOTHERMIA

In spite of abundant animal data showing that reduction in temperature of 2 to 6°C favorably alters biologic processes involved in brain injury, and results in neuroprotection following ischemia or hypoxia-ischemia, there remain important challenges to demonstrating efficacy in a randomized clinical trial. Encephalopathy is the clinical marker for infants that have had hypoxia-ischemia of a severity that may lead to brain injury. Encephalopathy represents a nonspecific response of the brain to multiple casual pathways, many of which are not amenable to therapy (eg, brain malformation, inborn error of metabolism, genetic disorders, etc). Encephalopathy of a hypoxic-ischemic origin (HIE) represents approximately 30% of all causes for encephalopathy based on a population case-control study[54] and may be amenable to therapy.

The first challenge is whether inclusion and exclusion criteria are robust enough to identify infants with HIE and distinguish other causes of encephalopathy. The second challenge is to identify infants at risk in a timely manner in view of the concept of a therapeutic window, even though the duration of the latter is not known for human newborns. The third challenge is the recognition that clinicians have a limited ability to time when a hypoxic-ischemic event occurred during the perinatal period. Although sentinel events (cord avulsion, ruptured uterus, acute abruptio placenta, etc) may lend to accurate timing, it may be harder to estimate timing of more insidious hypoxia-ischemia heralded by nonreassuring fetal heart rate patterns or some other measure of fetal well-being. The fourth challenge is that the duration of the insult in clinical practice may be heterogeneous. Animal studies have demonstrated efficacy for hypothermia following acute ischemia or hypoxia-ischemia under controlled laboratory conditions. In clinical practice, hypoxia-ischemia may be acute, chronic, or acute superimposed on chronic. In spite of these challenges, the successful laboratory demonstration of neuroprotection achieved with 2 to 6°C temperature reductions provided strong rationale for rigorous clinical testing.

CLINICAL TRIALS OF HYPOTHERMIA FOR NEWBORN ENCEPHALOPATHY

Multiple pilot studies were performed that established the feasibility of implementing hypothermia for newborns with HIE. Pilot studies were followed by five large randomized controlled trials to determine efficacy and safety of hypothermia for HIE. At present, two are published (CoolCap[55] and National Institute of Child Health and Human Development [NICHD] Body Cooling trials[56]), one has been completed and undergoing peer review (Total Body Cooling trail), and two have been stopped early because of recruitment issues (Infant Cooling Evaluation trial and European Network Induced Hypothermia trial).

The CoolCap and the NICHD Body Cooling trials were multicenter randomized controlled studies designed to determine if brain hypothermia reduced death or neurodevelopmental disability among infants with HIE who were greater than or equal to 36 weeks gestation. Inclusion criteria for each study was a stepwise process in which fulfillment of initial criteria (fetal acidemia, Apgars, need for resuscitation or ventilation) qualified infants to be evaluated for the presence or absence of moderate or severe encephalopathy using a modification of the Sarnat stages.[57] Infants meeting these criteria qualified for enrollment in the NICHD Body Cooling trail but infants in the Cool-Cap study also needed abnormalities on an amplitude-integrated electroencephalogram (aEEG). In both studies, infants (n = 234 for CoolCap, n = 208 for NICHD Body Cooling) were enrolled by 6 hours of age given the data of Gunn and colleagues.[35–37]

Brain hypothermia was induced for 72 hours in each study but the mode of cooling differed. Infants randomized to the intervention arm of the CoolCap trial underwent head cooling with a cap (initial water temperature 8–12°C, Olympic Medical, Seattle, Washington) combined with body cooling to a rectal temperature of 34 to 35°C by way of a radiant warmer and servo-control of abdominal skin temperature. Infants randomized to the control arm were cared for under radiant warmers using servo-control of the abdominal skin temperature to maintain rectal temperature at 36.8 to 37.2°C. In the NICHD Body Cooling trial, infants randomized to the intervention arm underwent whole-body cooling by lying on a cooling blanket interfaced with a Hyper-Hypothermia system (Cincinnati Subzero, Cincinnati, Ohio). Infants had an esophageal temperature probe positioned in the lower third of the esophagus, which was servo-controlled at 33.5°C by the cooling system. Infants assigned to the control arm were cared for under radiant warmers using servo-control of the abdominal skin temperature initially from 36.5 to 37°C and subsequent adjustments were made according to the usual protocol of each center. Infants in the control arm had esophageal temperature probes in place that were not used for clinical management. In both studies, infants were rewarmed after 72 hours of brain hypothermia at a rate of 0.5°C per hour.

The primary outcome was death or disability at 18 months in the CoolCap trial, and 18 to 22 months in the NICHD Body Cooling trial. In the CoolCap trial, disability was defined as severe and included any of the following: Bayley II mental developmental index of less than 70 (more than 2 standard deviations below the mean), Gross Motor Function Level III to V (from infants able to sit with support to infants that need adult assistance to move), or bilateral cortical visual impairment. In the NICHD Body Cooling trial, disability was defined as severe or moderate. Severe disability was similar to the CoolCap criteria except for the addition of hearing impairment requiring amplification. Moderate disability was defined as a mental development index score one to two standard deviations below the mean (ie, 70–84) in addition to one or more of the following: Gross Motor Function Level II (pull to stand and cruise holding on to support), hearing impairment not requiring amplification, or a seizure disorder present at the time of follow-up.

Characteristics of infants in each trial at the time of randomization are listed in **Table 1**. Infants were predominantly term, appropriate for gestational age, and enrollment occurred (on average) at an age of less than 5 hours. Given that outborn infants

Table 1
Brain hypothermia trials: characteristics at randomization

	CoolCap		NICHD Body Cooling	
	Control n = 118	Cool n = 116	Control n = 106	Cool n = 102
Postnatal age (h)	4.8	4.7	4.3	4.3
Gestational age (wk)	39±1[a]	39±2	39±2	39±2
Birth weight (kg)	3.5±0.6	3.4±0.7	3.4±0.6	3.4±0.7
Female (%)	51	45	37	50
Outborn (%)	—	—	42	47
Emergency cesarean section (%)	69	64	75	71
10-min Apgar <6(%)[b]	27	17	—	—
10-min Apgar <5(%)	—	—	77	84
pH[c]	6.9±0.2	6.9±0.2	6.8±0.2	6.9±0.2
Encephalopathy (%)				
Moderate	63	58	62	68
Severe	32	37	38	32
Seizures (%)				
Clinical	—	—	48	43
aEEG	64	59	—	—
aEEG (%)				
Moderate abnormal	64	54	—	—
Severe abnormal	27	36	—	—

[a] Data are mean ± SD.
[b] Apgar scores were reported for only 166 infants.
[c] pH values represent cord blood or within the first hour following birth.

accounted for approximately 45% of enrolled infants in the NICHD Body Cooling trial (this figure is not reported for the CoolCap study), pediatricians have an important role in recognition of at-risk infants and rapid referral to centers capable of implementing therapeutic hypothermia. As expected, high percentages of infants in both studies had depressed Apgar scores, fetal acidemia, and were delivered by emergency cesarean section. The proportions of infants with moderate and severe encephalopathy were comparable between the two studies. Rectal temperatures for infants in the CoolCap trial and esophageal and skin temperatures for infants in the NICHD Body Cooling trial are plotted in **Fig. 3**. The plots indicate that the majority of temperatures were in the targeted range of each study.

In the CoolCap trial, the primary outcome, death or disability (severe), was 66% in the control group and was reduced to 55% in the cooled group (odds ratio .61, 95% CI .34–1.09, $P = .10$). There was a chance imbalance between groups in the distribution of severity patterns of aEEG. Logistic regression adjusting for baseline-aEEG pattern, presence of seizures, and age at randomization indicated a possible effect for hypothermia (odds ratio, .57, 95% CI .32–1.01, $P = .05$). In the NICHD Body Cooling trial, death or disability (severe or moderate) was 62% in the control group and was reduced to 44% in the control group (relative risk, .72, 95% CI .54–.95, $P = .01$). The relative risk and CIs were unchanged after adjustment for center and level of encephalopathy (relative risk, .76, 95% CI .60–.97). Based on the NICHD Body Cooling trial, the number needed to treat was six infants to benefit one. In both trials, subgroup analysis suggested a more prominent effect of hypothermia on the primary outcome for infants with moderate compared with severe encephalopathy (NICHD Body Cooling), and for infants with intermediate compared with severe aEEG abnormalities (CoolCap).

Individual components of the primary outcome are listed for each trial in **Table 2**. There was a trend for fewer deaths in the hypothermic group of the NICHD Body Cooling trial that was not evident in the CoolCap trial. A concern of any new therapy is that infants destined to die without the therapy are salvaged, leaving more surviving infants with adverse neurodevelopment. Although not powered to discriminate differences

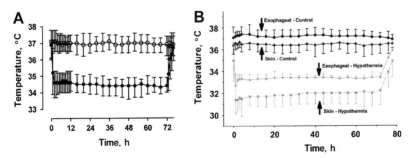

Fig. 3. The temperature profile is depicted over the 72-hour intervention and 6 hours following the intervention for each hypothermia trial. (*A*) The rectal temperatures of the control (*open circles*) and cooled infants (*circles*) of the CoolCap study. (*From* Wyatt JS, Gluckman PD, Liu PY, et al. Determinants of outcomes after head cooling for neonatal encephalopathy. Pediatrics 2007;119(5):912–21; with permission.) (*B*) The esophageal (*solid circles*) and skin (*triangles*) temperatures of control and cooled infants from the NICHD Body Cooling trial. (*From* Laptook A, Tyson J, Shankaran S, et al. Elevated temperature after hypoxic-ischemic encephalopathy: risk factor for adverse outcomes. Pediatrics 2008;122(3):491–99; with permission.)

Table 2
Secondary outcomes among survivors of brain hypothermia trials

	CoolCap		NICHD Body Cooling	
	Control n = 108[a]	Cool n = 110[a]	Control n = 103[a]	Cool n = 102
Survivors	68	72	68	78
Bayley mental developmental index <70	24 (39%)[b]	21 (30%)	24 (39%)	19 (25%)
Disabling cerebral palsy	21 (31%)	14 (19%)	19 (30%)	15 (19%)
Blindness	11 (17%)	7 (10%)	9 (14%)	5 (7%)
Hearing impairment	3 (5%)	5 (8%)	4 (6%)	3 (4%)

Some secondary outcomes are missing observations on all survivors.
[a] Number of infants are less than enrolled because of loss to follow-up.
[b] Number of infants (percent of survivors).

among secondary outcomes, the results are reassuring that therapeutic hypothermia did not increase the percent of infants with neurodevelopmental impairments relative to control infants. In both trials there were no differences in predefined adverse events between hypothermic and control groups.

IMPLEMENTATION AND DISSEMINATION OF THERAPEUTIC HYPOTHERMIA

There are important issues that have been recognized since publication of the Cool-Cap and NICHD Body Cooling trial that directly influence implementation and dissemination of therapeutic hypothermia. These include the deleterious effects of elevated temperatures, cooling on transport, early initiation of hypothermia, and late initiation of hypothermia.

Elevated Temperatures

In an observational analysis of the NICHD Body Cooling trial a broad range of esophageal temperatures were observed among infants in the noncooled control group.[58] Specifically 39% of infants had at least one esophageal temperature greater than or equal to 38°C. Of the 1690 temperatures recorded from infants in the noncooled control group (maximum of 19 temperatures per infant recorded over the 72-hour intervention), 8% of the values were greater than 38°C. Over this wide range of temperatures, relatively high esophageal temperatures were associated with increases in the odds of death or disability using logistic regression and adjusting for degree of encephalopathy, gender, race, and gestational age. The risk of death, or moderate or severe disability, was increased fourfold for every 1°C increase in the average of the highest quartile of esophageal temperatures. In secondary analyses of the CoolCap trial, elevated temperatures and similar associations with unfavorable outcome were reported.[59] Given that brain injury can be associated with disordered thermal regulation and elevated temperature,[60,61] it is unclear if the association between elevated temperature and adverse outcome is causal. In the absence of other data, core body temperatures should be monitored closely and timely interventions should be implemented to reduce elevated temperatures to normothermic values when hypothermia is not used (eg, during evaluations before initiation of hypothermia, if therapy is not available, or other contraindications to implementation).

Transport

Cooling on transport is a contentious issue and is advocated by some to allow earlier initiation of therapeutic hypothermia and potentially provide access to a therapy for centers that are geographically isolated. The CoolCap and NICHD Body Cooling trials did not provide cooling on transport. Cooling on transport has been used in a small randomized pilot trial of whole-body hypothermia (n = 65) performed by Eicher and colleagues.[62] The study intervention (hypothermia or normothermia) was initiated at the hospital of birth; for outborn infants the intervention was initiated by the transport team and continued on transport. Hypothermia was initiated with ice packs wrapped in wash cloths applied to the head and body for 2 hours and continued on a cooling blanket with a target temperature of 33°C (Cincinnati Sub-Zero, Cincinnati, OH). Two hours after enrollment the mean rectal temperature was 32.8 ± 1.4°C and target temperature was achieved by 5 hours in all hypothermic infants. Variability in rectal temperature was calculated as the average of the difference between the high and low temperatures; values were 2.5 ± 1.1°C and 1.6 ± .6°C at 2 to 24 hours and 25 to 48 hours, respectively. Implementation of hypothermia programs report the use of passive or active cooling on transport. In one report, 2 of 11 infants undergoing active cooling on transport without continuous rectal temperature monitoring had admission temperatures less than 30°C.[63]

Although these reports indicate that cooling can be performed and monitored on transport, the control of hypothermia and the effects of potentially fluctuating body and, therefore, brain temperature remain a concern. Requisites for adopting cooling on transport (active or passive) include a cooling mechanism that reliably cools infants in a systematic manner, continuous monitoring of temperature, absence of adverse effects, and associations with improved outcomes. The Infant Cooling Evaluation trial is an Australian cooling trial for HIE and may provide some of these answers. This study used cooling on transport for outborn patients to initiate therapy before 6 hours of age; enrolled infants (n = 110 hypothermic, n = 111 control) are currently in the follow-up phase.

Time to Initiate Therapy

Initiation of therapeutic hypothermia as early as possible is supported by most but not all animal data.[35–37,39] The challenge to initiating hypothermia shortly after birth relates to transitional physiologic events and verifying the presence of moderate or severe encephalopathy. Neonatal Resuscitation Program recommendations for resuscitation at birth are to minimize cold stress, which interferes with a successful transition from the placental-fetal circulation by preventing a fall in pulmonary vascular resistance. As indicated in **Table 2**, the majority of infants in the CoolCap and NICHD Body Cooling trials were enrolled between 3 and 6 hours of age; it remains unclear if cardio-pulmonary instability will be more frequent with earlier initiation of hypothermia. All hypothermia regimens include an assessment for the presence of neurologic abnormalities as part of the criteria to receive therapy. The neurologic examination in the hours after birth is a dynamic entity with the potential for improvement or deterioration over time. It is often difficult to perform a careful neurologic evaluation shortly after birth while critically ill infants are being stabilized. Of greater concern is whether early neurologic examinations (eg, at <1 or 2 hours after birth) can discriminate signs reflecting hypoxia-ischemia from maternal analgesia or anesthesia, or other nonhypoxic stressful events associated with labor and delivery. Severe encephalopathy is easier to recognize than moderate encephalopathy; whether practitioners in referring hospitals or transport team members have enough experience with neurologic examinations to reliably determine the presence of moderate encephalopathy is unclear. Early neurologic assessments may lead to treatment of infants who would not merit the intervention at 3 to 6 hours after birth.

Initiating therapeutic hypothermia after 6 hours of age is also a clinically important question. Some outborn infants cannot be transported to centers that provide therapeutic hypothermia because of geography or time of recognition. Other infants demonstrate progression of encephalopathy after 6 hours of age.[64] For human infants the duration of the therapeutic window is unknown and many variables such as nutritional state, hormonal status, extent of inflammation, and brain maturation may impact its length. A recent report describing how therapeutic hypothermia is being managed in the United Kingdom outside of a clinical trial indicates that a substantial number of infants have hypothermia initiated beyond 6 hours age.[65] A current NICHD study is attempting to study infants who merit hypothermia but do not present until after 6 hours of age by randomization to hypothermia or normothermic conditions and evaluating outcome at 18 to 22 months (ClinicalTrials.gov, CT00614744).

SUMMARY

The results of the CoolCap and NICHD Body Cooling trial are consistent and demonstrate beneficial effects of hypothermia in reducing death and adverse neurodevelopmental deficits in early childhood. Before these trials management of infants with HIE was best described as intensive supportive care; biochemical and physiologic abnormalities were corrected as adequately as possible and providers waited for brain function to improve without evolving to brain injury. Therapeutic hypothermia represents the only intervention which has been demonstrated to alter the outcome for term infants with HIE in randomized controlled trials. A workshop on hypothermia was conducted by the NICHD after publication of the CoolCap and Body Cooling trials to help clinicians put therapeutic hypothermia in perspective, recognize the knowledge gaps and limitations of the therapy, and urge centers that provide the therapy to follow a peer-reviewed protocol after proper training of providers.[66] Part of the rationale for these recommendations was to minimize the drift in adherence to clinical protocols and avoid adverse effects which may limit enthusiasm for what was termed a promising therapy. Pediatricians in community hospitals play an important role in determining access to therapeutic hypothermia for at-risk infants. Given that a high percentage of infants that receive therapeutic hypothermia are outborn, timely recognition of infants at risk, proper stabilization and attention to maintenance of normothermic temperatures, communication with referral centers with resources to provide this therapy, and proper care on transport will contribute to the benefits of this intervention.

REFERENCES

1. Narendran V, Hoath SB. Thermal management of the low birth weight infant: a cornerstone of neonatology. J Pediatr 1999;134(5):529–31.
2. Silverman WA, Fertig JW, Berger AP. The influence of the thermal environment upon the survival of newly born premature infants. Pediatrics 1958;22(5):876–86.
3. Jolly H, Molyneux P, Newell DJ. A controlled study of the effect of temperature on premature babies. J Pediatr 1962;60:889–94.
4. Day RL, Caliguiri L, Kamenski C, et al. Body temperature and survival of premature infants. Pediatrics 1964;34:171–81.
5. Buetow KC, Klein SW. Effect of maintenance of "normal" skin temperature on survival of infants of low birth weight. Pediatrics 1964;34:163–70.

6. Hey EN. The relation between environmental temperature and oxygen consumption in the new-born baby. J Physiol 1969;200(3):589–603.

7. Hill JR. The oxygen consumption of new-born and adult mammals. Its dependence on the oxygen tension in the inspired air and on the environmental temperature. J Physiol 1959;149:346–73.

8. Mahle WT, Clancy RR, Moss EM, et al. Neurodevelopmental outcome and lifestyle assessment in school-aged and adolescent children with hypoplastic left heart syndrome. Pediatrics 2000;105(5):1082–9.

9. Hope PL, Costello AM, Cady EB, et al. Cerebral energy metabolism studied with phosphorus NMR spectroscopy in normal and birth-asphyxiated infants. Lancet 1984;2(8399):366–70.

10. Lorek A, Takei Y, Cady EB, et al. Delayed ("secondary") cerebral energy failure after acute hypoxia-ischemia in the newborn piglet: continuous 48-hour studies by phosphorus magnetic resonance spectroscopy. Pediatr Res 1994;36(6):699–706.

11. Laptook AR, Corbett RJ, Uauy R, et al. Use of 31P magnetic resonance spectroscopy to characterize evolving brain damage after perinatal asphyxia. Neurology 1989;39(5):709–12.

12. Robertson NJ, Cowan FM, Cox IJ, et al. Brain alkaline intracellular pH after neonatal encephalopathy. Ann Neurol 2002;52(6):732–42.

13. Johnston MV, Trescher WH, Ishida A, et al. Neurobiology of hypoxic-ischemic injury in the developing brain. Pediatr Res 2001;49(6):735–41.

14. Siesjo BK, Bengtsson F. Calcium fluxes, calcium antagonists, and calcium-related pathology in brain ischemia, hypoglycemia, and spreading depression: a unifying hypothesis. J Cereb Blood Flow Metab 1989;9(2):127–40.

15. Fellman V, Raivio KO. Reperfusion injury as the mechanism of brain damage after perinatal asphyxia. Pediatr Res 1997;41(5):599–606.

16. Mehmet H, Yue X, Squier MV, et al. Increased apoptosis in the cingulate sulcus of newborn piglets following transient hypoxia-ischaemia is related to the degree of high energy phosphate depletion during the insult. Neurosci Lett 1994;181(1–2):121–5.

17. Tan WK, Williams CE, During MJ, et al. Accumulation of cytotoxins during the development of seizures and edema after hypoxic-ischemic injury in late gestation fetal sheep. Pediatr Res 1996;39(5):791–7.

18. Gluckman PD, Guan J, Williams C, et al. Asphyxial brain injury—the role of the IGF system. Mol Cell Endocrinol 1998;140(1–2):95–9.

19. Liu XH, Kwon D, Schielke GP, et al. Mice deficient in interleukin-1 converting enzyme are resistant to neonatal hypoxic-ischemic brain damage. J Cereb Blood Flow Metab 1999;19(10):1099–108.

20. Laptook AR, Corbett RJ, Sterett R, et al. Quantitative relationship between brain temperature and energy utilization rate measured in vivo using ^{31}P and ^{1}H magnetic resonance spectroscopy. Pediatr Res 1995;38(6):919–25.

21. Thoresen M, Satas S, Puka-Sundvall M, et al. Post-hypoxic hypothermia reduces cerebrocortical release of NO and excitotoxins. Neuroreport 1997;8(15):3359–62.

22. Edwards AD, Yue X, Squier MV, et al. Specific inhibition of apoptosis after cerebral hypoxia-ischaemia by moderate post-insult hypothermia. Biochem Biophys Res Commun 1995;217(3):1193–9.

23. Bergstedt K, Hu BR, Wieloch T. Postischaemic changes in protein synthesis in the rat brain: effects of hypothermia. Exp Brain Res 1993;95(1):91–9.

24. Yamashita K, Eguchi Y, Kajiwara K, et al. Mild hypothermia ameliorates ubiquitin synthesis and prevents delayed neuronal death in the gerbil hippocampus. Stroke 1991;22(12):1574–81.

25. Akisu M, Huseyinov A, Yalaz M, et al. Selective head cooling with hypothermia suppresses the generation of platelet-activating factor in cerebrospinal fluid of newborn infants with perinatal asphyxia. Prostaglandins Leukot Essent Fatty Acids 2003;69(1):45–50.

26. Lee YJ, Miyake S, Wakita H, et al. Protein SUMOylation is massively increased in hibernation torpor and is critical for the cytoprotection provided by ischemic pre-conditioning and hypothermia in SHSY5Y cells. J Cereb Blood Flow Metab 2007; 27(5):950–62.

27. Thoresen M, Penrice J, Lorek A, et al. Mild hypothermia after severe transient hypoxia-ischemia ameliorates delayed cerebral energy failure in the newborn piglet. Pediatr Res 1995;37(5):667–70.

28. Miller JA. Factors in neonatal resistance to anoxia. I. Temperature and survival of newborn guinea pigs under anoxia. Science 1949;110(2848):113–4.

29. Miller JA Jr, Miller FS, Westin B. Hypothermia in the treatment of asphyxia neona-torum. Biol Neonat 1964;6:148–63.

30. Cordey R, Chiolero R, Miller JA Jr. Resuscitation of neonates by hypothermia: report on 20 cases with acid-base determination on 10 cases and the long-term development of 33 cases. Resuscitation 1973;2(3):169–81.

31. Mann TP. Hypothermia in the newborn: a new syndrome? Lancet 1955;1:613–4.

32. Elliott RI, Mann TP. Neonatal cold injury due to accidental exposure to cold. Lancet 1957;272(6962):229–34.

33. American Academy of Pediatrics, American Heart Association. Neonatal resuscitation textbook. 5th edition. Elk Grove Village (IL): American Academy of Pediatrics; 2006.

34. Busto R, Dietrich WD, Globus MY, et al. Small differences in intraischemic brain temperature critically determine the extent of ischemic neuronal injury. J Cereb Blood Flow Metab 1987;7(6):729–38.

35. Gunn AJ, Gunn TR, de Haan HH, et al. Dramatic neuronal rescue with prolonged selective head cooling after ischemia in fetal lambs. J Clin Invest 1997;99(2): 248–56.

36. Gunn AJ, Gunn TR, Gunning MI, et al. Neuroprotection with prolonged head cooling started before postischemic seizures in fetal sheep. Pediatrics 1998;102(5): 1098–106.

37. Gunn AJ, Bennet L, Gunning MI, et al. Cerebral hypothermia is not neuroprotective when started after postischemic seizures in fetal sheep. Pediatr Res 1999; 46(3):274–80.

38. Iwata O, Iwata S, Thornton JS, et al. "Therapeutic time window" duration decreases with increasing severity of cerebral hypoxia-ischaemia under normo-thermia and delayed hypothermia in newborn piglets. Brain Res 2007;1154: 173–80.

39. Taylor DL, Mehmet H, Cady EB, et al. Improved neuroprotection with hypothermia delayed by 6 hours following cerebral hypoxia-ischemia in the 14-day-old rat. Pediatr Res 2002;51(1):13–9.

40. Laptook AR, Corbett RJ, Sterett R, et al. Modest hypothermia provides partial neuroprotection when used for immediate resuscitation after brain ischemia. Pediatr Res 1997;42(1):17–23.

41. Haaland K, Loberg EM, Steen PA, et al. Posthypoxic hypothermia in newborn piglets. Pediatr Res 1997;41(4 Pt 1):505–12.

42. Laptook AR, Corbett RJ, Burns DK, et al. A limited interval of delayed modest hypothermia for ischemic brain resuscitation is not beneficial in neonatal swine. Pediatr Res 1999;46(4):383–9.
43. Carroll M, Beek O. Protection against hippocampal CA1 cell loss by post-ischemic hypothermia is dependent on delay of initiation and duration. Metab Brain Dis 1992;7(1):45–50.
44. Coimbra C, Wieloch T. Moderate hypothermia mitigates neuronal damage in the rat brain when initiated several hours following transient cerebral ischemia. Acta Neuropathol 1994;87(4):325–31.
45. Colbourne F, Corbett D. Delayed and prolonged post-ischemic hypothermia is neuroprotective in the gerbil. Brain Res 1994;654(2):265–72.
46. Iwata O, Thornton JS, Sellwood MW, et al. Depth of delayed cooling alters neuro-protection pattern after hypoxia-ischemia. Ann Neurol 2005;58(1):75–87.
47. O'Brien FE, Iwata O, Thornton JS, et al. Delayed whole-body cooling to 33 or 35 degrees C and the development of impaired energy generation consequential to transient cerebral hypoxia-ischemia in the newborn piglet. Pediatrics 2006; 117(5):1549–59.
48. Laptook AR, Shalak L, Corbett RJ. Differences in brain temperature and cerebral blood flow during selective head versus whole-body cooling. Pediatrics 2001; 108(5):1103–10.
49. Thoresen M, Simmonds M, Satas S, et al. Effective selective head cooling during posthypoxic hypothermia in newborn piglets. Pediatr Res 2001;49(4):594–9.
50. Trescher WH, Ishiwa S, Johnston MV. Brief post-hypoxic-ischemic hypothermia markedly delays neonatal brain injury. Brain Dev 1997;19(5):326–38.
51. Dietrich WD, Busto R, Alonso O, et al. Intraischemic but not postischemic brain hypothermia protects chronically following global forebrain ischemia in rats. J Cereb Blood Flow Metab 1993;13(4):541–9.
52. Wagner BP, Nedelcu J, Martin E. Delayed postischemic hypothermia improves long-term behavioral outcome after cerebral hypoxia-ischemia in neonatal rats. Pediatr Res 2002;51(3):354–60.
53. Colbourne F, Corbett D. Delayed postischemic hypothermia: a six month survival study using behavioral and histological assessments of neuroprotection. J Neurosci 1995;15(11):7250–60.
54. Badawi N, Kurinczuk JJ, Keogh JM, et al. Intrapartum risk factors for newborn encephalopathy: the Western Australian case-control study. BMJ 1998; 317(7172):1554–8.
55. Gluckman PD, Wyatt JS, Azzopardi D, et al. Selective head cooling with mild systemic hypothermia after neonatal encephalopathy: multicentre randomised trial. Lancet 2005;365(9460):663–70.
56. Shankaran S, Laptook AR, Ehrenkranz RA, et al. Whole-body hypothermia for neonates with hypoxic-ischemic encephalopathy. N Engl J Med 2005;353(15): 1574–84.
57. Sarnat HB, Sarnat MS. Neonatal encephalopathy following fetal distress. A clinical and electroencephalographic study. Arch Neurol 1976;33(10):696–705.
58. Laptook A, Tyson J, Shankaran S, et al. Elevated temperature after hypoxic-ischemic encephalopathy: risk factor for adverse outcomes. Pediatrics 2008; 122(3):491–9.
59. Wyatt JS, Gluckman PD, Liu PY, et al. Determinants of outcomes after head cooling for neonatal encephalopathy. Pediatrics 2007;119(5):912–21.
60. Mellergard P, Nordstrom CH. Intracerebral temperature in neurosurgical patients. Neurosurgery 1991;28(5):709–13.

61. Rossi S, Roncati Zanier I, Mauri I, et al. Brain temperature, body core temperature, and intracranial pressure in acute cerebral damage. J Neurol Neurosurg Psychiatry 2001;71:448–54.
62. Eicher DJ, Wagner CL, Katikaneni LP, et al. Moderate hypothermia in neonatal encephalopathy: efficacy outcomes. Pediatr Neurol 2005;32(1):11–7.
63. Zanelli SA, Naylor M, Dobbins N, et al. Implementation of a 'Hypothermia for HIE' program: 2-year experience in a single NICU. J Perinatol 2008;28(3):171–5.
64. Shalak LF, Laptook AR, Velaphi SC, et al. Amplitude-integrated electroencephalography coupled with an early neurologic examination enhances prediction of term infants at risk for persistent encephalopathy. Pediatrics 2003;111(2):351–7.
65. Azzopardi D, Strohm B, Edwards AD, et al. Treatment of asphyxiated newborns with moderate hypothermia in routine clinical practice: how cooling is managed in the UK outside a clinical trial. Arch Dis Child Fetal Neonatal Ed 2008; [epub ahead of print].
66. Higgins RD, Raju TN, Perlman J, et al. Hypothermia and perinatal asphyxia: executive summary of the National Institute of Child Health and Human Development workshop. J Pediatr 2006;148(2):170–5.

Regionalization and Mortality in Neonatal Intensive Care

Scott T. Holmstrom, BA[a,b], Ciaran S. Phibbs, PhD[a,b,c,d,e,*]

KEYWORDS

- Neonatal care • Infant mortality • Neonatal intensive care units
- Regional health planning • Health policy

According to the latest data from the American Academy of Pediatrics, there were more than 850 neonatal ICUs (NICUs) and 4300 neonatologists in the United States in 2008.[1] This growth is remarkable for a field that in 1960 consisted of a handful of pediatricians who were starting to focus on the care of neonates and an even smaller number of units that were providing special care. Truly "intensive" care was not actually provided until the mid-1960s. Rapid growth in expenditures has come with this growth in neonatal care. The March of Dimes estimated that $45 billion was spent on care for preterm and low birth weight infants in 2001.[2] The costs of this care are highly concentrated: a recent study looking at all deliveries in California found that slightly more than 1% of all newborns incurred more than half of all neonatal-related costs.[3] These costs are further concentrated among extremely premature infants. Schmitt and colleagues[4] reported that very low birth weight (VLBW, < 1500 g) infants incurred about one third of all infant costs. Most of the remaining high-cost cases are infants who have serious congenital anomalies requiring surgical treatment.

Although neonatal intensive care is expensive, it also is one of the great successes of modern medicine and is cost effective.[5] The neonatal mortality rate has dropped from 2.60% in 1960 to 0.69% in 2007.[6] Almost all this decline has resulted from declines in birth weight–specific mortality rates that coincide with the introduction of and advances in neonatal intensive care.[7,8] In fact, in recent years the number of

[a] Health Economics Resource Center, VA Palo Alto Health Care System, 795 Willow Road, Menlo Park, CA 94025, USA
[b] Center for Health Care Evaluation, VA Palo Alto Health Care System, 795 Willow Road, Menlo Park, CA 94205, USA
[c] Department of Pediatrics, Stanford University School of Medicine, 750 Welch Road, Suite 315, Stanford, CA 94304, USA
[d] Department of Health Research and Policy, HRP Redwood Building, Stanford University School of Medicine, Stanford, CA 94305, USA
[e] Center for Primary Care Outcomes Research, Stanford University School of Medicine, 117 Encina Commons, Stanford, CA 94305, USA
* Corresponding author. Health Economics Resource Center, VA Palo Alto Health Care System, 795 Willow Road, Menlo Park, CA 94025.
E-mail address: cphibbs@stanford.edu (C.S. Phibbs).

Pediatr Clin N Am 56 (2009) 617–630
doi:10.1016/j.pcl.2009.04.006
0031-3955/09/$ – see front matter. Published by Elsevier Inc.

pediatric.theclinics.com

extremely preterm births actually has increased in the United States. Preterm deliveries accounted for 12.8% of all births in 2006, a 20% increase since 1990.[9] **Table 1** shows neonatal mortality rates for various groups of infants over time. Of specific note is a marked decline in neonatal mortality during the first half of the 1990s that is attributable largely to two technologies: the advent of surfactant replacement therapy and the increased use of antenatal corticosteroid therapy in cases of suspected premature labor.[8,10]

From the perspective of health care policy, there is at this time (Spring, 2009) a reasonable chance for significant health policy reform in the near future. If there is health care reform, it is almost certain that there will be increased efforts to control costs. Given its effectiveness, it is unlikely that there will be any efforts to limit access to neonatal intensive care, but the large expenditures for neonatal intensive care make it likely that there will be efforts to control the costs of neonatal care and to improve the efficiency of the delivery system. Even if a major health care reform bill is not passed, there will be considerable pressure to control health care costs.

One potential for increasing the efficiency of neonatal intensive care is better regionalization, which has had a mixed history in the United States. As noted earlier, the increased use of technology associated with the introduction of neonatal intensive care in the late 1960s and the early 1970s contributed to a marked decline in infant mortality.[7] Early shortages of trained personnel and facilities led to the concentration of perinatal services in select hospitals, usually large, academic medical

Table 1
Infant mortality rates according to birth weight

Birth Weight	1960	1980	1990	1995	2000	2005
All birth weights	26.0	12.6	9.2	7.60	6.90	6.90
Less than 2500 g	190.3	—	78.1	65.3	60.2	57.6
Less than 1500 g	—	—	317.6	270.7	246.9	245.7
Less than 500 g	1000.0	1000.0	898.2	904.9	847.9	857.2
500–999 g	899.1	695.2	440.1	351.0	313.8	305.1
1000–1499 gr	553.4	223.7	97.9	69.6	60.9	58.1
1500–1999 grams	223.0	73.5	43.8	33.5	28.7	27.0
2000–2499 grams	61.0	26.0	17.8	13.7	11.9	10.9
2500 g or more	—	—	3.7	3.0	2.5	2.3
2500–2999 g	19.0	8.9	6.7	5.5	4.6	4.2
3000–3499 g	10.1	4.8	3.7	2.9	2.4	2.2
3500–3999 g	8.0	3.5	2.6	2.0	1.7	1.5
4000 g or more	—	—	2.4	2.0	1.6	1.6
4000–4499 g	8.3	3.4	2.2	1.8	1.5	1.5
4000–4999 g	—	—	2.5	2.2	2.1	2.2
5000 g or more	—	—	9.8	8.5	6.1[a]	4.6[a]
%VLBW (< 1500 g)	1.03	1.15	1.27	—	1.43	1.49
%LBW (2500 g)	6.82	6.84	6.97	—	7.57	8.19

[a] Considered unreliable because of small sample size.

Data from Buehler JW, Kleinman JC, Hogue CJ, et al. Birth weight-specific infant mortality, United States, 1960 and 1980. Public Health Rep 1987;102(2):151–61; and Health, United States, 2008. Hyattsville (MD): US Department of Health and Human Services, National Center for Health Statistics; 2008.

centers and/or children's hospitals, and to efforts to regionalize perinatal care formally.[11] The correlation of decreased infant mortality with well-equipped medical centers led to the later formal designation of tertiary (regional or level III) and intermediate (level II) NICUs.[12] Regional NICUs offer the most complex care available, whereas intermediate-level facilities are designed for infants weighing more than 1500 g who do not need assisted ventilation for more than brief durations. Facilities providing neonatal care are formally designated with guidelines about which types of services may be provided. Lower-level facilities maintain contractual relationships with higher-level units to ensure that high-risk births can be referred to tertiary care facilities.[13] This arrangement is the basis for the regionalized perinatal network originally proposed by the March of Dimes Birth Defects Foundation in 1976.[14] Since then, these guidelines have been revised and expanded to account better for the wide diversity of care that can now be provided.[15]

EFFECTS OF REGIONALIZATION

A large body of literature shows that better regionalization of neonatal care is associated with better outcomes. Numerous studies have shown that neonatal mortality is lower in hospitals with higher-level NICUs, especially among VLBW infants (< 1500 g).[16–35] Some selected key papers for regionalization are summarized in **Table 2**. A smaller but still significant body of literature has reported that mortality is lower in higher-volume hospitals, with volume variously defined by the number of deliveries, by the number of NICU discharges or patient days, and by the number of VLBW infants treated.[18,20,24,28,36] A few of these studies have jointly examined the effects of level of

Table 2
Results of selected studies of the effects of regionalization

Study	Result	Statistic
Phibbs, et al (2007)[28]	Lower levels of care and lower volumes are associated with significantly higher odds ratios for death	Odds ratio ranged from 1.19 to 2.72 when compared with high-level, high-volume facilities
Phibbs, et al (1996)[24]	Patients born in higher-level hospitals with higher volume had significantly better risk-adjusted neonatal mortality	Odds ratio ranged from 1.40 to 1.59 when compared with high-volume level III hospitals
Menard, et al (1998)[21]	Race- and birth weight–adjusted neonatal mortality is higher when the patient is born at lower-level hospitals	Adjusted relative risk for infants born in a level I or II versus a level III hospital was 1.66
Gortmaker, et al (1985)[35]	Hospitals with a level III NICU showed significantly better survival rates for VLBW infants than other hospitals	Survival was better for infants weighing 1000–1500 g ($P < .0001$); similar but smaller differences existed for infants weighing 750–1000 g
Warner, et al (2004)[29]	VLBW infants born in hospitals lacking subspecialty perinatal care units have significantly worse mortality than those born in hospitals with such units	Odds ratio 2.64 when controlling for demographic characteristics; odds ratio 1.96 when controlling for practice characteristics

care and patient volume and have found that both matter.[18,24,28] It is difficult to separate the effects of volume and level of care, because all the very large NICUs also are tertiary facilities, and none of the true tertiary centers are low volume. Although the authors have not published their results, they did attempt to investigate this correlation in conjunction with their recent paper in the *New England Journal of Medicine*.[28] Although the results are not conclusive, they suggest that volume may be more important than level of care for small to moderate volumes where there are many levels of care with similar volumes.

There is some inconsistency across the studies that examine the effects of levels of care and patient volume. Many, but not all, studies use the level of care and/or the patient volume at the delivery hospital, rather than the highest level of care received. The authors have looked specifically at this issue several times and have found consistently that the level of care and patient volume at the delivery hospital are a much more important determinant of outcome than the highest level received.[18,24,28] Other studies have examined the issue of antenatal versus neonatal transfer and found that antenatal transfer is associated with better outcomes.[34,37–40] The transfer of VLBW infants also has been shown to correlate with increased incidence of severe intraventricular hemorrhage, respiratory distress syndrome, patent ductus arteriosus, and nosocomial infections.[17,41] This finding makes intuitive sense, because optimal care starting before delivery can prevent a cascade of complications, leading to both better outcomes and shorter lengths of stay. It is also supported by some studies that have shown adverse effects associated with neonatal transfer.[17,37,41,42] Lee and colleagues[43] found that significant physiologic decline occurred during transfer.

There also is limited evidence that regionalization potentially could save money. Phibbs and colleagues[24] reported that high-risk deliveries in hospitals with high-volume, tertiary NICUs had lower costs, as well as lower mortality rates. This finding is consistent with the well-established principle of economy of scale.

One limitation of many studies that support regionalization is that their reliance on vital statistics data, essentially limiting the risk adjustment to birth weight and gestational age. As a result, studies that use only vital records data have a systematic bias against the big tertiary centers, because they cannot adjust for the selective referral of cases at higher risk resulting from factors not included in the risk model, such as serious congenital anomalies. Some of the more recent studies have used data that link the vital records data with hospital discharge abstracts, allowing much more complete risk adjustment.[18,24,28,44] The authors' work with these linked data indicate that the bias resulting from using only vital statistics data can be quite large, with changes of up to 65% in the odds ratios.[45] Although these studies are limited by the coding classifications in the International Classification of Diseases (ICD-9), these linked data do allow much more complete risk adjustment. Given the direction of the observed bias, and because the risk adjustment with the linked data studies is still imperfect, it is very likely that even these studies underestimate the potential gains from regionalization.

Most of the studies that have examined the effects of level of care or patient volume on neonatal outcomes have focused on the effects on mortality. The effects on other outcomes have very important policy implications. In addition to the large costs associated with neonatal intensive care, the long-term complications of neonatal intensive care are associated with significant societal costs.[46,47] Unanswered questions are whether the higher survival rates for deliveries at the big tertiary centers result in the survival of more infants who have serious long-term morbidity or whether better care reduces both mortality and the rates of serious complications. The ability to study this issue is limited by the availability of data: although the linked vital records–discharge abstract data do include the ICD-9 codes for the major outcomes that need to be monitored (eg, intraventricular hemorrhage, necrotizing enterocolitis, bronchopulmonary dysplasia, retinopathy of prematurity), the ICD-9 coding for these conditions gives limited information about the severity of the conditions. In their work using California data, the authors have observed negative associations between level of care and patient volume and these outcomes, but, because of the data limitations, they have not published their observations. Using the more detailed data available from the Canadian Neonatal Network, Synnes and colleagues[48] have reported that incidence of intraventricular hemorrhage was lower for deliveries occurring at big tertiary centers. Although there is not yet a definitive answer about the effect of neonatal care on the overall incidence of serious disabilities, the preliminary data seem to indicate that better regionalization would reduce the number of infants who have serious disabilities. More research is needed to provide a definitive answer to this important question.

Although it is clear that the level-of-care effects are driven by the availability of specific services, the reason why NICU patient volume matters is less clear cut. There are two relevant issues with respect to volume. First, sufficient volume is needed to develop adequate systems and to maintain the skills of all the skilled personnel who care for these infants, not only neonatologists. This consideration is particularly important for the nursing staff. Second, there are structural differences, because smaller units simply cannot provide certain types and levels of services. The clearest example is an obstetric service: a fairly large volume of deliveries is needed to make dedicated, continuous, on-the-unit, anesthesia coverage for the delivery service economically feasible. This coverage is important, because it greatly reduces the time needed to perform emergency cesarean sections, which can convert potential fetal deaths into live births and deliver in better condition those infants who would have survived with a longer time to delivery.[49] A dedicated anesthesia service is only one example of a long list of services that become economically feasible only when there is a sufficient demand for the services.

TRENDS IN DEREGIONALIZATION

Given the strong evidence that neonatal outcomes are better when care is regionalized effectively, what has happened with regionalized neonatal care in the United States is a policy puzzle. As noted earlier, as NICUs were developed in the 1960s and early 1970s, there were serious efforts to set up regionalized systems of care to provide access to the limited number of providers. As the number of neonatologist increased, it became feasible to open more NICUs, and this technology was diffused into an increasing number of community hospitals. Initially many of the NICUs in community hospitals were intermediate-level facilities. Over time, in addition to increasing in number, NICUs, have increased in size and in the sophistication of the care they provide, with many NICUs in community hospitals offering tertiary-level services.[27,28] Although some of the diffusion of NICUs was driven by a need for these services, many studies have shown that this deregionalization of neonatal care has resulted in a large increase in the proportion of high-risk newborns receiving care in low-volume units offering midlevel care[24,25,28,44,50–52] and a decrease in referrals to regional NICUs.[25,42,44] Although California may not be reflective of the entire country, by 2000 only 21.5% of the VLBW infants were being delivered in hospitals with a large, tertiary-level NICU.[28]

Although it is clear that some of the expansion of NICUs was needed to allow reasonable geographic access, a very large share of this expansion has been in urbanized areas within reasonable distance of an existing tertiary-level facility. In California in 1990 more than 80% of the smaller, lower-level NICUs were within 25 miles of an existing large tertiary facility, and this trend has only intensified over time.[24] This proliferation of NICUs also has meant that in many moderate-sized communities there are two or more smaller NICUs instead of a single large facility. In California in 2000 the authors found that 92% of VLBW deliveries occurred in geographic areas with at least 100 VLBW infants.[28] Although not everywhere is as urbanized as California, if treating 50 VLBW infants is considered as the threshold for a high-volume NICU, most VLBW deliveries (and other high-risk deliveries) occur in geographic areas where regionalization is feasible.

WHY HAS DEREGIONALIZATION OCCURRED?

Deregionalization has occurred for many reasons, and it would be very difficult, if not impossible to try to determine the actual causes and their relative influences. The authors believe that the community-level NICU expansion was fueled largely by the confluence of the increased availability of advanced technology and neonatologists, economic forces, liability concerns, and policy decisions. Community hospitals have multiple incentives to install new NICUs and to upgrade existing facilities, including the desire to provide better care for the infants who are born in their hospitals. In all likelihood, all the reasons discussed in later sections had an effect, as did some factors that are not discussed here. It also is likely that the relative effects of these various factors varied by region. The authors believe that concerns regarding professional liability played a major role in the diffusion of NICUs. Although most deliveries do not result in a NICU admission, obstetric practice standards and the legal environment have resulted in the recommendation that at least a level II NICU be available for backup for 25% to 33% of deliveries.[53] To avoid potential litigation issues, obstetric physicians in urban areas began demanding that the hospitals where they practiced open an NICU or face losing their practice altogether to hospitals that had an NICU. In addition to retaining existing deliveries, the opening of a NICU would strengthen the hospital's reputation and therefore would help increase the overall patient volume across all services. Additionally, NICUs have the potential to bring in substantial sums of money, given that a very large share of all hospitalizations in the United States are delivery related (each delivery results in at least two hospitalizations, more for multiple births). Thus, the logical course of action for many hospitals was to open an NICU, to increase revenue from birthing operations and simultaneously to raise the overall profile of the hospital.

The opening of an NICU in a community hospital can set off a cascade of expansion. Most NICUs in the United States make money. The general level of financial pressure that hospitals in the United States have experienced for many years has created strong incentives to expand profitable services. This increased profit can be used to support other, less profitable services that can further strengthen the reputation of the hospital. Thus, once a community hospital opens an NICU, the hospital has further financial incentives to expand/upgrade the NICU to generate more profit. A hospital with a higher-level NICU will draw more complex cases with higher reimbursement rates as well as less complex cases for which a backup NICU is advised.

Well-intentioned changes in public policy also have facilitated the growth of NICUs in community hospitals. The best example probably is the Medicaid disproportionate share program in many states. Because this additional reimbursement is tied to the share of a hospital's patients that are Medicaid or uninsured patients, these programs can create incentives for hospitals to attempt to expand their share of these patients. This incentive is especially strong for hospitals that are close to the thresholds for participation in disproportionate share programs. Because births account for the majority of Medicaid hospitalizations, expanding obstetric/neonatal programs is an easy way for hospitals to increase their share of Medicaid patients. A study of the introduction of a Medicaid disproportionate share program in California found an associated expansion of obstetric and neonatal programs.[54]

SUMMARY OF THE PROS AND CONS OF REGIONALIZATION

Because one cannot conduct a randomized trial to assess the effects of regionalization/deregionalization, it is not possible to make definitive conclusions. The available evidence does provide some indications, however. A reasonable question is whether the proliferation of NICUs into community hospitals has had a positive effect on patient outcomes, independent of the huge mortality effect of NICUs. The literature consistently shows that mortality is lower when high-risk deliveries occur in hospitals with any NICU, even a low-level, low-volume NICU, than when such deliveries take place in hospitals with no NICU. Thus, there is clearly some potential benefit of NICUs in community hospitals. The evidence also clearly shows that these infants would be much better off if they were delivered in hospitals with high-volume, high-level NICUs. Although one can argue that new technologies such as surfactant replacement therapy can narrow the gap between large- and small-volume facilities, this effect has not been demonstrated, and postsurfactant studies still show large mortality gradients.

The policy question comes down to a trade-off between better geographic access with more NICUs versus potentially lower mortality rates but less geographic access with a more regionalized system. As noted previously, at least in California, it would be feasible with reorganization to provide reasonable geographic access to hospitals with high-volume, tertiary-level NICUs for most VLBW (and other high-risk) deliveries. The real question is where the high-risk cases would deliver if the community hospital did not have an NICU. The available evidence indicates that virtually all of the VLBW infants that deliver in community hospitals after they open or upgrade an NICU were cases that previously would have delivered in a hospital with a high-volume, high-level NICU.[44,55] Baker and Phibbs[55] used a model to examine the mortality effect of opening low- to moderate-volume, mid-level NICUs in community hospitals and found that they resulted in a net increase in mortality for VLBW infants. Even though there is a large reduction in mortality for VLBW infants that previously would have delivered in a hospital with no NICU, the net effect is more deaths because so many of the VLBW deliveries previously would have delivered in a lower-mortality tertiary center.

Thus, unless geographic access is an issue, the limited evidence available indicates that lower neonatal mortality rates can be achieved with more regionalized systems of care. Phibbs and colleagues[28] estimated that, if 90% of the VLBW deliveries in the urban areas of California with at least 100 VLBW deliveries per year could be shifted to hospitals that treated at least 100 VLBW infants, VLBW mortality could be reduced by more than 20%. It has also been suggested that eliminating small NICUs would not limit the bed supply in most metropolitan statistical areas.[52] This solution would help the remaining NICUs maintain optimal volume.

IS IT FEASIBLE TO REGIONALIZE VERY LOW BIRTH WEIGHT DELIVERIES?

Given the evidence discussed in the previous sections, is it really feasible to concentrate all of the VLBW deliveries at a select number of hospitals? Such an effort would require a large increase in the transfer of mothers before delivery. The current situation dictates more frequent transfer of VLBW infants, which admittedly is hazardous. Given the shorter distances and travel times, it probably is possible to shift almost all VLBW deliveries within urban areas to large tertiary centers that have sufficient volume to support such a center. The only real exception would be when a women presents to the hospital so late in labor that she cannot be moved safely, and this situation could be minimized through appropriate protocols for the emergency medical transport systems. It is feasible to concentrate very large shares of the VLBW or extremely preterm deliveries in large, tertiary centers. The highest level of regionalization for a geographic area that the authors know of is found in unpublished data from Western Australia for 1996–2005, where about 95% of such deliveries occur in large tertiary centers.

LOW-RISK DELIVERIES

So far this discussion has focused on regionalization for high-risk deliveries. There is some limited evidence from Europe of a volume–outcome relationship for term, low-risk deliveries. Because mortality rates for term, low-risk deliveries are low, these studies, one from Norway, and one from the State of Hesse, Germany, are low-power studies.[56,57] Even so, both studies found a statistically significant increased mortality risk for term, low-risk deliveries that occurred in hospitals with low delivery volumes. These studies need to be replicated with much larger samples, and in North America, before any North American policy implications can be considered. If the findings are replicated, the policy implications are radical: that all deliveries—not just the highest-risk deliveries—should be regionalized. Given the medico-legal environment in the United States, if United States studies replicate these findings, it may be very difficult for small-volume delivery services to remain open except where geographic access is an issue. Such a consolidation would have radical implications for how neonatal care is organized: there is no point in having small to mid-sized NICUs in hospitals that do not have delivery services.

FEASIBILITY OF CONSOLIDATING NEONATAL ICUs

As noted earlier, most of the deregionalization of neonatal care has occurred in urban areas. This trend extends beyond the larger urban areas that have big tertiary centers; many moderate-size urban areas have sufficient volume to support one large tertiary center, but this volume is split among two or more hospitals that almost always are within a few miles of each other. Thus, there is the potential for consolidating NICUs into a smaller number of larger, possibly higher-level, NICUs, with minimal effect on geographic access. The existing evidence indicates that such a consolidation potentially could save many lives[28] and probably would reduce the rates of serious complications (eg, intraventricular hemorrhage[48]) and reduce costs.[24] Although there are many potential barriers to such a consolidation, the adverse impact on hospital finances for those that lose NICUs is probably the biggest obstacle. A simple way around this financial barrier would be to have the hospitals set up a joint venture to share the profits of a consolidated service. For example, say a mid-sized city has about 120 VLBW deliveries per year, spread across four hospitals. These four hospitals could form a joint venture for high-risk obstetric and neonatal care and could consolidate all such care at a single facility. This consolidation almost certainly would require new construction to expand one of the units to sufficient size. The shares of the joint venture could be determined by the current market shares for VLBW deliveries. Similar mechanisms could be used to facilitate the consolidation of smaller NICUs in larger urban areas.

In considering the potential for improved regionalization, it is important to remember that even if the system of perinatal care is fully re-regionalized, the overall demand for NICU patient days and neonatologists would remain basically the same because there still would be the same number of neonates to treat. This stable population makes the consolidation feasible. Increased regionalization could have some impact on the demand for care at the margin, but it is uncertain in which direction the change would move. Because most preterm infant deaths occur in the first days after birth, reductions in preterm-associated mortality will increase the demand for NICU care. Conversely, because it is likely that larger units will, on average, have lower complication rates, there also would be some reduction in demand for NICU care. The potential for increased efficiencies in large units also could reduce marginally the demand for neonatologists and neonatal nurses. The estimates of these offsetting effects are too imprecise to make any accurate projection about the net effect, but it is likely that any net change in demand will be small.

LOOKING TO THE FUTURE

Given the very strong evidence that outcomes for high-risk newborns are much better when the births occur in large tertiary centers, several policy aspects need to be considered. These considerations will be influenced both by possible policy changes and by the emergence of new technologies. The following sections discuss three areas that could have significant affects on neonatal care.

PERFORMANCE MEASUREMENT AND OUTCOMES REPORTING

For several years various organizations have tried to facilitate the production, dissemination, and use of data on the quality and value of health care. Medicare's Hospital Compare Web site is providing ever-increasing amounts of information about hospitals.[58] The National Quality Forum (NQF) and the Leapfrog Group have established various measures of hospital and health plan quality, including measures for neonatal intensive care.[59,60] Although reporting of these measures is voluntary, participation in some of them is quite high. The Joint Commission on the Accreditation of Healthcare Organizations also has developed various standards and is in the process of developing a comprehensive set of performance measures for pregnancy and newborn care. One of the authors (CSP) has seen the draft set of Joint Commission measures, and they include a measure on the appropriateness of high-risk deliveries at hospitals with lower-level NICUs. Given the Joint Commission's accrediting function, hospitals will have to report these data, but it is unclear at this time how much of information will be released to the public. Even if the data are not released to the public initially, the information could be released at some future date, given the trend toward increased public reporting. It is almost certain that over time there will be increased public reporting of hospital performance measures. For neonatology, these reports almost certainly will include process measures, such as whether the delivery of various types of high-risk infants (eg, < 32 weeks' gestation) should have occurred at particular hospitals, as well as outcomes measures, such as risk-adjusted mortality. To date, the reporting of risk-adjusted outcomes measures has been constrained by the limits of risk-adjustment methodology, but more outcomes measures are being reported every year.

The increased availability of performance data about hospitals could have significant effects on the organization of neonatal care. There almost certainly will be more public reporting that labels as inappropriate the delivery of at least some of the high-risk cases in hospitals that are not large tertiary centers. The current NQF measures for delivery have such a measure for infants with a birth weight of less than 1500 g. How the public and policy makers will react to this information is uncertain, but it could lead to increased pressure for these cases to deliver in "appropriate" settings, and that pressure could lead to better regionalization of neonatal care.

PAYMENT INCENTIVES

Many of the proposals for health care reform include various types of payment reform. One suggestion that is receiving a lot of attention is tying payment to performance. There are many different proposals in this arena, so the outcome is uncertain. Because the performance measures include measures about where high-risk deliveries occur, it is quite conceivable payment incentives or penalties could be associated with where high-risk deliveries occur. Thus, payment reform also could be used as a mechanism to improve regionalization of neonatal care. Some payment incentives are in place already: most notably, Medicare no longer pays hospitals higher diagnosis-related group payments for many nosocomial complications.

At least one perinatal policy group has suggested extending the Medicare mechanism to high-risk deliveries. Guidelines would be established for where the highest-risk infants should be born. The obvious candidates are VLBW/extremely preterm deliveries, but the guideline could be expanded to other conditions over time. Although the evidence supports higher levels of concentration, the draft that one author (CSP) has seen proposed that all such deliveries occur in a hospital with an established high-risk obstetric service (including at least one perinatologist based at that hospital) and an NICU that treats at least 50 VLBW infants per year. When any such delivery occurs at a hospital that does not meet this standard, there is a payment penalty (eg, 30%) for both the hospital and the physician. Obviously, there would have to be exceptions to the policy to allow for cases when it is not feasible to move the mother. These exceptions would need to include all cases in which the delivery occurred within a short period after the mother first presented to the hospital (eg, 2 hours), with adjustments based on travel time for rural areas. There also would need to be exceptions when other factors, such as weather, prevented a transport.

There also are payment proposals that have financial incentives instead of penalties. For example, it has been noted that obstetricians in community hospitals lose revenue if they refer a high-risk pregnancy to a tertiary center and the delivery occurs at the other hospital. There is some evidence that total costs for these high-risk deliveries are lower if the deliveries occur in high-volume, tertiary-level facilities, so there is a potential for savings that could be used to create financial incentives for appropriate maternal referral/transfers. If an obstetrician in a community hospital referred an expectant mother in preterm labor to a nearby tertiary center, and the woman actually delivered a preterm infant, the obstetrician could receive an explicit payment for making an appropriate referral.

There are many different proposals for linking payment to performance, both in terms of quality and in terms of efficiency. Regardless of what happens with health care reform, it is very likely that new payment mechanisms will be introduced, and these mechanisms could have significant impact on how neonatal care is organized and produced.

POTENTIAL PREVENTION OF PRETERM LABOR

The treatment of preterm infants represents the majority of NICU patient days. What if new technologies succeed in preventing most types of preterm labor? If most preterm labor could be prevented, the number of NICU patient days would drop by more than half. The result would be a dramatic reduction in the need for NICUs and neonatologists. Although it is not possible to identify the time frame, there is a very real possibility that in the not-too-distant future technologies will exist to prevent a significant amount of preterm labor. A trial already has showed a significant reduction in repeat preterm labor in a group of women at high risk for a repeat preterm delivery.[61]

If new treatments do succeed in reducing many preterm deliveries, the dramatic reductions in the demand for NICU patient days will require a major restructuring of the delivery systems for neonatal care. If no action is taken, the result would be a reduction in the patient volumes for all NICUs, which almost certainly would have adverse effects on patient outcomes over time. Basically, any reduction in the demand for NICU patient days will make the need to improve the regionalization of neonatal care more urgent. Given this potential, it is all the more imperative to move now to improve the regionalization of neonatal care. It will be far easier to consolidate NICUs if the demand is constant than it will be in the face of falling demand, which will result in the loss of jobs.

The potential to prevent preterm labor poses an important policy question: are too many neonatologists being trained? Some body such as the American Academy of Pediatrics needs to establish a committee to monitor this situation. It is better to start too early than too late, given that each trained neonatologist will have a long post-training career. Because the expansion of the number of neonatologists certainly has contributed to the deregionalization of neonatal care,[50,51] a good case can be made that the number of neonatologists being trained should be reduced as soon as possible. A moderate reduction in the supply might ease the pressures for deregionalization and would ease the potential oversupply that is likely to occur in the relatively near future. If too many neonatologists are being trained, action is needed to start reducing the number of neonatal training slots. This reduction will be a difficult process, because trainees provide relatively low-cost physician labor, but, it is a process that should begin soon.

SUMMARY

Health care reform is currently on the political agenda. The extent to which health care reform will affect the delivery of neonatal care will depend on the details of any reforms that emerge from the political process. The economic pressures for health care reform are large and growing; the economy simply cannot tolerate the increasing burdens of the current system of financing and delivering health care. Regardless of the outcome of the effort to reform the health care system, it is likely that there will be increased efforts to improve its efficiency. The current lack of fully regionalized neonatal care in most parts of the country clearly offers opportunities for improved efficiency. Any of the ideas expressed in this article, plus many others not discussed, could be imposed on the delivery system in an effort to improve the efficiency and/or to reduce the costs of neonatal care.

REFERENCES

1. In: Database Committee Report on 2008 United States & Canada Newborn Intensive Care Units (NICUs), Neonatologists, Perinatologists & Neonatal Nurse Practitioners (NNPs), 35. Newsletter of the Section on Perinatal Pediatrics American Academy of Pediatrics; 2009. p. 12–14.
2. Russell RB, Green NS, Steiner CA, et al. Cost of hospitalization for preterm and low birthweight infants in the United States. Pediatrics 2007;120(1):e1–9.
3. Schmitt SK, Sneed L, Phibbs CS. Costs of newborn care in California: a population-based study. Pediatrics 2006;117(1):154–60.

4. Phibbs C, Williams R, Phibbs R. Newborn risk factors and the costs of neonatal intensive care. Pediatrics 1981;68:313–21.
5. Cutler DM, Meara E. The technology of birth: is it worth it? In: Garber A, editor, Frontiers in health policy research, 3. Cambridge (MA): MIT Press; 2000. p. 33–67.
6. Health, United States, 2008. Hyattsville (MD): US Department of Health and Human Services, National Center for Health Statistics; 2008.
7. Wiliams RL, Chen PM. Identifying the sources of the recent decline in perinatal mortality rates in California. N Engl J Med 1982;306:207–14.
8. Horbar JD, Badger GJ, Carpenter JH, et al. Trends in mortality and morbidity for very low birth weight infants, 1991–1999. Pediatrics 2002;110(1 Pt 1):143–51.
9. Martin JA, Hamilton BE, Sutton PD, et al. Births, final data for 2006. National Vital Statistics Reports 2009;57(7).
10. Fanaroff AA, Wright LL, Stevenson DK, et al. Very-low-birth-weight outcomes of the National Institute of Child Health and Human Development Neonatal Research Network, May 1991 through December 1992. Am J Obstet Gynecol 1995;173(5):1423–31.
11. Merkatz IR, Johnson KG. Regionalization of perinatal care for the United States. Clin Perinatol 1976;3(2):271–6.
12. McCormick MC, Shapiro S, Starfield BH. The regionalization of perinatal services. Summary of the evaluation of a national demonstration program. JAMA 1985; 253(6):799–804.
13. Stark AR. Levels of neonatal care. Pediatrics 2004;114(5):1341–7.
14. Committee on Perinatal Health. Towards improving the outcome of pregnancy: recommendations for the regional development of maternal and perinatal health services. White Plains (NY): March of Dimes Birth Defects Foundation; 1977.
15. Committee on Perinatal Health. Toward improving the outcome of pregnancy: the 90s and beyond. White Plains (NY): March of Dimes Birth Defects Foundation; 1993.
16. Bode MM, O'Shea TM, Metzguer KR, et al. Perinatal regionalization and neonatal mortality in North Carolina, 1968–1994. Am J Obstet Gynecol 2001;184(6): 1302–7.
17. Chien LY, Whyte R, Aziz K, et al. Improved outcome of preterm infants when delivered in tertiary care centers. Obstet Gynecol 2001;98(2):247–52.
18. Cifuentes J, Bronstein J, Phibbs CS, et al. Mortality in low birth weight infants according to level of neonatal care at hospital of birth. Pediatrics 2002;109(5): 745–51.
19. Johansson S, Montgomery SM, Ekbom A, et al. Preterm delivery, level of care, and infant death in Sweden: a population-based study. Pediatrics 2004;113(5): 1230–5.
20. Mayfield JA, Rosenblatt RA, Baldwin LM, et al. The relation of obstetrical volume and nursery level to perinatal mortality. Am J Public Health 1990;80(7): 819–23.
21. Menard MK, Liu Q, Holgren EA, et al. Neonatal mortality for very low birth weight deliveries in South Carolina by level of hospital perinatal service. Am J Obstet Gynecol 1998;179(2):374–81.
22. Paneth N, Kiely J, Wallenstein S, et al. The choice of place of delivery. Effect of hospital level on mortality in all singleton births in New York City. Am J Dis Child 1987;141:60–4.
23. Paneth N, Kiely JL, Wallenstein S, et al. Newborn intensive care and neonatal mortality in low-birth-weight infants: a population study. N Engl J Med 1982; 307(3):149–55.

24. Phibbs C, Bronstein J, Buxton E, et al. The effect of patient volume and level of care at the hospital of birth on neonatal mortality. JAMA 1996;276:1054–9.

25. Powell S, Holt V, Hickok D, et al. Recent changes in delivery site of low-birth-weight infants in Washington: impact on birth weight-specific mortality. Am J Obstet Gynecol 1995;173:1585–92.

26. Verloove-Vanhorick S, Verwey R, Ebeling M, et al. Mortality in very preterm and very low birth weight infants according to place of birth and level of care: results of a national collaborative survey of preterm and very low birth weight infants in the Netherlands. Pediatrics 1988;81:404–11.

27. Yeast J, Poskin M, Stockbauer J, et al. Changing patterns in regionalization of perinatal care and the impact on neonatal mortality. Am J Obstet Gynecol 1998;178:131–5.

28. Phibbs CS, Baker LC, Caughey AB, et al. Level and volume of neonatal intensive care and mortality in very-low-birth-weight infants. N Engl J Med 2007;356(21): 2165–75.

29. Warner B, Musial MJ, Chenier T, et al. The effect of birth hospital type on the outcome of very low birth weight infants. Pediatrics 2004;113(1 Pt 1):35–41.

30. Williams RL. Measuring the effectiveness of perinatal medical care. Med Care 1979;17(2):95–110.

31. Samuelson JL, Buehler JW, Norris D, et al. Maternal characteristics associated with place of delivery and neonatal mortality rates among very-low-birthweight infants, Georgia. Paediatr Perinat Epidemiol 2002;16(4):305–13.

32. Sanderson M, Sappenfield WM, Jespersen KM, et al. Association between level of delivery hospital and neonatal outcomes among South Carolina Medicaid recipients. Am J Obstet Gynecol 2000;183(6):1504–11.

33. Rosenblatt RA, Mayfield JA, Hart LG, et al. Outcomes of regionalized perinatal care in Washington state. West J Med 1988;149(1):98–102.

34. Kirby R. The role of hospital of birth. J Perinatol 1996;16:43–9.

35. Gortmaker S, Sobol A, Clark C, et al. The survival of very low-birth weight infants by level of hospital of birth: a population study of perinatal systems in four states. Am J Obstet Gynecol 1985;152:517–24.

36. Kahn JM, Goss CH, Heagerty PJ, et al. Hospital volume and the outcomes of mechanical ventilation. N Engl J Med 2006;355(1):41–50.

37. Bowman E, Doyle LW, Murton LJ, et al. Increased mortality of preterm infants transferred between tertiary perinatal centres. BMJ 1988;297(6656):1098–100.

38. Empana JP, Subtil D, Truffert P. In-hospital mortality of newborn infants born before 33 weeks of gestation depends on the initial level of neonatal care: the EPIPAGE study. Acta Paediatr 2003;92(3):346–51.

39. Harris TR, Isaman J, Giles HR. Improved neonatal survival through maternal transport. Obstet Gynecol 1978;52(3):294–300.

40. Modanlou HD, Dorchester W, Freeman RK, et al. Perinatal transport to a regional perinatal center in a metropolitan area: maternal versus neonatal transport. Am J Obstet Gynecol 1980;138(8):1157–64.

41. Towers CV, Bonebrake R, Padilla G, et al. The effect of transport on the rate of severe intraventricular hemorrhage in very low birth weight infants. Obstet Gynecol 2000;95(2):291–5.

42. Paneth N, Keily J, Susser M. Age at death used to assess the effect of interhospital transfer of newborns. Pediatrics 1984;73:854–61.

43. Lee SK, Zupancic JA, Pendray M, et al. Transport risk index of physiologic stability: a practical system for assessing infant transport care. J Pediatr 2001; 139(2):220–6.

44. Haberland CA, Phibbs CS, Baker LC. Effect of opening midlevel neonatal intensive care units on the location of low birth weight births in California. Pediatrics 2006;118(6):e1667–79.
45. Phibbs CS. Regionalization and birth outcomes. Presented at the Robert Wood Johnson Foundation "The Secrets of Information for State Health Policy and Practice" Meeting. Atlanta, October, 1997.
46. Behrman RE, Butler AS. Preterm birth: causes, consequences, and prevention. Washington DC: National Academy Press; 2007.
47. Mangham LJ, Petrou S, Doyle LW, et al. The cost of preterm birth throughout childhood in England and Wales. Pediatrics 2009;123(2):e312–27.
48. Synnes AR, Macnab YC, Qiu Z, et al. Neonatal intensive care unit characteristics affect the incidence of severe intraventricular hemorrhage. Med Care 2006;44(8): 754–9.
49. Phibbs C, Baker L, Caughey A, et al. Level and volume of neonatal intensive care and mortality in very-low-birth-weight infants. N Engl J Med 2007;356(21): 2165–75. Available at: http://content.nejm.org/cgi/content/full/356/21/2165/DC1 Accessed May 24, 2007.
50. Goodman DC, Fisher ES, Little GA, et al. Are neonatal intensive care resources located according to need? Regional variation in neonatologists, beds, and low birth weight newborns. Pediatrics 2001;108(2):426–31.
51. Goodman DC, Fisher ES, Little GA, et al. The relation between the availability of neonatal intensive care and neonatal mortality. N Engl J Med 2002;346(20): 1538–44.
52. Howell EM, Richardson D, Ginsburg P, et al. Deregionalization of neonatal intensive care in urban areas. Am J Public Health 2002;92(1):119–24.
53. Phibbs C, Mark D, Luft H, et al. Choice of hospital for delivery: a comparison of high-risk and low-risk women. Health Serv Res 1993;28:201–22.
54. Duggan MG. Hospital ownership and public medical spending. Q J Econ 2000; 115(4):1343–73.
55. Baker L, Phibbs C. Managed care, technology adoption, and health care: the adoption of neonatal intensive care. Rand Journal of Economics 2002;33:524–48.
56. Heller G, Richardson DK, Schnell R, et al. Are we regionalized enough? Early-neonatal deaths in low-risk births by the size of delivery units in Hesse, Germany 1990–1999. Int J Epidemiol 2002;31(5):1061–8.
57. Moster D, Lie RT, Markestad T. Relation between size of delivery unit and neonatal death in low risk deliveries: population based study. Arch Dis Child Fetal Neonatal Ed 1999;80(3):F221–5.
58. Hospital compare—a quality tool provided by Medicare. Available at: http://www. hospitalcompare.hhs.gov. Accessed April 1, 2009.
59. The National Quality Forum. Available at: http://www.qualityforum.org/. Accessed April 1, 2009.
60. The Leapfrog Group. Available at: http://www.leapfroggroup.org/. Accessed April 1, 2009.
61. Meis PJ, Klebanoff M, Thom E, et al. Prevention of recurrent preterm delivery by 17 alpha-hydroxyprogesterone caproate. N Engl J Med 2003;348(24):2379–85.

Neurodevelopmental Outcome of the Premature Infant

Bonnie E. Stephens, MD[a,b,*], Betty R. Vohr, MD[a,b]

KEYWORDS

- Prematurity • Outcomes • Neurodevelopment • ELBW
- Late preterm

Advances in antenatal medicine and neonatal intensive care, including more aggressive delivery room resuscitation, surfactant use, antenatal corticosteroid utilization, improved ventilatory techniques, and nutritional management have successfully resulted in improved survival rates of preterm infants.[1–11] These improvements have been most dramatic in infants born extremely low birth weight (ELBW, ≤1000 g) and at the limits of viability (22 to 25 weeks).[1–3,5–8] But improvements in survival have not been accompanied by proportional reductions in the incidence of disability in this population.[2,4–7,9–15] Thus, survival is not an adequate measure of success in these infants who remain at high risk for neurodevelopmental and behavioral morbidities. The primary outcome of most neonatal clinical trials is long-term neurodevelopmental outcome.[16] Numerous authors have reported on the developmental outcomes of ELBW infants in infancy and early childhood[2,4–7,9–15,17–21] and there is now increasing evidence of sustained adverse outcomes into school age and adolescence,[22–49] not only for ELBW infants but for infants born late preterm.

EXTREMELY LOW BIRTH WEIGHT AND VERY LOW BIRTH WEIGHT INFANT SURVIVAL RATES

Survival rates for very low birth weight (VLBW; ≤1500 g) and ELBW infants consistently improved during the 1980s and 1990s.[1–4,6,9–11] The National Institute of Child Health and Human Development (NICHD) Neonatal Research Network reported an improvement in the survival of all VLBW infants from 77% in 1987/1988 to 86% in 1999/2000 in their multicenter network.[1] ELBW infants in the NICHD had similar improvements in survival from 37% in 1991 to 1994 to 43% in 1995 to 1998,[3] and in a single-center report from 49% in 1982 to 1989 to 67% in 1990 to 1998.[4,12] In the early 2000s survival rates have stabilized at approximately 85% for VLBW and 70% for ELBW infants.[12,50]

[a] Department of Pediatrics, Women and Infants Hospital, The Warren Alpert Medical School of Brown University, 101 Dudley Street, Providence, RI 02905, USA
[b] Neonatal Follow-up Program, Women and Infants Hospital, 101 Dudley Street, Providence, RI 02905, USA
* Corresponding author.
E-mail address: bstephens@wihri.org (B.E. Stephens).

Pediatr Clin N Am 56 (2009) 631–646
doi:10.1016/j.pcl.2009.03.005
0031-3955/09/$ – see front matter © 2009 Elsevier Inc. All rights reserved.

Survival remains directly proportional to gestational age and birth weight.[1,2,8,10,11,19,50–54] Although most early follow-up studies reported the outcomes of low birth weight infants weighing less than 2500 g, the improvement in survival has shifted the focus to VLBW infants weighing less than 1500 g, ELBW infants weighing less than 1000 g, and micropremies weighing less than 750 g. From 1987/1988 to 1999/2000, survival of infants weighing 500 to 750 g improved from 44% to 65%; for infants weighing 751 to 1000 g survival improved from 66% to 88%; and for 1001- to 1500-g infants from 87% to 93%, in the NICHD Neonatal Research Network.[1,8] Single centers have reported similar trends. One center reported improved survival of infants born weighing 500 to 749 g from 27% (1982 to 1989) to 48% (1990 to 1998) and infants born weighing 750 to 999 g from 66% to 85%.[4] Another center saw improvements from presurfactant use (1979 to 1985) to universal surfactant use (1989 to 1991) for all ELBW infants proportional to birth weight (500 to 599 g: 26% to 38%, 600 to 699 g: 23% to 62%, 700 to 799 g: 47% to 75%, 800 to 899 g: 63% to 82%, and 900 to 999 g: 83% to 87%). Again, survival rates have stabilized in the early 2000s, and remain directly proportional to gestational age. In a more recent NICHD report, these rates were 55% for 501- to 750-g infants, 88% for 751- to 1000-g infants, 94% for 1001- to 1250-g infants, and 96% for 1251- to 1500-g infants born 1997 to 2002.[50]

As the methodology for assessing gestational age has improved, there have been an increasing number of reports evaluating the effects of prematurity, rather than low birth weight. Preterm is defined as less than 37 weeks', very preterm is less than 32 weeks', and extremely preterm is defined as less than 28 weeks' gestation. Survival has continued to improve for even the tiniest preterm infants born at the limits of viability (22 to 25 weeks, < 800 g).[1,2,5,6] Emsley and colleagues[5] reported an increase in survival of 23- to 25-week infants from 27% (1984 to 1989) to 42% (1990 to 1994). O'Shea and colleagues[6] reported survival at 501 to 800 g improved from 20% (1979 to 1984) to 36% (1984 to 1989) to 59% (1989 to 1994) over a similar time period. In the NICHD Neonatal Research Network from 1987/1988 to 1999/2000, survival at 23 weeks improved from 23% to 30%, at 24 weeks from 34% to 59%, and at 25 weeks from 54% to 70%. For infants born weighing 501 to 600 g, survival increased from 21% to 39%; 601 to 700 g from 33% to 59%; and 701 to 800 g from 53% to 77%.[1] These survival rates vary worldwide, according to reviews of the world literature in 2000 by Hack and Fanaroff[2] and by Lorenz and colleagues.[7] Hack and Fanaroff report a range of survival at 23 weeks from 2% to 35%, at 24 weeks from 17% to 62%, and at 25 weeks from 35% to 72%; survival by birth weight varied similarly, with survival at less than 500 g ranging from 4% to 38%, 500 to 599 g from 4% to 38%, and at 600 to 699 g from 27% to 63%.[2] Lorenz and colleagues[7] reported ranges of survival by gestational age less than 26 weeks (14% to 76%) and birth weight less than 800 g (4% to 81%). Factors related to the variability in survival rates include differences in reporting (inclusion/exclusion of fetal deaths, survival to discharge home versus inclusion of postdischarge deaths), and differences in aggressiveness of antenatal and neonatal management (antenatal steroid use, cesarean section rates, delivery room resuscitation).[2] Survival rates are also consistently higher in girls than boys.[1,2,9,50,51,53] But these documented improvements in survival of VLBW and ELBW infants over the past 20 years have not been accompanied by proportional reductions in the incidence of disability in this population.[2,4–7,9–15]

NEURODEVELOPMENTAL OUTCOME

It has been almost universally accepted that neurodevelopmental outcome after preterm birth is the most important measure of neonatal ICU (NICU) success. Most large clinical trials in the field of neonatology now include a measure of neurodevelop-mental outcome. But no one optimal age of assessment has been agreed on. Because of the administrative challenges of long-term follow-up including cost, tracking, and feasibility, most authors have published data on shorter long-term outcomes (18 to 22 months corrected age). But there is now increasing evidence of adverse outcomes into school age and adolescence.[22-49]

NEURODEVELOPMENTAL IMPAIRMENT

Most published reports of neurodevelopmental outcome in infancy focus primarily on the incidence of severe disability, often defined as mental retardation, cerebral palsy, epilepsy, blindness, and/or moderate to severe hearing impairment.[2] This has histor-ically been the neurodevelopmental outcome of interest owing to the severity of the developmental impact of these severe and often combined morbidities. Unlike mortality rates, the incidence of these moderate to severe disabilities has not changed significantly over the past 20 years.[2,4-7,9-15] Rates are highest in ELBW populations, and like mortality rates, rates of disability generally increase with decreasing gesta-tional age and birth weight.[2,4-6,15,17,20] Hack and Fanaroff[2] report worldwide rates of severe disability in infants of 23 to 25 weeks' gestation of 34%, with rates at 24 weeks ranging from 22% to 45%, rates at 25 weeks ranging from 12% to 35%, and rates in infants born of less than 800-g birthweight of 9% to 37%. Lorenz and colleagues'[7] rates were slightly lower, with 22% disability at less than 26 weeks and 24% at less than 800 g. Factors related to the variability in reported rates of disability include vari-able rates of survival and neonatal complications, socioeconomic status of the popu-lation reported on, reporting on chronologic versus corrected age, variability in the definition of disability or in its clinical diagnosis, the child's age at follow-up, and vari-ability in follow-up rates.

In the NICHD Neonatal Research Network, rates of neurodevelopmental impairment (NDI) (defined as the presence of any of the following: moderate to severe cerebral palsy, cognitive or motor scores that fall more than 2 standard deviations below the population mean on standardized testing, bilateral hearing impairment requiring amplification or bilateral blindness) in Network Centers in the 1990s ranged from 28% to 40% in infants born at 27 to 32 weeks and 45% to 50% in infants born at 22 to 26 weeks.[15] Only 21% of all ELBW infants had no impairments (no cerebral palsy, normal cognitive and motor scores, no visual or hearing impairment) at 18 months.[13] Regional and local studies in the 1990s report similar wide ranges of major neurodevelopmental impairment rates, from 20% to 48%.[4,6,9,10,12,17,37]

Center variability in outcomes is related to rates of neonatal morbidities such as sepsis, necrotizing enterocolitis, grade 3-4 intraventricular hemorrhage, and broncho-pulmonary dysplasia and differences in management style including rates of adminis-tration of antenatal steroids, postnatal steroids, antibiotics, cesarean section rate, and use of ventilators.[21,55]

COGNITIVE OUTCOMES

The most common severe impairment seen in VLBW and ELBW infants at 18 and 30 months is cognitive impairment, defined as scores that are more than 2 standard devi-ations below the mean on standardized cognitive testing. Most follow-up studies of ELBW infants use the Bayley Scales of Infant Development II as the measure of cogni-tive functioning between 6 months and 3 years.[56] The Bayley has a mean score of 100 with a standard deviation of ± 15. Scores of less than 70 (more than 2 standard deviations below the mean) are considered severely impaired. When scoring a preterm infant using this assessment, corrected age (chronologic age − weeks of prematurity) is most often used until 30 months of age. Average score for ELBW infants at 18 to 22 months corrected age in the NICHD is 76[20] but varies from center to center with a range of 70 to 83.[21] Center and regional reports cite higher average MDIs. Wilson-Costello and Hack[4,10,12] report average MDIs of 84 to 86 in their cohort of infants weighing less than 1000 g born from 1982 to 2002 and 83 to 89 in a subset of infants weighing less than 750 g at 20-month follow-up. Wood and colleagues[57] reported similar results at 30 months corrected age in a cohort of 20- to 25-week infants in the United Kingdom whose average MDI was 84.

Like rates of neurodevelopmental impairment, rates of cognitive impairment vary worldwide, and are inversely proportional to gestational age and birth weight. World-wide rates of cognitive impairment throughout childhood range from 14% to 39% at 24 weeks, 10% to 30% at 25 weeks,[2] 4% to 24% at less than 26weeks, and 11% to 18% at less than 29 weeks.[5,14] In infants born weighing less than 800 g, rates of cognitive impairment range from 13% to 50%,[2,6,7,14,19] and at less than 1250 g the rate is 26%.[14] In the NICHD, rates of cognitive impairment are reported at 37% to 47% in 22- to 26-week infants,[13,15] 23% to 30% in 27- to 32-week infants,[15] and 34% to 37% in all infants weighing less than 1000 g.[20,58] Wilson-Costello and Hack[4,10,12] site 20% to 26% rates of cognitive impairment in their cohort of ELBW infants at 18 months. At 30 months corrected age, 30% of Wood and colleagues'[57] cohort had cognitive impairment.

But cognitive functioning in infancy may not be predictive of cognitive functioning later in life. The assessment of an infant's cognitive function is highly dependent on motor, language, and social-emotional development. Thus, cognitive assessment in infancy is not as accurate as cognitive assessment later in life. In fact, Hack and colleagues[30] found that MDI at 20 months corrected age was not predictive of cognitive functioning at 8 years of age in their cohort of 330 ELBW infants. Although mean MDI at 20 months was 76, mean cognitive score at 8 years was 88. Rates of cognitive impairment dropped from 39% at 20 months to 16% at 8 years. The positive predictive value of having a low cognitive score at 8 years (<70) given a low cognitive score at 20 months (<70) was only 0.37. Ment and colleagues[33] had similar findings in a cohort of VLBW infants. Mean expressive language scores increased from 88 at 3 years to 99 at 8 years of age and full-scale IQ increased from 90 to 96.

At school age, cognitive functioning is assessed using a variety of different measures including the Stanford Binet Intelligence Scale–4th edition, the Wechsler Preschool and Primary Scales of Intelligence–3rd edition (WPPSI), the Wechsler Intelligence Scale for Children (WISC-III), the Woodcock-Johnson Psycho-Educational Battery–Revised, the Differential Abilities Scales, the McCarthy Scales of Children's Abilities, the British Abilities Scale, and the Kaufman Assessment Battery of Child-hood. Each of these assessments provides an intelligence quotient (IQ) and subtest scores that allow for a limited assessment of specific areas of strengths and weak-nesses. These tests, like the Bayley, have a mean of 100 with a standard deviation of 15 in the general population. Mean IQ for VLBW and ELBW infants at school age (5 to 14 years) ranges from 82 to 105.[22–24,26,27,30,33,34,41–43] Although the mean IQ is within the average or low average range for children born ELBW or VLBW, they have significantly lower IQ scores than their normal birth weight peers (0.5 to 1.0 SD lower)[22,23,26,27,31,34,41–43] and significantly higher rates of cognitive impairment.[23–25] Cognitive scores are significantly correlated with gestational age and birth weight.[22,26,28,41] Although environmental factors such as type of health insurance, bilingual household, income level, single parent, teenage mother, and level of maternal education are known to have an impact on intelligence, differences in IQ between preterm and term controls persist after adjustment for these confounders.[59]

Although measures of intelligence in children at school age provide a reliable assessment of general cognitive functioning, they do not identify specific learning disabilities. In addition to impairments in global cognitive functioning, more subtle cognitive impairments are often detected in school age. These higher prevalence, lower severity dysfunctions reportedly occur in 50% to 70% of children born VLBW.[37] Children born VLBW or ELBW have relative impairments of executive functioning,[29,41,60,61] visual-motor skills,[61] and memory,[29,41] especially verbal memory.[32] They score lower on tests of academic achievement,[29,30,42] perceptual-organizational skills,[31,41] visual processing tasks,[31,41] and adaptive functioning[29,41] compared with their normal birth weight peers. Even ELBW infants without neurosensory or cognitive impairment have higher rates of learning disabilities,[26,27] especially in math,[31,41,43,62] ranging from 25% to 40%.[26,31]

Thus, it is not a surprise that ELBW infants have higher rates of academic underachievement and need for special education services.[25,26,34] While ELBW infants have mean scores on formal tests of academic achievement that fall within the normal range (94 to 105), they score lower than normal birth weight peers.[26,34] Teachers of VLBW infants report rates of below average school performance in all academic areas, ranging from 24% to 41%.[25,26,38,42] Approximately 25% of VLBW infants and 25% to 62% of ELBW infants receive special education services.[25,34,35,40,41,45] Between 15% and 34% required grade repetition.[35,36,41,43]

An increasing number of investigators have reported on cognitive and academic abilities of former VLBW and ELBW teenagers and young adults.[24,28,29,32,35,41,61,63] ELBW teens continue to have mean cognitive scores in the average to low average range but persist in having significantly lower cognitive and academic scores than teens born normal birth weight,[44–46] and significantly higher rates of cognitive impairment.[45,46] Cognitive differences are greatest in areas of visual-perceptual tasks.[44] Academic differences are seen in reading and mathematics.[44] As a result, only 56% to 74% of preterm children, significantly fewer than normal birth weight teens, graduate from high school.[45,46] Hack and colleagues'[46] report on a single-center cohort of VLBW infants showed significant gender differences in graduation rates: 66% of VLBW males compared with 75% for term males and 81% for VLBW females compared with 90% for term females.

MOTOR OUTCOMES

Another outcome of major concern is cerebral palsy. Extremely preterm infants are born during a period of active brain development and maturation, placing them at extremely high risk for brain injury from hypoxia, ischemia, undernutrition, and infection, which are associated with both intraventricular hemorrhage (IVH) and periventricular leukomalacia (PVL). PVL is injury to the periventricular white matter as a result of hypoperfusion and infarction. It is visualized radiographically as echolucency, echodensity, or cystic degeneration. Although IVH, ventriculomegaly at term, and cystic PVL are all associated with cerebral palsy, cystic PVL is the strongest predictor.[64]

Cerebral palsy is typically defined as a disorder of movement and posture that involves abnormalities in tone, reflexes, coordination and movement, delay in motor milestone achievement, and aberration in primitive reflexes.[64] Rates of cerebral palsy in ELBW vary from 5% to 30%[2,4–7,10,12–15,17–21,23,24,57,64,65] but are most commonly sited at 15% to 23%.[13,15,17,20,23,24,57,64,65] The most common form of cerebral palsy in this population is spastic diplegia, accounting for 40% to 50%

of all cases, followed by spastic quadriplegia, and hemiplegia.[17,57,64] This is not surprising, as PVL lesions involve injury to the white matter that contains the descending motor tracts for the lower extremities. More extensive lesions also involve upper extremity motor tracts.

Arguably more important than the location of impairment is the functional level of the affected infant. Level of gross motor function can be assessed and categorized using Palisano's Gross Motor Function Classification System.[66] This system was developed as a method for assessment of a child's motor function by direct observation of the child's gross motor performance. It describes a child's function, not the fluidity of his or her movements. Palisano's system classifies gross motor function on a 5-point scale. Normal function at 18 to 24 months is defined as Level 0 and involves the ability to walk at least 10 steps independently. An infant at Level 1 can sit with hands free, creep or crawl on hands and knees, pull to stand, and cruise or walk with hands held. Those at Level 2 use their hands for sitting support, creep on their stomach, and may pull to stand; those at Level 3 require external support to sit, roll, and may creep; and those at Level 4 maintain head control in a supported sitting position and can roll prone to supine. Level 5 is the inability to maintain antigravity movements of the head and trunk.[64,66] Although 27% of a cohort of ELBW infants diagnosed with cerebral palsy at 18 to 22 months had moderate to severe gross motor function (Level 3 to 5), 28% had gross motor function consistent with level 0 or 1 and were ambulatory.[64] It is important to remember that a diagnosis of cerebral palsy includes a wide spectrum of motor performance.

Although cerebral palsy is the most well known and potentially most disabling motor abnormality associated with prematurity, infants born preterm often demonstrate less severe differences in their neurologic development. During the first year of life, transient dystonia is a common deviation in the motor development of VLBW infants.[67–69] Transient dystonia was first described in 1972 by Drillien[68] as transient abnormalities on neurologic examination in close to half of all low birth weight infants (<2000 g) in the first year of life. The motor features described included increased extensor tone of the trunk and lower extremities and increased adductor tone in the lower extremities leading to shoulder retraction and hip rotation, persistent primitive reflexes, head lag on pull to sit, and delayed supportive responses. These signs disappear gradually between 8 and 12 months of age in 80% of infants in which they occur. The other 20% often go on to be diagnosed with cerebral palsy. More recently these transient findings have been re-described as occurring in 21% to 36% of preterm infants with a peak incidence at 7 months corrected age.[67,69] The presence of findings consistent with dystonia increases the risk of later cognitive and motor problems including cerebral palsy but have a low specificity, as they are transient in most infants.

At school age, low birth weight infants are more likely to have subtle neurologic impairment than their normal birth weight peers.[61,70] On exam, 10% to 11% of low birth weight infants have neurologic soft signs, a twofold increased risk compared with their normal birth weight peers.[23,71] Soft signs are defined as deviations in speech, balance, coordination, gait, tone, or fine motor or visual motor tasks that do not signify localized brain dysfunction. These soft signs are associated with an increased the risk of subnormal IQ, learning disabilities, attention deficit disorder, and internalizing and externalizing behaviors at 6 and 11 years.[71]

Assessment of motor outcomes should be performed at each follow-up visit with a formal neurologic exam. Many centers use a variation of the Amiel-Tison neurologic assessment.[72] This assessment includes a standardized evaluation of muscle tone, strength, reflexes, joint angles, and posture.

NEUROSENSORY OUTCOMES

Although much less common than cognitive and motor disabilities, rates of neurosensory disabilities are higher in ELBW infants than the general population. Unilateral or bilateral blindness occurs in 1% to 10% of ELBW infants.[2,4,6,7,10,12–15,17,19–21,57] Milder visual impairments including myopia and strabismus occur at rates of 9% to 25%.[5,20,21,57]

Hearing impairment requiring amplification is reported in 1% to 9% of ELBW infants.[2,4,5,10,12–15,17,19–21,57] Milder hearing impairment has been reported in 11% to 13%,[20,57] and when transient conductive or unilateral hearing loss is included, rates of milder impairment are as high as 28%.[21] These rates of neurosensory impairment persist at school age.[23,24,40] with some studies reporting even higher rates of hearing impairment of 14%.[30]

BEHAVIORAL AND PSYCHOLOGICAL SEQUELAE

Evaluations of behavior are routinely obtained in infancy and childhood by parent, teacher, or subject interviews with standardized measures of behavior, attention, adaptive skills, and depression. The Child Behavior Checklist[73] is a questionnaire designed to describe social competencies and emotional/behavioral issues of children and is commonly used in follow-up studies. It has a version for 1.5- to 5-year-olds and a version for ages 4 to 18, which has scores that were derived for withdrawn, somatic complaints, anxious/depressed, social problems, thought problems, attention problems, delinquent behavior, aggressive behavior, and the presence of any behavior problem. The Conners Rating Scales[74,75] are questionnaires designed for parents or teachers to describe symptoms of inattention, hyperactivity, and oppositionality in school-age children. Multiple different measures of childhood depression exist and have been studied in this population.

VLBW has been associated with a wide variety of behavioral and psychological diagnoses and disabilities. Recent concern has arisen that rates of Autism Spectrum Disorder (ASD) may be higher in ELBW infants than previously thought. Although low birth weight (< 2500 g) may result in a two- to threefold increase in the risk of ASD,[76,77] true risk of ASD in very preterm infants is unknown. Two prior studies have investigated rates of autistic characteristics in children born VLBW (<1500g). Indredavik and colleagues[48] demonstrated a trend toward higher scores on the Autism Spectrum Screening Questionnaire in a population of 56 children at 14 years of age who were born VLBW compared with full-term controls. Limperopoulos and colleagues[78] recently reported 25% of VLBW infants screen positive on the Modified Checklist for Autism in Toddlers (M-CHAT). However, the M-CHAT was developed for use in the general population and not for a high-risk population such as VLBW infants. In addition, no diagnostic confirmation was performed.[78] Further studies are needed to determine the true risk of autism in this population.

At school age (8 to 12 years old), parents and teachers of VLBW/ELBW infants report higher rates of inattention and hyperactivity,[22,25–27,36,39,41,47,48] with rates of 23% to 27% in VLBW and 33% to 37% in ELBW infants.[25,27,47,48] One quarter to one half of VLBW/ELBW infants have symptoms of anxiety and/or social withdrawal,[25,27] and at 12 to 14 years old, 8% to 14% meet criteria for generalized anxiety disorder, compared with 1% to 4% of peers.[47,48] At 12 to 14 years old, 25% to 28% of VLBWs meet criteria for a psychiatric disorder compared with 7% to 10% of peers.[47,48] At 17 and 20 years of age, ELBWs continue to score higher on measures of inattention, anxiety/depression, withdrawn behavior, and social problems.[44,49]

At 14 and 17 years of age, VLBW children score significantly lower on measures of self-esteem.[43,44] They report less confidence in their athletic, school, romantic, and job-related abilities.[44] At the age of 20 years, VLBW adults report lower rates of alcohol and drug use, sexual activity, and pregnancy than adults born normal birth weight.[46,49]

FUNCTIONAL OUTCOMES

A practical and clinically relevant approach to evaluating a child's neurodevelopment is to provide information on functional skills in daily living and health care status. Functional assessment is the process of determining a child's ability to perform the tasks of daily living and to fulfill the social roles expected of a physically and emotionally healthy child of the same age and culture. This includes tasks of feeding, dressing, bathing, maintaining continency, mobility, communication, play, and social interaction. The social roles expected include involvement with peers.

As a result of the high rates of cognitive, motor, neurosensory, and behavioral difficulties seen in children who were born VLBW, even in those without severe impairments, these children have higher rates of functional limitations than children who were born normal birth weight.[40]

Four functional outcome measures are currently available:[79–81] the Pediatric Evaluation of Disability Inventory (PEDI) for children 6 months to 7.5 years;[79] the Functional Independence Measure for Children (WeeFIM)[80,81] for children with and without disabilities through age 8 years; the Vineland Adaptive Behavior Scale (VABS), which measures communication, daily living, socialization, and motor skills in children birth to 18 years;[82] and the Battelle Developmental Inventory for children age 0 to 8 years.[83,84]

Although 93% of ELBW infants achieve sitting balance, 83% walk, and 86% feed themselves independently by 18 to 22 months corrected age, more subtle functional deficits become apparent later in life.[20] At 10 to 14 years of age, 27% of children who were VLBW and 32% of those who were ELBW report restricted physical activity; and 24% of VLBW and 29% of ELBW report they are unable to participate in sports.[40] Functional outcomes are considered particularly important by parents.

FACTORS ASSOCIATED WITH OUTCOME

Recent studies support that a combination of biologic and environmental factors contribute to survival and outcome of preterm infants. Tyson and colleagues[85] evaluated the effects of both low gestational age and gender on outcomes of ELBW infants. In a cohort of 4192 22- to 25-week gestation infants for whom the outcome was known at 18 to 22 months, 73% had died or had NDI. Factors significantly associated with an increased likelihood of a favorable outcome for infants 22- to 25-weeks' gestation who received intensive care were higher gestational age, higher birth weight, female gender, singleton, and antenatal steroids, all factors present at birth.

Multiple birth is an important risk factor for both death and NDI among VLBW infants.[18,86] In a recent NICHD Neonatal Network study, ELBW twins born from 1997 to 2005 were at increased risk of moderate to severe cerebral palsy (8.4% versus 6.3%), MDI less than 70 (39% versus 29.9%), NDI (45.1% versus 36.0%), and death or NDI (64% versus 53%) compared with singletons.[87]

Common neonatal morbidities, including bronchopulmonary dysplasia (BPD), retinopathy of prematurity, necrotizing enterocolitis, and infection, have also been associated with poor cognitive function and academic abilities in infancy and at school age.[55,88–94] Rates of neurodevelopmental impairment at 18 to 22 months corrected age is directly proportional to duration of need for mechanical ventilation in the

NICU.[18,55] BPD has been implicated as a risk factor for cerebral palsy in multiple studies.[91–93] It also has an independent negative effect on motor outcome at 3 years.[88]

Cranial ultrasound abnormalities including severe intraventricular hemorrhage (IVH), hydrocephalus, and periventricular leukomalacia (PVL) are the strongest predictors of cerebral palsy.[91–95] Multiple authors have reported a two- to sixfold increased risk of cerebral palsy associated with grade 3 to 4 IVH,[13,15,19,93,96,97] and a 3- to 10-fold increased risk of cerebral palsy associated with cystic PVL.[13,15,19,97] The presence of hydrocephalus may increase the risk by 12.2 times,[93] and the presence of PVL and hydrocephalus by 15.4 times.[97] According to results from the Indomethacin trial, 60% of ELBW infants with grade 3 to 4 IVH had cerebral palsy at 5 years of age and 92% required special services.[98]

Yet ultrasound, although helpful, lacks both sensitivity and specificity. In fact, IVH grade has been shown to account for only 5% of the variance in predicting major handicap.[92] Additionally, 6% to 9% of ELBW infants who demonstrate no abnormalities on cranial ultrasound have cerebral palsy at 18 to 22 months corrected age.[18,99] Recent studies have suggested that MRI may be more predictive of neurodevelopmental outcomes in preterm infants than cranial ultrasound.[100,101] But although MRI identifies more subtle white matter lesions than cranial ultrasound, it remains controversial whether MRI is superior in predicting outcomes.[102–105] In addition, MRI is expensive and less practical, requiring transportation and often sedation of the infant. Thus, more investigation into the identification of those individual infants who will most benefit from intervention services is needed.

LATE PRETERM

Although most neonatal outcomes research has focused on the ELBW infant, more recent studies have brought a long neglected population of infants to our attention, the late preterm population. During the 1990s the rates of delivery at 40 or more weeks' gestation decreased while rates of deliveries between 34 and 36 weeks increased steadily.[106] From 1990 to 2005 the rate of late preterm births increased from 7.3% to 9.1% of all births.[107] Compared with term infants, these late preterm infants have higher mortality rates.[108–110] They also have higher rates of neonatal morbidities such as respiratory distress, temperature instability, hypoglycemia, kernicteris, apnea, seizures, infection, and feeding problems.[107–109,111,112] All of these morbidities have the potential to have long-term neurodevelopmental sequelae. In addition, the brain of the late preterm infant is more immature than the term infant's brain. At 34 weeks there are significantly fewer gyri and sulci, and the brain weighs an estimated 60% of that of a term infant.[111] Although there is a large body of literature that addresses the neurodevelopmental outcome of VLBW and ELBW infants, there is a paucity of information published about the neurodevelopmental sequelae of late preterm birth. Infants born at 34 to 36 weeks are 3.39 times as likely as term infants to develop cerebral palsy and 1.25 times as likely to have cognitive impairment.[113] They are more likely to qualify for special needs preschool and are more likely to have problems with school readiness.[114] In kindergarten and first grade they have lower reading scores, teachers report math skills below those of their full-term peers, and they are more likely to qualify for special education services.[115]

SUMMARY

As more and more preterm infants are born and survive, more is known about their short- and long-term neurodevelopmental outcomes. Infants born preterm are at significantly higher risk for neonatal morbidities and subsequent adverse neurologic, developmental, learning, and behavioral sequelae.

REFERENCES

1. Fanaroff AA, Hack M, Walsh MC. The NICHD neonatal research network: changes in practice and outcomes during the first 15 years. Semin Perinatol 2003;27(4):281–7.
2. Hack M, Fanaroff AA. Outcomes of children of extremely low birthweight and gestational age in the 1990s. Semin Neonatol 2000;5(2):89–106.
3. Hintz SR, Poole WK, Wright LL, et al. Changes in mortality and morbidities among infants born at less than 25 weeks during the post-surfactant era. Arch Dis Child Fetal Neonatal Ed 2005;90(2):F128–33.
4. Wilson-Costello D, Friedman H, Minich N, et al. Improved survival rates with increased neurodevelopmental disability for extremely low birth weight infants in the 1990s. Pediatrics 2005;115(4):997–1003.
5. Emsley HC, Wardle SP, Sims DG, et al. Increased survival and deteriorating developmental outcome in 23 to 25 week old gestation infants, 1990–4 compared with 1984–9. Arch Dis Child Fetal Neonatal Ed 1998;78(2):F99–104.
6. O'Shea TM, Klinepeter KL, Goldstein DJ, et al. Survival and developmental disability in infants with birth weights of 501 to 800 grams, born between 1979 and 1994. Pediatrics 1997;100(6):982–6.
7. Lorenz JM, Wooliever DE, Jetton JR, et al. A quantitative review of mortality and developmental disability in extremely premature newborns. Arch Pediatr Adolesc Med 1998;152(5):425–35.
8. Lemons JA, Bauer CR, Oh W, et al. Very low birth weight outcomes of the National Institute of Child Health and Human Development Neonatal Research Network, January 1995 through December 1996. NICHD Neonatal Research Network. Pediatrics 2001;107(1):E1.
9. Blaymore-Bier J, Pezzullo J, Kim E, et al. Outcome of extremely low-birth-weight infants: 1980–1990. Acta Paediatr 1994;83(12):1244–8.
10. Hack M, Friedman H, Fanaroff AA. Outcomes of extremely low birth weight infants. Pediatrics 1996;98(5):931–7.
11. Piecuch RE, Leonard CH, Cooper BA, et al. Outcome of extremely low birth weight infants (500 to 999 grams) over a 12-year period. Pediatrics 1997;100(4):633–9.
12. Wilson-Costello D, Friedman H, Minich N, et al. Improved neurodevelopmental outcomes for extremely low birth weight infants in 2000–2002. Pediatrics 2007; 119(1):37–45.
13. Hintz SR, Kendrick DE, Vohr BR, et al. Changes in neurodevelopmental outcomes at 18 to 22 months' corrected age among infants of less than 25 weeks' gestational age born in 1993–1999. Pediatrics 2005;115(6):1645–51.
14. Vohr BR, Msall ME. Neuropsychological and functional outcomes of very low birth weight infants. Semin Perinatol 1997;21(3):202–20.
15. Vohr BR, Wright LL, Poole WK, et al. Neurodevelopmental outcomes of extremely low birth weight infants <32 weeks' gestation between 1993 and 1998. Pediatrics 2005;116(3):635–43.
16. Barrington KJ, Saigal S. Long-term caring for neonates. Paediatr Child Health 2006;11(5):265–6.
17. Hack M, Wilson-Costello D, Friedman H, et al. Neurodevelopment and predictors of outcomes of children with birth weights of less than 1000 g: 1992–1995. Arch Pediatr Adolesc Med 2000;154(7):725–31.

18. Laptook AR, O'Shea TM, Shankaran S, et al. Adverse neurodevelopmental outcomes among extremely low birth weight infants with a normal head ultrasound: prevalence and antecedents. Pediatrics 2005;115(3):673–80.
19. Shankaran S, Johnson Y, Langer JC, et al. Outcome of extremely-low-birth-weight infants at highest risk: gestational age < or =24 weeks, birth weight < or =750 g, and 1-minute Apgar < or =3. Am J Obstet Gynecol 2004;191(4):1084–91.
20. Vohr BR, Wright LL, Dusick AM, et al. Neurodevelopmental and functional outcomes of extremely low birth weight infants in the National Institute of Child Health and Human Development Neonatal Research Network, 1993–1994. Pediatrics 2000;105(6):1216–26.
21. Vohr BR, Wright LL, Dusick AM, et al. Center differences and outcomes of extremely low birth weight infants. Pediatrics 2004;113(4):781–9.
22. Bhutta AT, Cleves MA, Casey PH, et al. Cognitive and behavioral outcomes of school-aged children who were born preterm: a meta-analysis. JAMA 2002; 288(6):728–37.
23. Marlow N, Wolke D, Bracewell MA, et al. Neurologic and developmental disability at six years of age after extremely preterm birth. N Engl J Med 2005; 352(1):9–19.
24. Doyle LW, Anderson PJ. Improved neurosensory outcome at 8 years of age of extremely low birthweight children born in Victoria over three distinct eras. Arch Dis Child Fetal Neonatal Ed 2005;90(6):F484–8.
25. Horwood LJ, Mogridge N, Darlow BA. Cognitive, educational, and behavioural outcomes at 7 to 8 years in a national very low birthweight cohort. Arch Dis Child Fetal Neonatal Ed 1998;79(1):F12–20.
26. Anderson P, Doyle LW. Neurobehavioral outcomes of school-age children born extremely low birth weight or very preterm in the 1990s. JAMA 2003;289(24): 3264–72.
27. Whitfield MF, Grunau RV, Holsti L. Extremely premature (< or = 800 g) school-children: multiple areas of hidden disability. Arch Dis Child Fetal Neonatal Ed 1997;77(2):F85–90.
28. Taylor HG, Klein N, Hack M. School-age consequences of birth weight less than 750 g: a review and update. Dev Neuropsychol 2000;17(3):289–321.
29. Taylor HG, Klein N, Drotar D, et al. Consequences and risks of <1000-g birth weight for neuropsychological skills, achievement, and adaptive functioning. J Dev Behav Pediatr 2006;27(6):459–69.
30. Hack M, Taylor HG, Drotar D, et al. Poor predictive validity of the Bayley scales of infant development for cognitive function of extremely low birth weight children at school age. Pediatrics 2005;116(2):333–41.
31. Litt J, Taylor HG, Klein N, et al. Learning disabilities in children with very low birthweight: prevalence, neuropsychological correlates, and educational interventions. J Learn Disabil 2005;38(2):130–41.
32. Taylor GH, Klein NM, Minich NM, et al. Verbal memory deficits in children with less than 750 g birth weight. Child Neuropsychol 2000;6(1):49–63.
33. Ment LR, Vohr B, Allan W, et al. Change in cognitive function over time in very low-birth-weight infants. JAMA 2003;289(6):705–11.
34. Halsey CL, Collin MF, Anderson CL. Extremely low-birth-weight children and their peers. A comparison of school-age outcomes. Arch Pediatr Adolesc Med 1996;150(8):790–4.
35. Saigal S, den Ouden L, Wolke D, et al. School-age outcomes in children who were extremely low birth weight from four international population-based cohorts. Pediatrics 2003;112(4):943–50.

36. Klebanov PK, Brooks-Gunn J, McCormick MC. Classroom behavior of very low birth weight elementary school children. Pediatrics 1994;94(5):700–8.

37. Msall ME, Buck GM, Rogers BT, et al. Kindergarten readiness after extreme prematurity. Am J Dis Child 1992;146(11):1371–5.

38. O'Callaghan MJ, Burns YR, Gray PH, et al. School performance of ELBW children: a controlled study. Dev Med Child Neurol 1996;38(10):917–26.

39. Breslau N, Chilcoat HD. Psychiatric sequelae of low birth weight at 11 years of age. Biol Psychiatry 2000;47(11):1005–11.

40. Hack M, Taylor HG, Klein N, et al. Functional limitations and special health care needs of 10- to 14-year-old children weighing less than 750 grams at birth. Pediatrics 2000;106(3):554–60.

41. Taylor HG, Klein N, Minich NM, et al. Middle-school-age outcomes in children with very low birthweight. Child Dev 2000;71(6):1495–511.

42. Botting N, Powls A, Cooke RW, et al. Cognitive and educational outcome of very-low-birthweight children in early adolescence. Dev Med Child Neurol 1998; 40(10):652–60.

43. Rickards AL, Kelly EA, Doyle LW, et al. Cognition, academic progress, behavior and self-concept at 14 years of very low birth weight children. J Dev Behav Pediatr 2001;22(1):11–8.

44. Grunau RE, Whitfield MF, Fay TB. Psychosocial and academic characteristics of extremely low birth weight (< or =800 g) adolescents who are free of major impairment compared with term-born control subjects. Pediatrics 2004;114(6):e725–32.

45. Lefebvre F, Mazurier E, Tessier R. Cognitive and educational outcomes in early adulthood for infants weighing 1000 grams or less at birth. Acta Paediatr 2005; 94(6):733–40.

46. Hack M, Flannery DJ, Schluchter M, et al. Outcomes in young adulthood for very-low-birth-weight infants. N Engl J Med 2002;346(3):149–57.

47. Botting N, Powls A, Cooke RW, et al. Attention deficit hyperactivity disorders and other psychiatric outcomes in very low birthweight children at 12 years. J Child Psychol Psychiatry 1997;38(8):931–41.

48. Indredavik MS, Vik T, Heyerdahl S, et al. Psychiatric symptoms and disorders in adolescents with low birth weight. Arch Dis Child Fetal Neonatal Ed 2004;89(5): F445–50.

49. Hack M, Youngstrom EA, Cartar L, et al. Behavioral outcomes and evidence of psychopathology among very low birth weight infants at age 20 years. Pediatrics 2004;114(4):932–40.

50. Fanaroff AA, Stoll BJ, Wright LL, et al. Trends in neonatal morbidity and mortality for very low birthweight infants. Am J Obstet Gynecol 2007;196(2):147, e141–8.

51. El-Metwally D, Vohr B, Tucker R. Survival and neonatal morbidity at the limits of viability in the mid 1990s: 22 to 25 weeks. J Pediatr 2000;137(5):616–22.

52. Allen MC, Donohue PK, Dusman AE. The limit of viability–neonatal outcome of infants born at 22 to 25 weeks' gestation. N Engl J Med 1993;329(22):1597–601.

53. Costeloe K, Hennessy E, Gibson AT, et al. The EPICure study: outcomes to discharge from hospital for infants born at the threshold of viability. Pediatrics 2000;106(4):659–71.

54. Hack M, Horbar JD, Malloy MH, et al. Very low birth weight outcomes of the National Institute of Child Health and Human Development Neonatal Network. Pediatrics 1991;87(5):587–97.

55. Walsh MC, Morris BH, Wrage LA, et al. Extremely low birthweight neonates with protracted ventilation: mortality and 18-month neurodevelopmental outcomes. J Pediatr 2005;146(6):798–804.

56. Bayley N. Bayley scales of infant development-II. San Antonio (TX): Psychological Corporation; 1993.

57. Wood NS, Marlow N, Costeloe K, et al. Neurologic and developmental disability after extremely preterm birth. EPICure Study Group. N Engl J Med 2000;343(6): 378–84.

58. Stephens BE, Bann CM, Poole WK, et al. Neurodevelopmental impairment: predictors of its impact on the families of extremely low birth weight infants at 18 months. Infant Ment Health J 2009;29(6):570–87.

59. Breslau N, Johnson EO, Lucia VC. Academic achievement of low birthweight children at age 11: the role of cognitive abilities at school entry. J Abnorm Child Psychol 2001;29(4):273–9.

60. Anderson PJ, Doyle LW. Executive functioning in school-aged children who were born very preterm or with extremely low birth weight in the 1990s. Pediatrics 2004;114(1):50–7.

61. Marlow N, Hennessy EM, Bracewell MA, et al. Motor and executive function at 6 years of age after extremely preterm birth. Pediatrics 2007;120(4): 793–804.

62. Waber DP, McCormick MC. Late neuropsychological outcomes in preterm infants of normal IQ: selective vulnerability of the visual system. J Pediatr Psychol 1995;20(6):721–35.

63. Saigal S, Hoult LA, Streiner DL, et al. School difficulties at adolescence in a regional cohort of children who were extremely low birth weight. Pediatrics 2000;105(2):325–31.

64. Vohr BR, Msall ME, Wilson D, et al. Spectrum of gross motor function in extremely low birth weight children with cerebral palsy at 18 months of age. Pediatrics 2005;116(1):123–9.

65. Wood NS, Costeloe K, Gibson AT, et al. The EPICure study: associations and antecedents of neurological and developmental disability at 30 months of age following extremely preterm birth. Arch Dis Child Fetal Neonatal Ed 2005;90(2):F134–40.

66. Palisano R, Rosenbaum P, Walter S, et al. Development and reliability of a system to classify gross motor function in children with cerebral palsy. Dev Med Child Neurol 1997;39(4):214–23.

67. Bracewell M, Marlow N. Patterns of motor disability in very preterm children. Ment Retard Dev Disabil Res Rev 2002;8(4):241–8.

68. Drillien CM. Abnormal neurologic signs in the first year of life in low-birthweight infants: possible prognostic significance. Dev Med Child Neurol 1972;14(5): 575–84.

69. Pederson SJ, Sommerfelt K, Markestad T. Early motor development of premature infants with birth weight <2000g. Acta Paediatr 2000;89:1456–61.

70. Marlow N, Roberts BL, Cooke RW. Motor skills in extremely low birthweight children at the age of 6 years. Arch Dis Child 1989;64(6):839–47.

71. Breslau N, Chilcoat HD, Johnson EO, et al. Neurologic soft signs and low birthweight: their association and neuropsychiatric implications. Biol Psychiatry 2000;47(1):71–9.

72. Amiel-Tison C. Neuromotor status. In: Taeusch HW, Yogman MW, editors. Follow-up management of the high-risk infant. Boston: Little, Brown & Company; 1987. p. 115–26.

73. Achenbach TM. Manual for the child behavior checklist/4-18 and 1991 profile. Burlington (VT): University of Vermont Department of Psychiatry; 1991.

74. Gianarris WJ, Golden CJ, Greene L. The Conners' parent rating scales: a critical review of the literature. Clin Psychol Rev 2001;21(7):1061–93.

75. Goyette CH, Conners CK, Ulrich RF. Normative data on revised Conners parent and teacher rating scales. J Abnorm Child Psychol 1978;6(2):221–36.

76. Kolevzon A, Gross R, Reichenberg A. Prenatal and perinatal risk factors for autism: a review and integration of findings. Arch Pediatr Adolesc Med 2007; 161(4):326–33.

77. Schendel D, Bhasin TK. Birth weight and gestational age characteristics of children with autism, including a comparison with other developmental disabilities. Pediatrics 2008;121(6):1155–64.

78. Limperopoulos C, Bassan H, Sullivan NR, et al. Positive screening for autism in ex-preterm infants: prevalence and risk factors. Pediatrics 2008;121(4): 758–65.

79. Feldman AB, Haley SM, Coryell J. Concurrent and construct validity of the pediatric evaluation of disability inventory. Phys Ther 1990;70(10):602–10.

80. Msall ME, DiGaudio K, Duffy LC, et al. WeeFIM. Normative sample of an instrument for tracking functional independence in children. Clin Pediatr (Phila) 1994; 33(7):431–8.

81. Msall ME, DiGaudio K, Rogers BT, et al. The functional independence measure for children (WeeFIM). Conceptual basis and pilot use in children with developmental disabilities. Clin Pediatr (Phila) 1994;33(7):421–30.

82. Sparrow SS, Cicchetti DV. Diagnostic uses of the Vineland adaptive behavior scales. J Pediatr Psychol 1985;10(2):215–25.

83. Berls AT, McEwen IR. Battelle developmental inventory. Phys Ther 1999;79(8): 776–83.

84. Glascoe FP, Byrne KE. The usefulness of the Battelle developmental inventory screening test. Clin Pediatr (Phila) 1993;32(5):273–80.

85. Tyson JE, Parikh NA, Langer J, et al. Intensive care for extreme prematurity—moving beyond gestational age. N Engl J Med 2008;358(16):1672–81.

86. Pharoah PO. Neurological outcome in twins. Semin Neonatol 2002;7(3): 223–30.

87. Wadhawan R, Oh W, Perritt RL, et al. Twin gestation and neurodevelopmental outcome in extremely low birth weight infants. Pediatrics 2009;123: e220–7.

88. Singer L, Yamashita T, Lilien L, et al. A longitudinal study of developmental outcome of infants with bronchopulmonary dysplasia and very low birth weight. Pediatrics 1997;100(6):987–93.

89. Taylor HG, Klein N, Schatschneider C, et al. Predictors of early school age outcomes in very low birth weight children. J Dev Behav Pediatr 1998;19(4): 235–43.

90. Schmidt B, Asztalos EV, Roberts RS, et al. Impact of bronchopulmonary dysplasia, brain injury, and severe retinopathy on the outcome of extremely low-birth-weight infants at 18 months: results from the trial of indomethacin prophylaxis in preterms. JAMA 2003;289(9):1124–9.

91. Allan WC, Vohr B, Makuch RW, et al. Antecedents of cerebral palsy in a multicenter trial of indomethacin for intraventricular hemorrhage. Arch Pediatr Adolesc Med 1997;151(6):580–5.

92. Ambalavanan N, Nelson KG, Alexander G, et al. Prediction of neurologic morbidity in extremely low birth weight infants. J Perinatol 2000;20(8 Pt 1): 496–503.

93. Msall ME, Buck GM, Rogers BT, et al. Risk factors for major neurodevelopmental impairments and need for special education resources in extremely premature infants. J Pediatr 1991;119(4):606–14.

94. Wilson-Costello D, Borawski E, Friedman H, et al. Perinatal correlates of cerebral palsy and other neurologic impairment among very low birth weight children. Pediatrics 1998;102(2 Pt 1):315–22.

95. Pinto-Martin JA, Riolo S, Cnaan A, et al. Cranial ultrasound prediction of disabling and nondisabling cerebral palsy at age two in a low birth weight population. Pediatrics 1995;95(2):249–54.

96. Grether JK, Nelson KB, Emery ES 3rd, et al. Prenatal and perinatal factors and cerebral palsy in very low birth weight infants. J Pediatr 1996;128(3):407–14.

97. Ment LR, Bada HS, Barnes P, et al. Practice parameter: neuroimaging of the neonate: report of the Quality Standards Subcommittee of the American Academy of Neurology and the Practice Committee of the Child Neurology Society. Neurology 2002;58(12):1726–38.

98. Ment LR, Allan WC, Makuch RW, et al. Grade 3 to 4 intraventricular hemorrhage and Bayley scores predict outcome. Pediatrics 2005;116(6):1597–8, author reply 1598.

99. Aziz K, Vickar DB, Sauve RS, et al. Province-based study of neurologic disability of children weighing 500 through 1249 grams at birth in relation to neonatal cerebral ultrasound findings. Pediatrics 1995;95(6):837–44.

100. Woodward TS, Meier B, Cairo TA, et al. Temporo-prefrontal coordination increases when semantic associations are strongly encoded. Neuropsychologia 2006;44(12):2308–14.

101. Inder TE, Warfield SK, Wang H, et al. Abnormal cerebral structure is present at term in premature infants. Pediatrics 2005;115(2):286–94.

102. Dammann O, Leviton A. Neuroimaging and the prediction of outcomes in preterm infants. N Engl J Med 2006;355(7):727–9.

103. Hintz SR, O'Shea M. Neuroimaging and neurodevelopmental outcomes in preterm infants. Semin Perinatol 2008;32(1):11–9.

104. Mirmiran M, Barnes PD, Keller K, et al. Neonatal brain magnetic resonance imaging before discharge is better than serial cranial ultrasound in predicting cerebral palsy in very low birth weight preterm infants. Pediatrics 2004;114(4):992–8.

105. Woodward LJ, Anderson PJ, Austin NC, et al. Neonatal MRI to predict neurodevelopmental outcomes in preterm infants. N Engl J Med 2006;355(7):685–94.

106. Davidoff MJ, Dias T, Damus K, et al. Changes in the gestational age distribution among U.S. singleton births: impact on rates of late preterm birth, 1992 to 2002. Semin Perinatol 2006;30(1):8–15.

107. Engle WA, Tomashek KM, Wallman C. "Late-preterm" infants: a population at risk. Pediatrics 2007;120(6):1390–401.

108. Khashu M, Narayanan M, Bhargava S, et al. Perinatal outcomes associated with preterm birth at 33 to 36 weeks' gestation: a population-based cohort study. Pediatrics 2009;123(1):109–13.

109. McIntire DD, Leveno KJ. Neonatal mortality and morbidity rates in late preterm births compared with births at term. Obstet Gynecol 2008;111(1):35–41.

110. Tomashek KM, Shapiro-Mendoza CK, Davidoff MJ, et al. Differences in mortality between late-preterm and term singleton infants in the United States, 1995–2002. J Pediatr 2007;151(5):450–6, 456. e451.

111. Raju TN, Higgins RD, Stark AR, et al. Optimizing care and outcome for late-preterm (near-term) infants: a summary of the workshop sponsored by the National Institute of Child Health and Human Development. Pediatrics 2006;118(3):1207–14.

112. Bastek JA, Sammel MD, Pare E, et al. Adverse neonatal outcomes: examining the risks between preterm, late preterm, and term infants. Am J Obstet Gynecol 2008;199(4):367, e361–8.
113. Petrini JR, Dias T, McCormick MC, et al. Increased risk of adverse neurological development for late preterm infants. J Pediatr 2009;154(2):169–76.e3.
114. Adams-Chapman I. Neurodevelopmental outcome of the late preterm infant. Clin Perinatol 2006;33(4):947–64 [Abstract xi].
115. Chyi LJ, Lee HC, Hintz SR, et al. School outcomes of late preterm infants: special needs and challenges for infants born at 32 to 36 weeks gestation. J Pediatr 2008;153(1):25–31.

Commonly Encountered Surgical Problems in the Fetus and Neonate

Emily F. Durkin, MD[a], Aimen Shaaban, MD[b],*

KEYWORDS

- Surgery • Neonate • Fetus • Prenatal • Congenital • Review

Profound scientific and technical advances in perinatal and neonatal care allow critically ill fetal and neonatal patients to survive to the point where surgical intervention is possible. As a result, neonatal surgical care requires a current understanding of pre- and postnatal intervention for a myriad of congenital anomalies. The following article summarizes the recent advances and controversies surrounding commonly encountered fetal and neonatal surgical problems. An attempt has been made to expand the discussion in certain areas where uncertainty persists and to offer traditional guidance in other areas. The authors hope that this article provides a useful tool for those unfamiliar with fetal and neonatal surgical care as well as a focus for discussion among those with such expertise.

NONCARDIAC THORACIC SURGERY
Congenital Cystic Adenomatous Malformation and Bronchopulmonary Sequestration

Congenital cystic adenomatoid malformation (CCAM) and bronchopulmonary sequestration (BPS) are relatively rare fetal pulmonary malformations that are most frequently and easily diagnosed on routine prenatal ultrasound imaging. Either lesion usually presents in the fetus as a space occupying, echodense and/or cystic mass in the fetal thorax. Grossly, a CCAM represents a multicystic mass of pulmonary tissue with proliferation of bronchial elements.[1] These lesions may result from a failure of maturation of bronchiolar structures or focal pulmonary dysplasia arising in the fifth or sixth week of gestation. Histologic examination reveals overgrowth of terminal respiratory bronchioles that form cysts of various sizes with rapid vascular and

[a] Department of Surgery, University of Wisconsin, School of Medicine and Public Health, H4/325 Clinical Science Center, 600 Highland Avenue, Madison, WI 53798, USA
[b] Department of Surgery, University of Iowa, Carver College of Medicine, 1500 JCP, 200 Hawkins Drive, Iowa City, IA 52242, USA
* Corresponding author.
E-mail address: aimen-shaaban@uiowa.edu (A. Shaaban).

Pediatr Clin N Am 56 (2009) 647–669
doi:10.1016/j.pcl.2009.05.001
0031-3955/09/$ – see front matter © 2009 Elsevier Inc. All rights reserved.

epithelial growth within the tumor.[2,3] By definition, a CCAM communicates with the bronchopulmonary tree and has a normal arterial supply, though variations have been described.[4–6] In contrast, a BPS is a mass of nonfunctioning, histologically normal lung tissue that is supplied by an anomalous systemic artery and does not have a connection to the native tracheobronchial tree. A BPS can be diagnosed prenatally if a systemic arterial supply to the lesion is detected by color Doppler. However, if this finding is not seen, a BPS may be indistinguishable from a CCAM.

The incidence of CCAM occurs equally in both lungs but more commonly in the lower lobes.[7] Gender distribution is nearly equal. Associated anomalies are common and include renal agenesis or dysgenesis, truncus arteriosus, tetralogy of Fallot, jejunal atresia, congenital diaphragmatic hernia (CDH), hydrocephalus, and skeletal anomalies. Because of the potential for dramatic growth, serial ultrasounds are recommended once a prenatal diagnosis of CCAM has been made. Physiologic consequences of fetal CCAMs are related to the size of the lesion and typically occur secondary to mediastinal compression and shift.[5,8–10] In the most severe cases, this can result in fetal hydrops and demise. Postnatal complications typically result from pulmonary hypoplasia and present as tachypnea and respiratory distress. Previous studies have demonstrated that Stocker classification or micro- versus macrocystic appearance is unreliable in predicting fetal outcome. A more consistent correlation exists between survival and the CAM volume ratio (CVR).[8] The CVR if defined as the estimated volume of the lesion based on the volume of an ellipsoid (length $\times$ width $\times$ height $\times$ 0.52) divided by the head circumference (cm). A CVR less than 1.6 is associated with a survival rate of 94% and a less than 3% risk of developing fetal hydrops.[5] Peak growth is reached near the end of the second trimester and usually reaches a plateau by 28 weeks. Thereafter, fetal growth typically outpaces the growth of the lesion and the CVR decreases. Prenatal intervention is reserved for cases of a large CCAM and fetal hydrops. Treatment options include percutaneous cyst–amniotic shunt placement, maternal betamethasone administration, or open fetal resection.[5,9–15] Beyond 32 weeks, urgent delivery is usually performed where delivery and resection by ex utero intrapartum treatment (EXIT) can provide for a safe transition. Ultimately, these rare cases of CCAM complicated by fetal hydrops should be referred to a regional fetal treatment center for evaluation and consideration for betamethasone therapy or open fetal resection.

With careful pre- and postnatal care, outcomes for the vast majority cases of CCAM are quite good.[16] Long-term risks for unresected CCAMs include a high incidence of chronic pulmonary infection and a small but finite risk of rhabdomyosarcoma and bronchoalveolar carcinoma arising in the second and third decades of life.[3,17–21] As such, resection is recommended at all ages. In the case of an uncomplicated prenatal diagnosis, resection is planned at 2–3 months after birth depending on the size and cystic nature of the lesion and the presence of comorbidity. Newborns who have larger lesions should be observed overnight in the intensive care nursery as air-trapping can occur within the lesion after birth. Although most CCAMs are not directly visualized, a plain chest radiograph should be performed on the first day of life to gauge the degree of air-trapping and mediastinal shift. In rare cases, a risk for compromised breathing warrants resection in the neonatal period.

Because of a high degree of suspected multicentricity and recurrence, complete lobectomy is undertaken in most cases of CCAM. Segmental or wedge resection may be appropriate in small peripheral lesions. However, the benefit of preserving a small amount of normal lung tissue must be weighed against the risk of recurrent disease, uncertainty about long-term cancer risk and compromise of the lobar or segmental bronchus. Conversely, infant lobectomy in this setting has excellent short- and long-term outcomes. Minimally invasive resection for a CCAM has limited outcome data to support its benefit in most cases.

Bronchopulmonary sequestrations are the second most commonly diagnosed cystic congenital lung lesion in neonates. Similar to CCAM, prenatal ultrasound can provide excellent visualization of BPS. As mentioned previously, a BPS is defined by relatively normal lung histology, the absence of a true connection to the broncho-pulmonary tree and blood supply via an anomalous connection with the aorta. An ex-tralobar BPS is separate from the remainder of the lung and contained within its own pleural envelope. An intralobar BPS can be more difficult to distinguish prenatally from a CCAM. In addition, "hybrid" lung masses that display clinicopathologic features of both CCAM and BPS have been described suggesting a common embryologic basis for some of these lesions.[3,22,23] Axial CT imaging postnatally demonstrates the rela-tionship of the BPS to the adjacent structure and delineates the blood supply to assist in operative planning. Resection is always indicated for BPS for the same reasons as described for CCAM and includes the risk of hemorrhage and arteriovenous shunting associated with the aberrant vasculature. The potential for a hybrid lesions and uncer-tainty regarding the neoplastic potential of this entity calls for the same risk–benefit analysis as described above for CCAM resection. Extralobar sequestrations are best treated by simple excision. A minimally invasive approach is particularly well-suited for these cases because simple widening of a single thoracoscopic port facil-itates delivery of the mass. Alternatively, intralobar sequestrations are contained within the visceral pleural envelope of the adjacent lung and typically require an open operation with lobectomy. Careful attention must be paid intraoperatively to controlling the anomalous systemic arterial supply.

Congenital Diaphragmatic Hernia

CDH is a particularly challenging neonatal condition. The primary anatomic anomaly is a hernia in the diaphragm. The hernia occurs most often as a posteriolateral defect in the left hemidiaphragm (88%).[24] The defect arises in the right hemidiaphragm in 10% of cases and bilaterally in 2%. Herniation of the intra-abdominal viscera results in compression of thoracic structures beginning in the second half of the first trimester. Compression of the lung during the pseudoglandular stage of lung development (8 to 16 weeks' gestation) appears to disrupt the normal process of branching morphogen-esis.[25] As a result, the arborization of the ipsilateral bronchus is dramatically and irre-versibly impaired. Consequently, pulmonary hypoplasia with associated pulmonary hypertension develops. The incidence ranges from 1 in 3000 to 5000 live births and, despite advances in neonatal care of these children, the overall mortality rate remains at 20–30%.[26] Significant morbidity can be expected in 50% of survivors.[27,28] The inci-dence in boys is three times higher than in girls. Nearly all cases of CDH are sporadic with the exception of a few reports of familial CDH. No distinct mode of inheritance has been defined, but the risk of CDH in a subsequent sibling may be as high as 2%.[7] Associated anomalies are seen in 25%–57% of all cases of CDH and 95% of stillborns and include congenital heart defects, hydronephrosis, renal agenesis, intestinal atresia, extralobar sequestrations, and neurologic defects including hydrocephalus, anencephaly, and spina bifida.[25,29] Chromosomal anomalies including trisomy 21, 18, and 15 occur in association with CDH in 10% to 20% of cases diagnosed prena-tally. Reported associations with maternal ingestion of thalidomide, benedectin, gui-nine, and antiepileptic drugs have not been thoroughly examined.[7]

The prenatal diagnosis of CDH is usually made at midgestational ultrasound screening. In severe cases, however, polyhydramnios may signal the presence of CDH. Polyhydramnios may arise from kinking of the displaced duodenum resulting in gastric dilatation and more severe pulmonary hypoplasia. This proposed mechanism could explain the relationship between polyhydramnios and a worsening prognosis with CDH.[30] Critical ultrasound findings include the presence of viscera in either the right or left hemithorax above the level of the inferior margin of the scapula or at the level of the four-chamber view of the heart.[31] The hypoechoic signal of the fluid-filled stomach and bowel can be easily distinguished from the hyperechoic signal of the fetal lung. A small ipsilateral lung, a defect in the ipsilateral diaphragm, and a shift of the mediastinum away from the affected side are other common findings. The diagnosis of a right-sided CDH can be particularly elusive. In these cases, the liver, which is usually the only herniated organ, is difficult to distinguish from the fetal lung due to their similar echodensities. Identification of the diaphragm does not exclude the possibility of CDH because some portions of the diaphragm are usually present.[32] The differential diagnosis includes Type I CCAM, bronchogenic cysts, neurenteric cysts, and cystic mediastinal teratoma, which may mimic herniated bowel. Identification of a normal upper abdominal anatomy and presence of peristalsis in herniated bowel loops helps to distinguish other diagnoses from CDH.

In the most severe cases, the liver and the stomach are present in the thorax. Bowing of the umbilical segment of the portal vein to the left of the midline or coursing of the portal branches to the lateral segment of the left lobe of the liver toward or above the diaphragm are the best predictors of liver herniation.[33] Color Doppler exam usually reveals the direction of flow in these vessels. As well, the presence of the stomach (easily seen in contrast to the more echogenic fetal lung) in a posterior or midthoracic location is a good predictor of liver herniation.

A number of other findings have also been correlated with the ultimate prognosis. As stated previously, associated polyhydramnios signals a more severe form of CDH and may explain the increased mortality associated with this finding. Similarly, diagnosis at an early age suggests a larger degree of visceral herniation and pulmonary hypoplasia.[34,35] Evidence of fetal cardiac ventricular disproportion due to compression of the heart from herniated viscera is an excellent predictor of fetal mortality.[36] The lung area (cross-sectional area of the contralateral lung measured at the level of the four-chamber view)–to–head circumference ratio (LHR) has been widely used to risk-stratify fetuses who have CDH. Previous retrospective studies demonstrated survival rates directly proportional to increased LHR ($>1.5 = 100\%$; $0.6–1.5 = 60\%$; $<0.6 = 0\%$).[31] More recent studies correlating the LHR with outcomes in prenatally diagnosed CDH display a less consistent relationship.[37,38] Other less studied prognostic indices include the degree of mediastinal shift, the right-lung-to-thorax diameter ratio, and various metrics of fetal pulmonary blood flow.[39,40]

As a result of the relative rarity of this entity and the absence of a clearly superior treatment, the management of CDH has evolved slowly over the past 50 years. Current ventilatory strategies include conventional or high frequency ventilation aimed at avoiding barotrauma by balancing the peak or mean airway pressure (< 30 mm Hg or < 17 mm Hg, respectively) with the lowest acceptable level of oxygenation ($> 88\%$ SaO_2). Hypercapnia is accepted and pH is buffered (> 7.25).[41] This gentle ventilation, or "gentilation," strategy has yielded the largest increases yet in survival for newborns who have CDH. Additionally, although previous studies revealed inhaled nitric oxide exerts only a transient effect,[42] other pharmacologic approaches have recently shown promise in the sustained reduction of pulmonary vascular resistance in cases of newborn CDH.[43]

Selection criteria for the use of extracorporeal membrane oxygenation (ECMO) in cases of CDH remain poorly defined. Even less clear is the optimal timing for hernia repair with ECMO, ie, early, late, or after ECMO. A few multicenter studies are underway to address these questions. Until these issues are resolved, the approach to each patient should be individualized and the treatment plan should include a risk–benefit analysis for all available resources. As such, all cases of CDH should be delivered and treated at a tertiary care facility where these treatment options are available.

Operative repair of CDH consists of gentle manual reduction of the herniated viscera from the chest followed by repair of the diaphragmatic defect via primary closure or use of a prosthetic graft. This is typically accomplished via an open laparotomy. Recently, some authors have proposed treatment of CDH via either the laparoscopic, thoracoscopic, or even robotic approach.[44–49] In the last few years, there has been increasing interest in attempting minimally invasive repair for neonates who have CDH; however, selection criteria remain poorly developed. Yang and colleagues[47] reviewed a series of infants selected for thoracoscopic repair who were required to have a preoperative peak inspiratory pressure (PIP) less than 24 mmHg and demonstration of the nasogastric tube tip within the abdomen. The rationale for the former requirement was to include only subjects with some pulmonary reserve that would tolerate an applied pneumothorax during the procedure. The latter requirement predicted an intact esophageal hiatus, enhancing the feasibility of completing the repair thoracoscopically without the use of a patch. Using this approach, the authors were able to complete the thoracoscopic repair in all of the subjects (n = 7) without significant complications. Other investigators advocate a far more aggressive approach to minimally invasive repair, even if a large diaphragmatic patch is needed. Clearly not all patients who have CDH would be good candidates for thoracoscopic repair and prospective controlled trials are needed to help define selection criteria and document outcomes.

Currently, the authors' preference is to attempt thoracoscopic repair in any newborn with stable ventilation and hemodynamics without ECMO who may be safely transported to the operating room for repair. The chest and abdomen are prepped in case conversion to a laparotomy is needed. The thoracoscopy is performed with minimal applied pneumothorax (pressure of 2–3 mm Hg; flow rate of 1 liter/minute) and 3 mm ports. The diaphragm is mobilized from the posterior abdominal wall as usual and repair is performed with standard suture. Knots may be tied using an intra- or extracorporeal technique and a small or large patch may be used in some cases. Conversion to laparotomy should be considered when the defect is quite large, the esophageal hiatus is absent, a muscular flap is preferred, or cardiopulmonary instability is encountered. Lastly, the benefits of minimally invasive repair must be tempered with the hypothermia and edema that results following a 3- or 4-hour operation.

Given the high morbidity and mortality associated with CDH, there may be a role for prenatal treatment of this condition in select cases in which severe pulmonary hypoplasia not consistent with life after birth is likely to develop. However, two large prospective single institution controlled trials of open fetal tracheal occlusion failed to show improvement in infant survival at 90 days postdelivery.[50,51] Subsequent studies on fetal endoscopic tracheal occlusion (FETO) were reported, but failed to show a survival benefit above that reported in numerous North American series on the treatment of CDH with conventional postnatal therapies.[52–54] Currently, efforts are underway through the North American Fetal Treatment Network (NAFTNet) to organize a multicenter study of balloon tracheal occlusion for cases of large fetal CDH. Ongoing challenges include risk-stratification for inclusion or exclusion and standardization of technique.

Esophageal Atresia and Tracheoesophageal Fistula

Esophageal atresia with or without associated tracheoesophageal fistula (EA/TEF) has an incidence of about 1 in 3000 to 5000 live births.[55] Despite a polygenetic hereditary pattern, EA/TEF is frequently associated with trisomy 18 and 21. Other associated diseases include Holt-Oram syndrome, DiGeorge, and Pierre Robin sequences.[56] Prenatal diagnosis of the most common type of EA/TEF is rare and relies on a high index of suspicion coupled with the identification of a dilated proximal esophageal pouch.[57,58] Conversely, pure EA without a fistula is readily suggested by the nonspecific findings of polyhydramnios and the sonographic absence of a stomach bubble.[59,60] Fetal magnetic resonance imaging is a useful diagnostic adjunct to confirm suspicious ultrasound findings and plan delivery at a center where definitive care can be provided.[61,62]

The majority of cases of isolated EA/TEF are diagnosed in the newborn period after failing to feed on the first few attempts. The afflicted infant will reproducibly choke and spit with every swallow. The preferred diagnostic test for EA is the careful passage of an orogastric tube with demonstration of coiling in the esophagus on the babygram. The presence of gas-filled intestine below the level of the diaphragm confirms the presence of an associated TEF, whereas a gasless abdomen indicates an isolated EA. Infants who have suspected EA/TEF should be transferred promptly to a pediatric surgical center. Commonly associated anomalies include the VACTERL (vertebral, anorectal, cardiac, tracheal–esophageal, renal, and limb) and CHARGE (coloboma, hearing, atresia choanae, retardation, genitourinary, esophageal) associations. Following resuscitation and a preoperative echocardiogram, primary surgical repair should be expedited unless a significant comorbidity takes precedence. Elective preoperative endotracheal intubation or CPAP should be avoided if possible. While waiting in the intensive care nursery, a Replogle suction tube positioned in the proximal esophageal pouch decreases the aspiration of secretions. Reverse Trendelenburg positioning and peptic acid blockade helps to reduce reflux pneumonitis. A dose of prophylactic antibiotic (ampicillin and gentamicin) is usually given on a scheduled basis.

Rigid bronchoscopy is performed immediately after induction of anesthesia to confirm the anatomy, to evaluate for a proximal fistula and to control the distal fistula with a 4 Fr or 5 Fr Fogarty balloon catheter inflated in the distal esophagus. Following bronchoscopy, an endotracheal tube is positioned in the trachea and the patient is prepped for repair. The placing of the tube usually requires a right posteriolateral thoracotomy. The fistula is ligated first and every attempt is made to perform a primary repair of the esophagus. In the case of a long-gap EA without fistula, primary repair is deferred and a simple gastrostomy is performed following bronchoscopy. The patient is fed via gastrostomy and studied radiographically. Definitive repair for isolated EA is typically attempted 4 to 6 weeks later.

Following surgery, infants are cared for in the neonatal intensive care unit with intravenous fluid resuscitation, broad-spectrum antibiotics, and weaned from the ventilator. Orogastric tube feedings are initiated on postoperative day #2 and steadily advanced. Following a confirmatory esophogram on postoperative day #5, the orogastric tube is removed and oral feedings begun. H2 blockers are continued after discharge and for the first few years of life to reduce esophagitis in the relatively insensate and dysmotile distal esophagus.[63–65] A single follow-up esophogram 4 to 6 weeks later helps to identify any early stricture formation that may benefit from dilatation prior to the initiation of solid foods.

Patent Ductus Ateriosus

Patent ductus arteriosus (PDA) remains the most common cardiovascular condition encountered in neonates.[66] Hemodynamically significant or symptomatic PDA results in significant left-to-right shunting and pulmonary overcirculation, which can lead to prolonged ventilatory requirements, bronchopulmonary dysplasia, and possibly even necrotizing enterocolitis from poor systemic perfusion. For these reasons, closure of symptomatic PDA is strongly advocated even in very–low–birth–weight (VLBW) infants. Although the optimal treatment for PDA closure has not been clearly elucidated, a role exists for surgical intervention in infants who fail medical treatment with non-steroidal therapy (indomethacin) or who are not candidates for medical therapy due to other risk factors such as intraventricular hemorrhage. Additionally, there may be a role for prophylactic surgical closure to reduce the incidence of necrotizing enterocolitis.[66–69]

Video-assisted thoracoscopic surgical (VATS) ligation of the patent ductus is safe and effective, even in VLBW infants, resulting in shorter operative time, recovery time, and length of stay.[70–73] Additionally, VATS closure has also recently been compared with catheter-based approaches and found to have equivalent, if not superior, results.[74] Although these results seem promising, this report and others exclude subjects with large ductal diameters and VLBW premature infants with hemodynamic instability.[73] Additionally, the application of this approach in older children must take into consideration the excellent results seen with coil occlusion. Therefore, VATS PDA ligation seems to be best suited for hemodynamically stable infants and older children who may be at high risk for complications following coil occlusion.

ABDOMINAL SURGERY
Necrotizing Enterocolitis

Necrotizing enterocolitis (NEC) remains a significant source of both morbidity and mortality in this population and one of the leading causes for gastrointestinal surgery in the neonate. Advancements in the resuscitation and survival of the more preterm infants have likely led to the increase in the number of infants at risk for developing NEC. As a result, the incidence and mortality rate of NEC remains relatively unchanged over the last 20 years, with fewer infants dying of respiratory failure but succumbing instead to the complications associated with NEC.[75] These patients often require prolonged hospitalization and suffer the consequences of intestinal loss, such as catheter-based infections, short bowel syndrome, parenteral nutrition-associated cholestasis, growth and developmental delay, and nutritional deficiency. Multiple overlapping theories have been put forth to explain the pathophysiology of NEC, including (1) an exaggerated intestinal inflammatory/immune response to injury; (2) intestinal ischemia aggravated by a disordered balance in the production of nitric oxide and endothelin-1; (3) abnormal gut colonization with pathogenic bacteria; (4) high levels of intestinal lipopolysaccharide; and (5) deficient epidermal growth factor production. Conclusive evidence exists demonstrating that the use of formula rather human milk in VLBW infants are associated with a higher incidence of NEC.[76–86]

The clinical presentation of NEC can range from feeding intolerance and abdominal distension to a fulminant abdominal catastrophe with hypotension and abdominal wall changes. Although Bell's criteria[87] and their modifications provide an initial risk-stratification strategy for affected neonates, the potential for rapid deterioration exists in every case. Ultimately, most infants diagnosed with NEC should be treated nonoperatively with intravenous fluids, broad-spectrum antibiotics, and bowel rest. Absolute indications for surgery include evidence for intestinal perforation or failure of medical treatment. These unfortunate infants have a mortality rate of 30%–40% in the acute phase and significant long-term morbidity in the survivors.[88,89] However, maintaining an aggressive surgical bias in cases of NEC may help to limit the severity of the disease and avoid devastating secondary complications and worse outcomes.

Numerous approaches are described for surgical management including laparotomy and resection, ostomy decompression, intestinal washout, peritoneal drainage, and silo decompression. Significant controversy exists regarding the use of peritoneal drainage versus laparotomy for the operative management of NEC in VLBW infants (<1000 g). The results from three large multicenter studies suggest that similar mortality rates for either approach can be expected. Despite the significant efforts of the investigators, each of these can be criticized for selection bias or inadequate power.[88–90] The analysis is further complicated by an incomplete assessment of the long-term neurodevelopmental outcome that has been shown to be quite poor in these subjects.[91,92] Nonetheless, an observed mortality rate approaching 40% in these patients suggests that survival should remain as the primary focus when considering various treatment options for an individual patient. At this time, categorical recommendations regarding the optimal operative treatment of VLBW infants who have NEC are not supported by the available literature. Perhaps the best current approach relies on an individualized process involving the judgment of an experienced pediatric surgeon in consultation with the neonatologist. Upcoming studies on the medical prevention and treatment of NEC through growth factor administration hold the greatest promise for meaningful advancement in this area.[93]

Abdominal Wall Defects

Abdominal wall defects exist within a spectrum of disorders that appear to be increasing in incidence.[94] Among these, gastroschisis and omphalocele are more common. Most cases are suspected by abnormal maternal serology and reliably diagnosed by fetal ultrasound. Ultrasound diagnosis in the late first trimester is possible as the physiologic return of the intestines to the peritoneal cavity is complete by 11 weeks of gestation.[95] The identifying sonographic features of gastroschisis are the findings of multiple loops of bowel floating freely in the amniotic fluid. Herniated bowel is typically seen to the right of the umbilical cord insertion. Omphalocele defects are centrally located and have a membranous covering of the bowel. The associated anomaly rate for gastroschisis ranges from 10% to 15% in various studies and includes other GI anomalies, central nervous system, cardiovascular, musculoskeletal, and genitourinary anomalies.[96] An infrequent association of gastroschisis with complex congenital heart disease suggests little benefit from routine echocardiography.[97] Because of the low incidence of chromosomal anomalies, the risks of amniocentesis are unwarranted in cases of isolated gastroschisis. In contrast, a strong association has been described between omphalocele and cardiovascular, genitourinary, and karyotypic anomalies. As a result, echocardiography is routinely performed and amniocentesis is offered in every case of omphalocele. Because several reports document a survival advantage for fetuses who have abdominal wall defects born in a center where both neonatal and surgical care can be provided, the positive correlation of maternal screening with the improved outcome of affected fetuses cannot be overstated.[95,98]

A rationale for prenatal intervention exists only in cases of gastroschisis. Significant and potentially irreversible injury of the herniated bowel resulting from exposure to the amniotic fluid or contracture of the umbilical ring may occur in gastroschisis. Indeed, the progression of injury can be tracked with serial ultrasound. Risk stratification of bowel injury in affected fetuses has been proposed based upon the ultrasound characteristics. Sonographic parameters include matting and dilatation of the bowel, loss of peristaltic activity, changes in bowel wall echogenicity, alterations in mesenteric blood flow, and changes in stomach position. Despite the ominous appearance of the anatomy, none of these parameters appear to correlate with postnatal outcomes.[99] Prospective studies of planned early delivery or amniotic fluid exchange have not been shown to be helpful.[100-104] A subset of newborns who have gastroschisis experience severe bowel injury during the third trimester that results in much of the long-term morbidity and mortality associated with this disease. The use of routine frequent follow-up ultrasound or amniotic fluid exchange currently provides no demonstrated advantage for these affected infants. Cesarean delivery has no demonstrated benefit in cases of prenatally diagnosed gastroschisis, but may help to prevent rupture of the membranous sac of a large omphalocele.[105-107] It is hoped that future research will more accurately identify these fetuses so that treatment may be optimized.

Despite multiple differences, gastroschisis and omphalocele share an increasingly convergent postnatal management strategy. The goals of surgical treatment include[1] safe reduction of the evisceration,[2] fascial closure with an acceptable cosmetic outcome,[3] identification of associated anomalies,[4] nutritional support,[5] and identification and treatment of complications. Initial therapy for infants who have abdominal wall defects includes nasogastric decompression and protection of the herniated intestinal contents, and, in the case of gastroschisis, prior transport of the neonate to the intensive care nursery. The infant should then be placed in a bowel bag that covers the entire torso, abdomen, and lower extremities, loosely secured around the chest just above the nipple line. This allows direct visualization of the bowel through the bag during transport. Bowel congestion can thus be easily identified and any kinking in the mesentery alleviated by repositioning through the bag. Next, the liberal administration of intravenous normal saline including at least one 20 mL/kg bolus is beneficial in nearly all cases of gastroschisis. An initial dose of ampicillin and gentamicin shortly after arrival in the nursery is also routine.

Depending on the size of the defect, either primary or staged reduction is undertaken. The medical literature is replete with studies of varying quality and opposite conclusions comparing early versus delayed (silo-assisted) staged closure of gastroschisis.[108-112] The short-term benefits of primary closure must be weighed against the risks of ventilatory compromise or bowel ischemia. Such risks are likely to be inappropriate in preterm infants or those with markedly edematous bowel. These risks are amplified when infants arrive at the operating room hypothermic and dehydrated after an incomplete resuscitation for an aggressive attempt at primary closure. Alternatively, if the abdominal defect is quite narrow or the status of the bowel and infant favorable, an attempt at primary repair following resuscitation and warming is sensible. Because these situations are relatively infrequent, it has been our practice to place the bowel in a preformed silo in the vast majority of cases of gastroschisis. Similarly, nearly all cases of omphalocele are managed with delayed repair and aseptic management of the sac.

Outcomes for infants who have abdominal wall defects have significantly improved. With survival rates now exceeding 90%–95% in most series, these infants have benefited from advances in general neonatal care and parenteral nutrition.[113] Associated complex cardiac and pulmonary anomalies portend a poorer overall prognosis and account for the majority of mortality in affected newborns.

Intestinal Atresia

The incidence of intestinal atresias range from 1 in 3000 live births for jejunoileal atresia to 1 in 5000 for duodenal atresia to 1 in 10,000 births for the rare colonic atresia. As a group, intestinal atresias are commonly diagnosed prenatally.[114,115] Polyhydramnios is a prominent feature of atresias of the duodenum or proximal jejunum and less so for atresias of the ileum and colon. A sonographic "double bubble" sign is diagnostic of duodenal atresia. Dilated small bowel loops with hyperperistalsis are more suggestive of a distal atresia. Sonographically visible peritoneal calcifications or ascites indicate a prenatal perforation. Roughly 40% of cases of duodenal atresia are associated with other anomalies that most commonly include trisomy 21, genitourinary, and cardiac anomalies.[115–118] Colonic atresia can be associated with syndactyly, polydactyly, clubfoot, absent radius, ocular and cardiac anomalies, abdominal wall defects, and Hirschsprung's disease.[118–120] Jejunal and ileal atresias are usually isolated problems; however, multiple atresias are frequently encountered.

Postnatally, intestinal atresia manifests early by obstructive symptoms of feeding intolerance, bilious emesis, abdominal distension, and failure to pass meconium. The differential diagnosis for a neonatal bowel obstruction most commonly includes intestinal atresia, midgut volvulus, meconium ileus (MI), meconium plug (MP), NEC, Hirschsprung's disease (HD), obstructions associated with an omphalomesenteric remnant, lower urinary tract obstruction (LUTO), anorectal malformation, intestinal duplication, and various tumors. An examination of the abdomen and perineum coupled with plain abdominal radiographs helps to identify the presence of a tumor, LUTO, or an anorectal malformation and enables the sorting of patients into proximal and distal bowel obstructions. The presence of a sign on a plain abdominal radiograph is almost always indicative of the presence of a duodenal atresia, especially in a patient who has features of trisomy 21. Most proximal obstructions should be operated upon directly without further studies and the potential hazards associated with them. Occasionally, significant comorbidities preclude prompt repair. In these cases, it is important to recognize that a midgut volvulus can be misdiagnosed as a duodenal or proximal jejunal atresia on a plain radiograph. As such, an upper gastrointestinal series or bedside ultrasound of the superior mesenteric vessels can exclude this possibility when delayed repair is in the patient's best interest.

Distal obstructions are more diagnostically challenging and include diseases such as ileal and colonic atresias, NEC, HD, MI, and MP. Operative treatment is not typically offered as a frontline therapy for some of these conditions. A family history of cystic fibrosis (CF) or HD helps to narrow the diagnostic spectrum. Physical exam findings of abdominal wall erythema, tenderness, and rigidity are found most commonly in NEC and less often in HD and MI. Findings of pneumatosis intestinalis and thrombocytopenia further support the diagnosis of NEC, whereas palpable and dilated intestinal loops with a soap-bubble appearance on plain abdominal radiographs are characteristic of MI. If ambiguity persists, patients in whom NEC can be ruled out may be safely studied for distal intestinal atresia by the use of contrast radiographic enemas.

Following a brief diagnostic evaluation, NG decompression, and resuscitation, operative repair should be done without unnecessary delay. The approach to repair varies according to the type of anatomic aberration. Because of their spatial relationship to the pancreas and ampulla of Vater, atresias of the duodenum are typically bypassed via a diamond-shaped duodenoduodenostomy.[121,122] Occasionally, a duodenal web is identified intraoperatively and managed with a duodenostomy and simple incision of the lateral two thirds of the web's wall. A markedly dilated proximal duodenal segment is probably best treated with a tapering enteroplasty at the time of the initial repair.[123] Atresias of the jejunum or ileum are frequently associated with a second or multiple intestinal atresias. This latter point underlines the need to closely examine the distal atrophic intestine at the time of repair. The spectrum of atresias range from a simple web or point atresia to those with large defects in the mesentery, multiple atresias, and associated loss of bowel length. As such, a number of possible operative techniques may be employed with these cases. The principles guiding operative management include (1) identification all intestinal defects; (2) limited resection or tapering of proximally dilated bowel; and (3) preservation of remaining intestinal length through multiple anastomoses as needed. Atresias of the colon are quite rare and are difficult to diagnose preoperatively. The finding of "white mucus" on rectal exam provides a clue to the presence of colonic atresia. Historically, a staged operation with a temporary or permanent proximal colostomy had been advocated. However, this approach has fallen out of favor with modern series reporting good results after primary anastomosis.[124,125] Care must be taken to exclude the possibility of associated HD (10%) at the time of primary anastomosis.

Overall outcomes for all forms of intestinal atresia are excellent with greater than 90% long-term survival. Morbidity and mortality relates to the presence of other anomalies or very low birthweights. In the absence of comorbidity, postoperative care focuses on nutritional management that frequently requires the use of elemental feeding or parenteral support. Prevention and control of central line sepsis and bacterial overgrowth coupled with the use of alternative TPN formulations greatly benefits marginally recovering infants during intestinal growth and adaptation.[126,127]

Intestinal Malrotation

Congenital intestinal malrotation exists as a spectrum of rotational anomalies. The vast majority of infants are diagnosed within the first year of life, and 80% of these are diagnosed within the first month of life.[128] Although the diagnosis of malrotation may not be straightforward in older children, newborns typically present with an acute onset of intermittent bilious emesis with or without associated signs of intestinal ischemia. The classical abdominal radiographic appearance of an infant with malrotation is that of a gasless abdomen with air present in the stomach and duodenum. Contrast upper gastrointestinal studies typically demonstrate the lack of a duodenal C-loop as the course of the duodenum remains to the right of the midline adjacent to the remainder of the small intestine. A lateral abdominal view reveals the absence of the normal retroperitoneal fixation of the second and third portion of the duodenum. An associated midgut volvulus is indicated by a corkscrew appearance of the distal duodenum and proximal jejunum.

As mentioned previously, ultrasound examination can be particularly helpful in determining the relationship of the major mesenteric vessels, and is a very sensitive and noninvasive way of diagnosing malrotation. Complications from malrotation can occur at any age and treatment outcomes are inferior in the nonneonatal age groups.[129] For these reasons, the authors recommend operative treatment in nearly all cases of malrotation. More specifically, symptomatic intestinal malrotation in an infant always requires operative intervention. The presence or suspicion of midgut volvulus is a true neonatal surgical emergency. In cases of heterotaxia, the severity of associated complex congenital heart disease must be considered in asymptomatic patients, whereas all symptomatic patients should undergo a Ladd procedure.[130,131] Operative management usually consists of a Ladd procedure via an open or minimally invasive approach. Laparoscopy should not be performed in cases in which midgut volvulus is suspected. Outcomes for neonates diagnosed promptly with malrotation or midgut volvulus are generally excellent. However, for infants in whom the diagnosis of intestinal ischemia is delayed, the result can be profound intestinal loss leading to short gut syndrome or death. Extensive injury associated with midgut volvulus is best managed with a limited resection of any perforated intestine and placement of a preformed silo. A second-look operation can be planned 24–48 hours later following further resuscitation and parental counseling.

Hirschsprung's Disease

HD results in retention of stool in the normal proximal colon resulting from an inability to empty into the aganglionic distal colon that does not reflexively relax. This occurs most commonly in the rectum or sigmoid colon, but total intestinal HD and ultra short-segment HD has also been described.[132] Abnormal development or migration of the enteric nervous system cells during fetal development are the likely cause of HD.[133-137] Underlying genetic factors likely play a strong role in the development of HD as evidenced by the increased incidence in boys, in those with affected siblings, and in association with certain genetic syndromes (ie, trisomy 21, multiple endocrine neoplasia type II, and neurofibromatosis).[138] Whereas genetic studies have demonstrated mutations associated with HD in several different genes, more than 20 different mutations in the RET proto-oncogene have been described. Improved awareness of the disease and its presentation, coupled with advances in neonatal care, has significantly improved outcomes in children diagnosed with HD.[139]

HD should be suspected in any neonate who fails to pass meconium within 48 hours of birth. Additional nonspecific findings include abdominal distension, bilious emesis, and feeding intolerance. As mentioned earlier, other acute forms of bowel obstruction, such as midgut volvulus or intestinal atresia, must first be excluded. A contrast enema can help to establish the diagnosis and suggest the location of a transition zone from ganglionic to aganglionic bowel. However, a significant false-negative rate prevents excluding the possibility of HD using contrast enema alone in neonates.[140,141] Presumptive treatment with rectal irrigations and antibiotics should begin immediately. The diagnosed is then confirmed by rectal suction biopsy identifying the absence of ganglion cells, hypertrophic nerve fibers, and enhanced acetylcholinesterase staining within the submucosa.

Following confirmation of HD, an operative strategy can be devised and tailored to the individual presentation. Whereas operative intervention for HD in the past involved two- and sometimes even three-stage operations, single-stage endorectal pull-through procedures in neonates are now commonly employed with excellent results.[139,142] These minimally invasive procedures can be used in infants or older children and have been found to reduce the length of stay, the time to full feedings, and overall reduced pain and postoperative bowel obstructions. However, cases that present with associated enterocolitis may benefit from an early leveling colostomy and a delayed pull-through.

Intestinal Duplication

Intestinal duplications are rare malformations of the alimentary tract that involve the mesenteric side of the associated alimentary tract and share a common blood supply with the native bowel. They can occur anywhere from the mouth to the anus and are best categorized as alimentary tract duplications, though they rarely involve a true doubling of the bowel and are much more commonly just enterogenous cysts.[143] The cause of intestinal duplications is not yet known, and several theories have been proposed, including intrauterine vascular accidents, persistence of embryonic diverticula, and even abortive twinning in some cases. Ileal duplications are the most common (31%), followed by duplication of the colon and appendix (30%), esophagus (17%), jejunum (13%), and the stomach and duodenum (8%).[144,145]

The sonographic appearance of intestinal duplications may be purely cystic or contain some solid components.[145] The differential diagnosis is extensive and includes ovarian cyst, hemangioma, teratoma, lymphangioma, mesenteric cyst, meconium cyst, choledochal cyst, LUTO, myelomeningocele, and various malignant and benign tumors of the abdominal viscera. Peristalsis may or may not be visualized in these loops of dilated bowel and the stomach and duodenum may also be dilated.[146–148] The cyst itself may demonstrate a "muscular" rim.[145] No prenatal intervention is typically offered for intestinal duplications, although large lesions may cause dystocia or respiratory compromise at birth. In these cases, fetal MRI may help to clarify the diagnosis and plan Cesarean delivery or an EXIT procedure.[149]

After birth, intestinal duplications may be diagnosed in neonates during the evaluation of a bowel obstruction or discovered incidentally at elective laparotomy. Abdominal pain and melena are the most common presenting symptoms in older children.[143] Heterotopic gastric mucosa is commonly present within the cyst and may lead to mucosal ulceration and bleeding. Foregut duplications can cause obstructive vomiting, whereas those in the small intestine can present with abdominal distension. Hindgut duplications frequently cause bleeding and constipation or overflow diarrhea and late signs of obstruction. Radiographic diagnosis of intestinal duplications may be somewhat difficult; however, ultrasound often gives excellent visualization of the lesion. Upper gastrointestinal and small bowel contrast studies are traditionally the gold standard for diagnosis. However, CT and MRI imaging and endoscopic ultrasound are emerging as superior modalities.[143] The mainstay of therapy for intestinal duplications is surgical extirpation of the lesion both for symptomatic relief and definitive diagnosis and pathologic review.

Meconium Ileus

MI is always associated with CF, and 6%–20% of infants who have CF will develop an MI as their first presenting symptom.[150,151] Inspissated meconium accumulates in the terminal ileum, causing a mechanical bowel obstruction. Nonspecific prenatal ultrasound findings of dilated hyperechoic bowel on routine ultrasound should prompt more detailed evaluation. If MI is suspected, the CF mutation carrier status should be determined in the parents. A confirmed prenatal diagnosis facilitates counseling and improves outcomes. As discussed previously, MI should be considered in every case of neonatal intestinal obstruction. No specific prenatal therapy is typically offered for MI. However, the availability of a new large-animal model of MI opens a new arena of investigation.[152]

Infants who have suspected MI should undergo nasogastric decompression and intravenous resuscitation, followed by a diagnostic water-soluble contrast enema under fluoroscopic guidance. Although surgical therapy is occasionally warranted, cathartic bowel cleansing and pancreatic enzyme supplementation remain the mainstay of therapy. Serial contrast enemas greatly enhance the clearance of the inspissated meconium. N–acetylcysteine may be simultaneously added to the bedside enemas.[153] Infants who fail to respond to a reasonable trial of medical therapy or who develop complicated MI associated with perforation should undergo prompt laparotomy. Primary catheter enterotomy, either in the terminal ileum or through the appendiceal stump, is the preferred approach for intraoperative irrigation of the intestine. Resection with or without enterostomy is reserved for infants with associated perforation.[150,154,155]

MP syndrome is primarily seen in lower birthweight infants and is rarely associated with CF.[156–159] Generally, these obstructions resolve with either simple digital rectal exam or a contrast enema. Importantly, a recent series of 77 infants over a 13-year period at a tertiary children's hospital identified HD in 13% of the subjects.[159] Subsequent stooling irregularities should prompt an evaluation for HD in these patients.

Biliary Atresia

Though a relatively rare clinical entity with a disease incidence of 1 in 8000 to 18,000, biliary atresia is a devastating congenital illness that may present relatively early in neonatal life.[160] Atresia of the biliary system appears to exist in two clinical phenotypes—embryonal and perinatal. The embryonal type presents early in association with other congenital abnormalities such as polysplenia, situs inversus, and cardiac abnormalities.[161–165] In these cases, primary maldevelopment of the biliary tree is the likely cause. The perinatal type is more common and often presents later in an otherwise normal infant. The pathophysiology in these infants may be acquired through infectious, ischemic, or autoimmune mechanisms.[166]

Direct hyperbilirubinemia persisting for more than 2 weeks should prompt an expedited diagnostic evaluation. Much research interest is currently directed into developing simple and effective screening methods to identify affected infants sooner.[162] Laboratory studies usually reveal a mixed hyperbilirubinemia (6–12 mg/dL, >50% direct) and elevated ductal enzymes. Abdominal ultrasound may show an enlarged liver and an absent or contracted gallbladder after a 4-hour fast. Percutaneous liver biopsy may show ductal proliferation with portal fibrosis. Whereas the use of ERCP is technically challenging in these infants, MRCP is emerging as a promising noninvasive study with a highly accurate diagnostic rate.[160,167,168] Ultimately, the diagnosis is clarified only by laparotomy and intraoperative cholangiogram. Ambiguity following these less invasive diagnostic measures is best elucidated in the operating room without significant delay.

The primary therapy for biliary atresia remains surgical in nature. Several factors have been shown to improve outcomes in children diagnosed with biliary atresia, but age at surgical intervention is likely most important. The current standard of care is to perform a portoenterostomy as originally described by Kasai.[169,170] In infants treated in the first 60 days of life, an early success rate approaching 70% can be expected.[171] Beyond 120 days of life, the success rate is quite poor. Many centers now perform a laparoscopic cholangiogram and then proceed with portoenterostomy if the cholangiogram demonstrates biliary atresia. Recently, the use of robotic instrumentation has been employed to improve visualization and instrument dexterity in this challenging operation.[172]

Although the short-term success rate of portoenterostomy is encouraging, long-term studies show 70%-80% of children ultimately require liver transplantation and the remaining 20%–30% survive with their native liver but develop cirrhosis.[173] Large series demonstrate that liver transplantation is an effective treatment for biliary atresia. However, organ shortages and technical challenges in small infants provide the impetus to consider portoenterostomy in every case of biliary atresia. Liver transplantation is typically reserved for children in whom biliary flow cannot be restored or who develop complications resulting from biliary cirrhosis. In the absence of a size-matched organ, the availability of a living related donor may provide a better outcome. A recent case series confirmed that live-donor liver transplantation following portoenterostomy is more effective and has fewer complications if done early during childhood.[174]

SUMMARY

The study of neonatal disease brings to mind Socrates' famous quote: *The more I learn, the more I learn how little I know.* However, developing a healthy multidisciplinary approach helps to illuminate the optimal care for the surgical neonate. The marriage of surgical, pediatric, and obstetrical disciplines ensures that everyone speaks the same language. The next decade will likely see an enormous expansion of centers where residents and fellows may receive crossdisciplinary training in the treatment of fetal and neonatal disease. Surgical neonates should benefit greatly from this evolution as the nonelective nature of neonatal surgery poses an enormous barrier to centralization of fetal and neonatal expertise.

REFERENCES

1. Stocker JT, Madewell JE, Drake RM. Congenital cystic adenomatoid malformation of the lung. Classification and morphologic spectrum. Hum Pathol 1977;8:155–71.
2. Cass DL, Quinn TM, Yang EY, et al. Increased cell proliferation and decreased apoptosis characterize congenital cystic adenomatoid malformation of the lung. J Pediatr Surg 1998;33:1043–6 [discussion: 1047].
3. Griffin N, Devaraj A, Goldstraw P, et al. CT and histopathological correlation of congenital cystic pulmonary lesions: a common pathogenesis? Clin Radiol 2008;63:995–1005.
4. Hubbard AM, Adzick NS, Crombleholme TM, et al. Congenital chest lesions: diagnosis and characterization with prenatal MR imaging. Radiology 1999;212:43–8.
5. Mann S, Wilson RD, Bebbington MW, et al. Antenatal diagnosis and management of congenital cystic adenomatoid malformation. Semin Fetal Neonatal Med 2007;12:477–81.
6. Peranteau WH, Merchant AM, Hedrick HL, et al. Prenatal course and postnatal management of peripheral bronchial atresia: association with congenital cystic adenomatoid malformation of the lung. Fetal Diagn Ther 2008;24:190–6.
7. Morin L, Crombleholme TM, D'Alton ME. Prenatal diagnosis and management of fetal thoracic lesions. Semin Perinatol 1994;18:228–53.
8. Crombleholme TM, Coleman B, Hedrick H, et al. Cystic adenomatoid malformation volume ratio predicts outcome in prenatally diagnosed cystic adenomatoid malformation of the lung. J Pediatr Surg 2002;37:331–8.
9. Adzick NS, Flake AW, Crombleholme TM. Management of congenital lung lesions. Semin Pediatr Surg 2003;12:10–6.
10. Wilson RD, Hedrick HL, Liechty KW, et al. Cystic adenomatoid malformation of the lung: review of genetics, prenatal diagnosis, and in utero treatment. Am J Med Genet A 2006;140:151–5.
11. Bouchard S, Johnson MP, Flake AW, et al. The EXIT procedure: experience and outcome in 31 cases. J Pediatr Surg 2002;37:418–26.
12. Wilson RD, Baxter JK, Johnson MP, et al. Thoracoamniotic shunts: fetal treatment of pleural effusions and congenital cystic adenomatoid malformations. Fetal Diagn Ther 2004;19:413–20.
13. Hedrick HL, Flake AW, Crombleholme TM, et al. The ex utero intrapartum therapy procedure for high-risk fetal lung lesions. J Pediatr Surg 2005;40: 1038–43 [discussion: 1044].
14. Merchant AM, Peranteau W, Wilson RD, et al. Postnatal chest wall deformities after fetal thoracoamniotic shunting for congenital cystic adenomatoid malformation. Fetal Diagn Ther 2007;22:435–9.
15. Peranteau WH, Wilson RD, Liechty KW, et al. Effect of maternal betamethasone administration on prenatal congenital cystic adenomatoid malformation growth and fetal survival. Fetal Diagn Ther 2007;22:365–71.
16. Kunisaki SM, Barnewolt CE, Estroff JA, et al. Large fetal congenital cystic adenomatoid malformations: growth trends and patient survival. J Pediatr Surg 2007; 42:404–10.

17. Ozcan C, Celik A, Ural Z, et al. Primary pulmonary rhabdomyosarcoma arising within cystic adenomatoid malformation: a case report and review of the literature. J Pediatr Surg 2001;36:1062–5.
18. Pai S, Eng HL, Lee SY, et al. Rhabdomyosarcoma arising within congenital cystic adenomatoid malformation. Pediatr Blood Cancer 2005;45:841–5.
19. Lantuejoul S, Nicholson AG, Sartori G, et al. Mucinous cells in type 1 pulmonary congenital cystic adenomatoid malformation as mucinous bronchioloalveolar carcinoma precursors. Am J Surg Pathol 2007;31:961–9.
20. Nur S, Badr R, Sandoval C, et al. Syndromic presentation of a pleuropulmonary blastoma associated with congenital cystic adenomatoid malformation. A case report. J Pediatr Surg 2007;42:1772–5.
21. Gutweiler JR, Labelle J, Suh MY, et al. A familial case of pleuropulmonary blastoma. Eur J Pediatr Surg 2008;18:192–4.
22. Morin C, Filiatrault D, Russo P. Pulmonary sequestration with histologic changes of cystic adenomatoid malformation. Pediatr Radiol 1989;19:130–2.
23. McLean SE, Pfeifer JD, Siegel MJ, et al. Congenital cystic adenomatoid malformation connected to an extralobar pulmonary sequestration in the contralateral chest: common origin? J Pediatr Surg 2004;39:e13–7.
24. Pober BR. Overview of epidemiology, genetics, birth defects, and chromosome abnormalities associated with CDH. Am J Med Genet C Semin Med Genet 2007; 15:158–71.
25. Kinane TB. Lung development and implications for hypoplasia found in congenital diaphragmatic hernia. Am J Med Genet C Semin Med Genet 2007;15:117–24.
26. Tsao K, Lally KP. The Congenital Diaphragmatic Hernia Study Group: a voluntary international registry. Semin Pediatr Surg 2008;17:90–7.
27. Friedman S, Chen C, Chapman JS, et al. Neurodevelopmental outcomes of congenital diaphragmatic hernia survivors followed in a multidisciplinary clinic at ages 1 and 3. J Pediatr Surg 2008;43:1035–43.
28. Lally KP, Engle W. Postdischarge follow-up of infants with congenital diaphragmatic hernia. Pediatrics 2008;121:627–32.
29. Stoll C, Alembik Y, Dott B, et al. Associated malformations in cases with congenital diaphragmatic hernia. Genet Couns 2008;19:331–9.
30. Adzick NS, Harrison MR. The developmental pathophysiology of surgical disease. Semin Pediatr Surg 1993;2:92–102.
31. Metkus AP, Filly RA, Stringer MD, et al. Sonographic predictors of survival in fetal diaphragmatic hernia. J Pediatr Surg 1996;31:148–51 [discussion: 151].
32. Shaaban AF, Kim HB, Milner R, et al. The role of ultrasonography in fetal surgery and invasive fetal procedures. Semin Roentgenol 1999;34:62–77.
33. Harrison MR, Adzick NS, Longaker MT, et al. Successful repair in utero of a fetal diaphragmatic hernia after removal of herniated viscera from the left thorax. N Engl J Med 1990;322:1582–4.
34. Neff KW, Kilian AK, Schaible T, et al. Prediction of mortality and need for neonatal extracorporeal membrane oxygenation in fetuses with congenital diaphragmatic hernia: logistic regression analysis based on MRI fetal lung volume measurements. AJR Am J Roentgenol 2007;189:1307–11.
35. Busing KA, Kilian AK, Schaible T, et al. MR lung volume in fetal congenital diaphragmatic hernia: logistic regression analysis–mortality and extracorporeal membrane oxygenation. Radiology 2008;248:233–9.
36. Flake AW. Fetal surgery for congenital diaphragmatic hernia. Semin Pediatr Surg 1996;5:266–74.

37. Arkovitz MS, Russo M, Devine P, et al. Fetal lung-head ratio is not related to outcome for antenatal diagnosed congenital diaphragmatic hernia. J Pediatr Surg 2007;42:107–10 [discussion: 110].

38. Ba'ath ME, Jesudason EC, Losty PD. How useful is the lung-to-head ratio in predicting outcome in the fetus with congenital diaphragmatic hernia? A systematic review and meta-analysis. Ultrasound Obstet Gynecol 2007;30:897–906.

39. Tsukimori K, Masumoto K, Morokuma S, et al. The lung-to-thorax transverse area ratio at term and near term correlates with survival in isolated congenital diaphragmatic hernia. J Ultrasound Med 2008;27:707–13.

40. Usui N, Okuyama H, Sawai T, et al. Relationship between L/T ratio and LHR in the prenatal assessment of pulmonary hypoplasia in congenital diaphragmatic hernia. Pediatr Surg Int 2007;23:971–6.

41. Boloker J, Bateman DA, Wung JT, et al. Congenital diaphragmatic hernia in 120 infants treated consecutively with permissive hypercapnea/spontaneous respiration/elective repair. J Pediatr Surg 2002;37:357–66.

42. Inhaled nitric oxide and hypoxic respiratory failure in infants with congenital diaphragmatic hernia. The Neonatal Inhaled Nitric Oxide Study Group (NINOS). Pediatrics 1997;99:838–45.

43. Noori S, Friedlich P, Wong P, et al. Cardiovascular effects of sildenafil in neonates and infants with congenital diaphragmatic hernia and pulmonary hypertension. Neonatology 2007;91:92–100.

44. Becmeur F, Jamali RR, Moog R, et al. Thoracoscopic treatment for delayed presentation of congenital diaphragmatic hernia in the infant. A report of three cases. Surg Endosc 2001;15:1163–6.

45. van der Zee DC, Bax NM. Laparoscopic repair of congenital diaphragmatic hernia in a 6-month-old child. Surg Endosc 1995;9:1001–3.

46. Arca MJ, Barnhart DC, Lelli JL Jr, et al. Early experience with minimally invasive repair of congenital diaphragmatic hernias: results and lessons learned. J Pediatr Surg 2003;38:1563–8.

47. Yang EY, Allmendinger N, Johnson SM, et al. Neonatal thoracoscopic repair of congenital diaphragmatic hernia: selection criteria for successful outcome. J Pediatr Surg 2005;40:1369–75.

48. Durkin ET, Shaaban AF. Recent advances and controversies in pediatric laparoscopic surgery. Surg Clin North Am 2008;88:1101–19.

49. Meehan JJ, Sandler A. Robotic repair of a Bochdalek congenital diaphragmatic hernia in a small neonate: robotic advantages and limitations. J Pediatr Surg 2007;42:1757–60.

50. Flake AW, Crombleholme TM, Johnson MP, et al. Treatment of severe congenital diaphragmatic hernia by fetal tracheal occlusion: clinical experience with fifteen cases. Am J Obstet Gynecol 2000;183:1059–66.

51. Harrison MR, Keller RL, Hawgood SB, et al. A randomized trial of fetal endoscopic tracheal occlusion for severe fetal congenital diaphragmatic hernia. N Engl J Med 2003;349:1916–24.

52. Deprest J, Gratacos E, Nicolaides KH. Fetoscopic tracheal occlusion (FETO) for severe congenital diaphragmatic hernia: evolution of a technique and preliminary results. Ultrasound Obstet Gynecol 2004;24:121–6.

53. Deprest J, Jani J, Gratacos E, et al. Fetal intervention for congenital diaphragmatic hernia: the European experience. Semin Perinatol 2005;29:94–103.

54. Jani J, Gratacos E, Greenough A, et al. Percutaneous fetal endoscopic tracheal occlusion (FETO) for severe left-sided congenital diaphragmatic hernia. Clin Obstet Gynecol 2005;48:910–22.

55. Depaepe A, Dolk H, Lechat MF. The epidemiology of tracheo-oesophageal fistula and oesophageal atresia in Europe. EUROCAT Working Group. Arch Dis Child 1993;68:743–8.

56. Pletcher BA, Friedes JS, Breg WR, et al. Familial occurrence of esophageal atresia with and without tracheoesophageal fistula: report of two unusual kindreds. Am J Med Genet 1991;39:380–4.

57. Pretorius DH, Drose JA, Dennis MA, et al. Tracheoesophageal fistula in utero. Twenty-two cases. J Ultrasound Med 1987;6:509–13.

58. Houben CH, Curry JI. Current status of prenatal diagnosis, operative management and outcome of esophageal atresia/tracheo-esophageal fistula. Prenat Diagn 2008;28:667–75.

59. Sparey C, Jawaheer G, Barrett AM, et al. Esophageal atresia in the northern region congenital anomaly survey, 1985–1997: prenatal diagnosis and outcome. Am J Obstet Gynecol 2000;182:427–31.

60. Sparey C, Robson SC. Oesophageal atresia. Prenat Diagn 2000;20:251–3.

61. Langer JC, Hussain H, Khan A, et al. Prenatal diagnosis of esophageal atresia using sonography and magnetic resonance imaging. J Pediatr Surg 2001;36:804–7.

62. Levine D, Barnewolt CE, Mehta TS, et al. Fetal thoracic abnormalities: MR imaging. Radiology 2003;228:379–88.

63. Spitz L, Kiely E, Brereton RJ. Esophageal atresia: five-year experience with 148 cases. J Pediatr Surg 1987;22:103–8.

64. Chittmittrapap S, Spitz L, Kiely EM, et al. Anastomotic leakage following surgery for esophageal atresia. J Pediatr Surg 1992;27:29–32.

65. Spitz L. Esophageal atresia and tracheoesophageal fistula in children. Curr Opin Pediatr 1993;5:347–52.

66. Malviya M, Ohlsson A, Shah S. Surgical versus medical treatment with cyclooxygenase inhibitors for symptomatic patent ductus arteriosus in preterm infants. Cochrane Database Syst Rev 2008;23(1):CD003951.

67. Mikhail M, Lee W, Toews W, et al. Surgical and medical experience with 734 premature infants with patent ductus arteriosus. J Thorac Cardiovasc Surg 1982;83:349–57.

68. Grosfeld JL, Chaet M, Molinari F, et al. Increased risk of necrotizing enterocolitis in premature infants with patent ductus arteriosus treated with indomethacin. Ann Surg 1996;224:350–5 [discussion: 355].

69. Mosalli R, Alfaleh K. Prophylactic surgical ligation of patent ductus arteriosus for prevention of mortality and morbidity in extremely low birth weight infants. Cochrane Database Syst Rev 2008;23(1):CD006181.

70. Burke RP, Wernovsky G, van der Velde M, et al. Video-assisted thoracoscopic surgery for congenital heart disease. J Thorac Cardiovasc Surg 1995;109:499–507 [discussion: 508].

71. Hines MH, Bensky AS, Hammon JW Jr, et al. Video-assisted thoracoscopic ligation of patent ductus arteriosus: safe and outpatient. Ann Thorac Surg 1998;66:853–8 [discussion: 858].

72. Vanamo K, Berg E, Kokki H, et al. Video-assisted thoracoscopic versus open surgery for persistent ductus arteriosus. J Pediatr Surg 2006;41:1226–9.

73. Nezafati MH, Soltani G, Vedadian A. Video-assisted ductal closure with new modifications: minimally invasive, maximally effective, 1300 cases. Ann Thorac Surg 2007;84:1343–8.

74. Dutta S, Mihailovic A, Benson L, et al. Thoracoscopic ligation versus coil occlusion for patent ductus arteriosus: a matched cohort study of outcomes and cost. Surg Endosc 2008;22:1643–8.

75. Henry MC, Moss RL. Neonatal necrotizing enterocolitis. Semin Pediatr Surg 2008;17:98–109.
76. Nowicki PT, Dunaway DJ, Nankervis CA, et al. Endothelin-1 in human intestine resected for necrotizing enterocolitis. J Pediatr 2005;146:805–10.
77. Gonzalez-Crussi F, Hsueh W. Experimental model of ischemic bowel necrosis. The role of platelet-activating factor and endotoxin. Am J Pathol 1983;112:127–35.
78. Nanthakumar NN, Fusunyan RD, Sanderson I, et al. Inflammation in the developing human intestine: A possible pathophysiologic contribution to necrotizing enterocolitis. Proc Natl Acad Sci U S A 2000;97:6043–8.
79. Chan KL, Ho JC, Chan KW, et al. A study of gut immunity to enteral endotoxin in rats of different ages: a possible cause for necrotizing enterocolitis. J Pediatr Surg 2002;37:1435–40.
80. Cetin S, Dunklebarger J, Li J, et al. Endotoxin differentially modulates the basolateral and apical sodium/proton exchangers (NHE) in enterocytes. Surgery 2004;136:375–83.
81. Qureshi FG, Leaphart C, Cetin S, et al. Increased expression and function of integrins in enterocytes by endotoxin impairs epithelial restitution. Gastroenterology 2005;128:1012–22.
82. Feng J, El-Assal ON, Besner GE. Heparin-binding epidermal growth factor-like growth factor reduces intestinal apoptosis in neonatal rats with necrotizing enterocolitis. J Pediatr Surg 2006;41:742–7 [discussion: 742].
83. Feng J, El-Assal ON, Besner GE. Heparin-binding epidermal growth factor-like growth factor decreases the incidence of necrotizing enterocolitis in neonatal rats. J Pediatr Surg 2006;41:144–9 [discussion: 144].
84. Grishin AV, Wang J, Potoka DA, et al. Lipopolysaccharide induces cyclooxygenase-2 in intestinal epithelium via a noncanonical p38 MAPK pathway. J Immunol 2006;176:580–8.
85. Leaphart CL, Cavallo J, Gribar SC, et al. A critical role for TLR4 in the pathogenesis of necrotizing enterocolitis by modulating intestinal injury and repair. J Immunol 2007;179:4808–20.
86. Gribar SC, Sodhi CP, Richardson WM, et al. Reciprocal expression and signaling of TLR4 and TLR9 in the pathogenesis and treatment of necrotizing enterocolitis. J Immunol 2009;182:636–46.
87. Bell MJ, Ternberg JL, Feigin RD, et al. Neonatal necrotizing enterocolitis. Therapeutic decisions based upon clinical staging. Ann Surg 1978;187:1–7.
88. Blakely ML, Lally KP, McDonald S, et al. Postoperative outcomes of extremely low birth-weight infants with necrotizing enterocolitis or isolated intestinal perforation: a prospective cohort study by the NICHD Neonatal Research Network. Ann Surg 2005;241:984–9 [discussion: 989].
89. Moss RL, Dimmitt RA, Barnhart DC, et al. Laparotomy versus peritoneal drainage for necrotizing enterocolitis and perforation. N Engl J Med 2006;354:2225–34.
90. Rees CM, Eaton S, Kiely EM, et al. Peritoneal drainage or laparotomy for neonatal bowel perforation? A randomized controlled trial. Ann Surg 2008;248:44–51.
91. Stevenson DK, Kerner JA, Malachowski N, et al. Late morbidity among survivors of necrotizing enterocolitis. Pediatrics 1980;66:925–7.
92. Hintz SR, Kendrick DE, Stoll BJ, et al. Neurodevelopmental and growth outcomes of extremely low birth weight infants after necrotizing enterocolitis. Pediatrics 2005;115:696–703.

93. Grave GD, Nelson SA, Walker WA, et al. New therapies and preventive approaches for necrotizing enterocolitis: report of a research planning workshop. Pediatr Res 2007;62:510–4.

94. Loane M, Dolk H, Bradbury I. Increasing prevalence of gastroschisis in Europe 1980-2002: a phenomenon restricted to younger mothers? Paediatr Perinat Epidemiol 2007;21:363–9.

95. David AL, Tan A, Curry J. Gastroschisis: sonographic diagnosis, associations, management and outcome. Prenat Diagn 2008;28:633–44.

96. Hunter AG, Stevenson RE. Gastroschisis: clinical presentation and associations. Am J Med Genet C Semin Med Genet 2008;148C:219–30.

97. Abdullah F, Arnold MA, Nabaweesi R, et al. Gastroschisis in the United States 1988–2003: analysis and risk categorization of 4344 patients. J Perinatol 2007; 27:50–5.

98. Quirk JG Jr, Fortney J, Collins HB II, et al. Outcomes of newborns with gastroschisis: the effects of mode of delivery, site of delivery, and interval from birth to surgery. Am J Obstet Gynecol 1996;174:1134–8.

99. Badillo AT, Hedrick HL, Wilson RD, et al. Prenatal ultrasonographic gastrointestinal abnormalities in fetuses with gastroschisis do not correlate with postnatal outcomes. J Pediatr Surg 2008;43:647–53.

100. Luton D, de Lagausie P, Guibourdenche J, et al. Effect of amnioinfusion on the outcome of prenatally diagnosed gastroschisis. Fetal Diagn Ther 1999;14: 152–5.

101. Huang J, Kurkchubasche AG, Carr SR, et al. Benefits of term delivery in infants with antenatally diagnosed gastroschisis. Obstet Gynecol 2002;100:695–9.

102. Ergun O, Barksdale E, Ergun FS, et al. The timing of delivery of infants with gastroschisis influences outcome. J Pediatr Surg 2005;40:424–8.

103. Logghe HL, Mason GC, Thornton JG, et al. A randomized controlled trial of elective preterm delivery of fetuses with gastroschisis. J Pediatr Surg 2005;40: 1726–31.

104. Midrio P, Stefanutti G, Mussap M, et al. Amnioexchange for fetuses with gastroschisis: is it effective? J Pediatr Surg 2007;42:777–82.

105. Moretti M, Khoury A, Rodriquez J, et al. The effect of mode of delivery on the perinatal outcome in fetuses with abdominal wall defects. Am J Obstet Gynecol 1990;163:833–8.

106. How HY, Harris BJ, Pietrantoni M, et al. Is vaginal delivery preferable to elective cesarean delivery in fetuses with a known ventral wall defect? Am J Obstet Gynecol 2000;182:1527–34.

107. Puligandla PS, Janvier A, Flageole H, et al. Routine cesarean delivery does not improve the outcome of infants with gastroschisis. J Pediatr Surg 2004; 39:742–5.

108. Jona JZ. The 'gentle touch' technique in the treatment of gastroschisis. J Pediatr Surg 2003;38:1036–8.

109. Kidd JN Jr, Jackson RJ, Smith SD, et al. Evolution of staged versus primary closure of gastroschisis. Ann Surg 2003;237:759–64.

110. Schlatter M, Norris K, Uitvlugt N, et al. Improved outcomes in the treatment of gastroschisis using a preformed silo and delayed repair approach. J Pediatr Surg 2003;38:459–64.

111. Chiu B, Lopoo J, Hoover JD, et al. Closing arguments for gastroschisis: management with silo reduction. J Perinat Med 2006;34:243–5.

112. Weinsheimer RL, Yanchar NL, Bouchard SB, et al. Gastroschisis closure—does method really matter? J Pediatr Surg 2008;43:874–8.

113. Schlatter M. Preformed silos in the management of gastroschisis: new progress with an old idea. Curr Opin Pediatr 2003;15:239–42.
114. Miro J, Bard H. Congenital atresia and stenosis of the duodenum: the impact of a prenatal diagnosis. Am J Obstet Gynecol 1988;158:555–9.
115. Haeusler MC, Berghold A, Stoll C, et al. Prenatal ultrasonographic detection of gastrointestinal obstruction: results from 18 European congenital anomaly registries. Prenat Diagn 2002;22:616–23.
116. Stoll C, Alembik Y, Dott B. Impact of routine fetal ultrasonographic screening on the prevalence of Down syndrome in non aged mothers. Ann Genet 1998; 41:27–30.
117. Stoll C, Alembik Y, Dott B, et al. Study of Down syndrome in 238,942 consecutive births. Ann Genet 1998;41:44–51.
118. Piper HG, Alesbury J, Waterford SD, et al. Intestinal atresias: factors affecting clinical outcomes. J Pediatr Surg 2008;43:1244–8.
119. Seo T, Ando H, Watanabe Y, et al. Colonic atresia and Hirschsprung's disease: importance of histologic examination of the distal bowel. J Pediatr Surg 2002; 37:E19.
120. Draus JM Jr, Maxfield CM, Bond SJ. Hirschsprung's disease in an infant with colonic atresia and normal fixation of the distal colon. J Pediatr Surg 2007;42:e5–8.
121. Kimura K, Tsugawa C, Ogawa K, et al. Diamond-shaped anastomosis for congenital duodenal obstruction. Arch Surg 1977;112:1262–3.
122. Kimura K, Mukohara N, Nishijima E, et al. Diamond-shaped anastomosis for duodenal atresia: an experience with 44 patients over 15 years. J Pediatr Surg 1990;25:977–9.
123. Adzick NS, Harrison MR, deLorimier AA. Tapering duodenoplasty for megaduodenum associated with duodenal atresia. J Pediatr Surg 1986;21:311–2.
124. Etensel B, Temir G, Karkiner A, et al. Atresia of the colon. J Pediatr Surg 2005; 40:1258–68.
125. Watts AC, Sabharwal AJ, MacKinlay GA, et al. Congenital colonic atresia: should primary anastomosis always be the goal? Pediatr Surg Int 2003;19:14–7.
126. Gura KM, Lee S, Valim C, et al. Safety and efficacy of a fish-oil-based fat emulsion in the treatment of parenteral nutrition-associated liver disease. Pediatrics 2008;121:e678–86.
127. Modi BP, Langer M, Ching YA, et al. Improved survival in a multidisciplinary short bowel syndrome program. J Pediatr Surg 2008;43:20–4.
128. von Flue M, Herzog U, Ackermann C, et al. Acute and chronic presentation of intestinal nonrotation in adults. Dis Colon Rectum 1994;37:192–8.
129. Durkin ET, Lund DP, Shaaban AF, et al. Age-related differences in diagnosis and morbidity of intestinal malrotation. J Am Coll Surg 2008;206:658–63.
130. Choi M, Borenstein SH, Hornberger L, et al. Heterotaxia syndrome: the role of screening for intestinal rotation abnormalities. Arch Dis Child 2005;90:813–5.
131. Tashjian DB, Weeks B, Brueckner M, et al. Outcomes after a Ladd procedure for intestinal malrotation with heterotaxia. J Pediatr Surg 2007;42:528–31.
132. Suita S, Taguchi T, Ieiri S, et al. Hirschsprung's disease in Japan: analysis of 3852 patients based on a nationwide survey in 30 years. J Pediatr Surg 2005; 40:197–201 [discussion: 201].
133. Fujimoto T, Hata J, Yokoyama S, et al. A study of the extracellular matrix protein as the migration pathway of neural crest cells in the gut: analysis in human embryos with special reference to the pathogenesis of Hirschsprung's disease. J Pediatr Surg 1989;24:550–6.

134. Newgreen DF, Southwell B, Hartley L, et al. Migration of enteric neural crest cells in relation to growth of the gut in avian embryos. Acta Anat 1996;157:105–15.

135. Hearn CJ, Murphy M, Newgreen D. GDNF and ET-3 differentially modulate the numbers of avian enteric neural crest cells and enteric neurons in vitro. Dev Biol 1998;197:93–105.

136. Heanue TA, Pachnis V. Enteric nervous system development and Hirschsprung's disease: advances in genetic and stem cell studies. Nat Rev Neurosci 2007;8:466–79.

137. Tobin JL, Di Franco M, Eichers E, et al. Inhibition of neural crest migration underlies craniofacial dysmorphology and Hirschsprung's disease in Bardet-Biedl syndrome. Proc Natl Acad Sci U S A 2008;105:6714–9.

138. Ikeda K, Goto S. Diagnosis and treatment of Hirschsprung's disease in Japan. An analysis of 1628 patients. Ann Surg 1984;199:400–5.

139. Langer JC, Durrant AC, de la Torre L, et al. One-stage transanal Soave pull-through for Hirschsprung disease: a multicenter experience with 141 children. Ann Surg 2003;238:569–83 [discussion: 583].

140. Taxman TL, Yulish BS, Rothstein FC. How useful is the barium enema in the diagnosis of infantile Hirschsprung's disease? Am J Dis Child 1986;140:881–4.

141. O'Donovan AN, Habra G, Somers S, et al. Diagnosis of Hirschsprung's disease. AJR Am J Roentgenol 1996;167:517–20.

142. Georgeson KE, Cohen RD, Hebra A, et al. Primary laparoscopic-assisted endorectal colon pull-through for Hirschsprung's disease: a new gold standard. Ann Surg 1999;229:678–82 [discussion: 682].

143. Stern LE, Warner BW. Gastrointestinal duplications. Semin Pediatr Surg 2000;9:135–40.

144. Ildstad ST, Tollerud DJ, Weiss RG, et al. Duplications of the alimentary tract. Clinical characteristics, preferred treatment, and associated malformations. Ann Surg 1988;208:184–9.

145. Segal SR, Sherman NH, Rosenberg HK, et al. Ultrasonographic features of gastrointestinal duplications. J Ultrasound Med 1994;13:863–70.

146. Teele RL, Henschke CI, Tapper D. The radiographic and ultrasonographic evaluation of enteric duplication cysts. Pediatr Radiol 1980;10:9–14.

147. Spottswood SE. Peristalsis in duplication cyst: a new diagnostic sonographic finding. Pediatr Radiol 1994;24:344–5.

148. Vijayaraghavan SB, Manonmani K, Rajamani G. Sonographic features of tubular duplication of the small bowel. J Ultrasound Med 2002;21:1319–22.

149. Hall NJ, Ade-Ajayi N, Peebles D, et al. Antenatally diagnosed duplication cyst of the tongue: modern imaging modalities assist perinatal management. Pediatr Surg Int 2005;21:289–91.

150. Beierle EA, Vinocur CD. Gastrointestinal surgery in cystic fibrosis. Curr Opin Pulm Med 1998;4:319–25.

151. Winfield RD, Beierle EA. Pediatric surgical issues in meconium disease and cystic fibrosis. Surg Clin North Am 2006;86:317–27.

152. Rogers CS, Stoltz DA, Meyerholz DK, et al. Disruption of the CFTR gene produces a model of cystic fibrosis in newborn pigs. Science 2008;321:1837–41.

153. Meeker IA Jr. Acetylcysteine used to liquefy inspissated meconium causing intestinal obstruction in the newborn. Surgery 1964;56:419–25.

154. Rescorla FJ, Grosfeld JL. Contemporary management of meconium ileus. World J Surg 1993;17:318–25.

155. Escobar MA, Grosfeld JL, Burdick JJ, et al. Surgical considerations in cystic fibrosis: a 32-year evaluation of outcomes. Surgery 2005;138:560–71 [discussion: 571].
156. Clatworthy HW Jr, Howard WH, Lloyd J. The meconium plug syndrome. Surgery 1956;39:131–42.
157. Van Leeuwen G, Glenn L, Woodruff C, et al. Meconium plug syndrome with aganglionosis. Pediatrics 1967;40:665–6.
158. Hajivassiliou CA. Intestinal obstruction in neonatal/pediatric surgery. Semin Pediatr Surg 2003;12:241–53.
159. Keckler SJ, St Peter SD, Spilde TL, et al. Current significance of meconium plug syndrome. J Pediatr Surg 2008;43:896–8.
160. Bassett MD, Murray KF. Biliary atresia: recent progress. J Clin Gastroenterol 2008;42:720–9.
161. Chandra RS. Biliary atresia and other structural anomalies in the congenital polysplenia syndrome. J Pediatr 1974;85:649–55.
162. Davenport M, Savage M, Mowat AP, et al. Biliary atresia splenic malformation syndrome: an etiologic and prognostic subgroup. Surgery 1993;113:662–8.
163. Ferdman B, States L, Gaynor JW, et al. Abnormalities of intestinal rotation in patients with congenital heart disease and the heterotaxy syndrome. Congenit Heart Dis 2007;2:12–8.
164. Karrer FM, Hall RJ, Lilly JR. Biliary atresia and the polysplenia syndrome. J Pediatr Surg 1991;26:524–7.
165. Carmi R, Magee CA, Neill CA, et al. Extrahepatic biliary atresia and associated anomalies: etiologic heterogeneity suggested by distinctive patterns of associations. Am J Med Genet 1993;45:683–93.
166. Mack CL. The pathogenesis of biliary atresia: evidence for a virus-induced autoimmune disease. Semin Liver Dis 2007;27:233–42.
167. Aabakken L, Aagenaes I, Sanengen T, et al. Utility of ERCP in neonatal and infant cholestasis. J Laparoendosc Adv Surg Tech A 2009;13:13.
168. Vegting IL, Tabbers MM, Taminiau JA, et al. Is endoscopic retrograde cholangiopancreatography valuable and safe in children of all ages? J Pediatr Gastroenterol Nutr 2009;48:66–71.
169. Kasai M. Treatment of biliary atresia with special reference to hepatic portoenterostomy and its modifications. Prog Pediatr Surg 1974;6:5–52.
170. Kasai M, Watanabe I, Ohi R. Follow-up studies of long-term survivors after hepatic portoenterostomy for "noncorrectible" biliary atresia. J Pediatr Surg 1975;10:173–82.
171. Meyers RL, Book LS, O'Gorman MA, et al. High-dose steroids, ursodeoxycholic acid, and chronic intravenous antibiotics improve bile flow after Kasai procedure in infants with biliary atresia. J Pediatr Surg 2003;38:406–11.
172. Dutta S, Woo R, Albanese CT. Minimal access portoenterostomy: advantages and disadvantages of standard laparoscopic and robotic techniques. J Laparoendosc Adv Surg Tech A 2007;17:258–64.
173. Shinkai M, Ohhama Y, Take H, et al. Long-term outcome of children with biliary atresia who were not transplanted after the Kasai operation: >20-year experience at a children's hospital. J Pediatr Gastroenterol Nutr 2009;48:443–50.
174. Chen CL, Concejero A, Wang CC, et al. Living donor liver transplantation for biliary atresia: a single-center experience with first 100 cases. Am J Transplant 2006;6:2672–9.

Identification of Neonates at Risk for Hazardous Hyperbilirubinemia: Emerging Clinical Insights

Jon F. Watchko, MD

KEYWORDS

- Jaundice • Kernicterus
- Glucose-6-phosphate dehydrogenase deficiency
- Late preterm gestation • Breast milk feeding
- East Asian ethnicity

Hyperbilirubinemia is the most common condition requiring evaluation and treatment in neonates, but for most newborns, it is a benign postnatal transitional phenomenon of no overt clinical significance. In a select few, however, the total serum bilirubin (TSB) may rise to hazardous levels that pose a direct threat of brain damage. Advanced phases of acute bilirubin encephalopathy may ensue, frequently evolving into chronic bilirubin encephalopathy (kernicterus), a devastating, disabling condition classically characterized by the clinical tetrad of choreoathetoid cerebral palsy, high-frequency central neural hearing loss, palsy of vertical gaze, and dental enamel hypoplasia as the result of bilirubin-induced cell toxicity.[1,2]

Originally described in newborns who had Rh hemolytic disease, kernicterus has been reported in apparently healthy term and late preterm gestation breastfed infants who do not have documented hemolysis.[3–5] Published reports of kernicterus in the United States[3–5] and abroad[6–8] have increased since the mid- to late-1980s. In the United States, a striking and sustained increase in breastfeeding prevalence[9] coupled with a concurrent progressive decline in birth hospitalization length of stay[10] appear to have unmasked a previously underappreciated potential to develop extreme levels of

Funding was received from Mario Lemieux Centers for Patient Care and Research of the Mario Lemieux Foundation.

Division of Newborn Medicine, Department of Pediatrics, University of Pittsburgh School of Medicine, Magee-Womens Research Institute, Magee-Womens Hospital, 300 Halket Street, Pittsburgh, PA 15213, USA

E-mail address: jwatchko@mail.magee.edu

Pediatr Clin N Am 56 (2009) 671–687
doi:10.1016/j.pcl.2009.04.005
0031-3955/09/$ – see front matter © 2009 Elsevier Inc. All rights reserved.

pediatric.theclinics.com

hyperbilirubinemia in some neonates (**Fig. 1**), the biologic basis of which is often multi-factorial.[11,12] This article highlights selected demographic, environmental, and genetic risk factors that may contribute to a neonate's predisposition to marked hyperbilirubi-nemia. It is meant not to be comprehensive in scope but to define among the myriad of potential contributors the salient ones that may merit special clinical attention and provide updated details regarding their possible etiopathogenic roles.

Although each selected factor holds the potential to be a singularly important, even sole, contributor to an infant's marked hyperbilirubinemia, risk factors are more often observed in combination with others.[11,12] In infants who had peak TSB levels of 25 mg/dL (428 μmol/L) or higher, 88% had a least two and 43% had three or more identified risk factors in one recent report,[11] and 58% who had peak TSB levels of 20 mg/dL (342 μmol/L) or higher had at least two risk factors in another report.[12] Data derived from risk instruments that incorporate several factors support the potential multifactorial etiopathogenesis of marked hyperbilirubinemia, albeit genetic contributors may go undetected and individual factors confer different degrees of risk.[11,13] These risk instruments further highlight the clinical importance of two specific risk factors in particular, namely late preterm gestational age and exclusive breast-feeding.[11,13,14] These two contributors are reviewed first, followed by six others of notable clinical impact: glucose-6-phosphate dehydrogenase (G6PD) deficiency, ABO hemolytic disease, East Asian ethnicity, jaundice observed in the first 24 hours of life, cephalohematoma or significant bruising, and history of a previous sibling treated with phototherapy.[15] Each contributor is characterized as a major risk factor for the development of severe hyperbilirubinemia in infants of 35 or more weeks' gestation in the 2004 American Academy of Pediatrics (AAP) clinical practice guideline on hyperbilirubinemia management (**Box 1**).[15] Also summarized is the emerging evidence that combining risk factors with predischarge TSB or transcutaneous bilirubin (TcB) levels improves hyperbilirubinemia risk prediction.[13,14,16] Practitioners

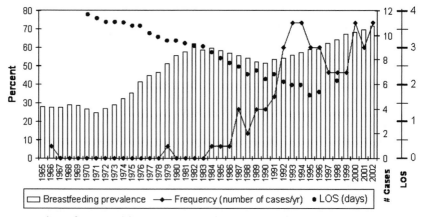

Fig. 1. Number of reported kernicterus cases by birth year from 1965 to 2002 (*solid dia-monds*)[4] in relation to annual prevalence of breastfeeding at birth hospitalization (*open bars, as percentage*)[9] and birth hospitalization length of stay (*solid circles, in days*).[10] An increase in reported cases of kernicterus is seen in conjunction with a sustained resurgence of breastfeeding initiation prevalence during birth hospitalization and concurrent decreased birth hospitalization length of stay (LOS). (*From* Watchko JF. Kernicterus and the molecular mechanisms of bilirubin-induced CNS injury in newborns. Neuromolecular Med 2006;8:515; with permission.)

Box 1
Major risk factors for development of severe hyperbilirubinemia in infants of 35 or more weeks' gestation

Gestational age 35 to 36 weeks

Exclusive breastfeeding, particularly if nursing is not going well and weight loss is excessive

Blood group incompatibility with positive direct antiglobulin test; other known hemolytic disease (eg, G6PD deficiency)

East Asian race

Jaundice observed in the first 24 hours

Cephalohematoma or significant bruising

Previous sibling received phototherapy

Predischarge TSB or TcB level in the high risk zone

From American Academy of Pediatrics. Management of hyperbilirubinemia in the newborn infant 35 or more weeks of gestation. Pediatrics 2004;114(1):297–316; with permission. Copyright © 2004, American Academy of Pediatrics.

---

are referred to the 2004 AAP guideline for specific evaluation, management, and treatment recommendations.[15]

LATE PRETERM GESTATION

Late preterm ($34^{0/7}$–$36^{6/7}$ weeks' gestation) and full-term infants become jaundiced by similar mechanisms, including (1) an increased bilirubin load on the hepatocyte as a result of decreased erythrocyte survival, increased erythrocyte volume, and the enterohepatic circulation of bilirubin; and (2) defective hepatic bilirubin conjugation.[17] Late preterm infants evidence a similar degree of red blood cell turnover and heme degradation as their full-term counterparts;[18] however, they differ from term newborns in how effectively they handle the resultant hepatic bilirubin load,[18] demonstrating a lower hepatic bilirubin conjugation capacity (uridine-diphosphate glucuronosyl transferase 1A1 [*UGT1A1*] enzyme activity).[18,19] Moreover, although there is a marked postnatal increase in *UGT1A1* enzyme activity in newborns, such maturation appears to be slower in late preterm neonates during the first week of life.[19] This exaggerated hepatic immaturity[18,19] contributes to the greater prevalence, severity, and duration of neonatal jaundice in late preterm infants.

Underscoring the importance of late preterm gestational age is the approximately eightfold increased risk of developing a TSB level of 20 mg/dL (342 μmol/L) or higher in infants born at 36 weeks' gestational age (5.2%) compared with those born at 41 and 42 or more weeks' gestation (0.7% and 0.6%, respectively).[20] This gestational age effect is even more evident when examined as a function of hour-specific TSB risk zones using the percentile-based nomogram described by Bhutani and colleagues[21] (**Fig. 2**).[13] It can be seen, for example, that coupling 36 weeks' gestation with a high risk zone ($\geq$95%) TSB is associated with a greater than 40% chance of developing a TSB level of 20 mg/dL (342 μmol/L) or higher.[13] Even a high-intermediate risk zone (75%–94%) TSB in a 36 weeks' gestation late preterm neonate is associated with a greater than 10% chance of developing a TSB level of 20 mg/dL (342 μmol/L) or higher, a risk greater than that for a full-term newborn who has a TSB level of 95% or greater.[13] In this regard, the reported difficulty in visually assessing jaundice in late preterm newborns[22] suggests that they should have a birth hospitalization TSB or

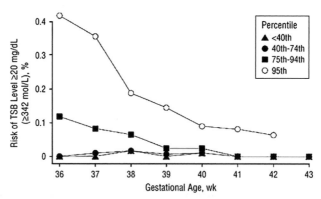

Fig. 2. Risk of developing a TSB level of 20 mg/dL (342 μmol/L) or higher as a function of gestational age and percentile-based TSB level using the Bhutani nomogram measured at 48 hours of age or less. wk, weeks. (*From* Newman TB, Liljestrand P, Escobar GJ. Combining clinical risk factors with serum bilirubin levels to predict hyperbilirubinemia in newborns. Arch Pediatr Adolesc Med 159(2):117. Copyright © 2005, American Medical Association. All rights reserved; with permission.)

TcB screen before discharge interpreted using the hour-specific nomogram to more fully ascertain their hyperbilirubinemia risk.

Late preterm infants are disproportionately overrepresented in the United States Pilot Kernicterus Registry, a database of voluntarily reported cases of kernicterus.[4,23] Moreover, the registry demonstrates that late preterm neonates evidence signs of bilirubin neurotoxicity at an earlier postnatal age than term newborns, indirectly suggesting a greater vulnerability to bilirubin-induced brain injury.[23] Clinical hyperbilirubinemia management guidelines for late preterm infants therefore recommend treatment at lower TSB thresholds than for term newborns, a distinction that is an important component of the 2004 AAP practice guideline on neonatal jaundice.[15] In this regard, it is important to note that the management of late preterm newborns born between $34^{0/7}$ and $34^{6/7}$ weeks' gestation is not addressed by the 2004 AAP guideline, and that infants born between $37^{0/7}$ and $37^{6/7}$ weeks' gestation, although strictly defined as term, are characterized in the 2004 AAP guideline as medium to higher risk and are to be managed as "late preterm" regarding phototherapy and exchange thresholds.[15]

Of the various clinical factors observed in conjunction with late preterm gestation hyperbilirubinemia risk, breast milk feeding has been identified most consistently (indeed almost uniformly) and therefore appears to be of paramount importance.[4,23] Late preterm neonates, because of their immaturity, often demonstrate less effective sucking and swallowing and may have difficulties achieving consistent nutritive breastfeeding,[24] phenomena that may predispose to varying degrees of lactation failure. Suboptimal feeding was the leading reason for discharge delay during birth hospitalization in late preterm neonates in one recent study.[24] Pediatricians, therefore, need to be alert to the potential of suboptimal breast milk feeding in late preterm neonates and not be misled by the seemingly satisfactory breastfeeding efforts of late preterm newborns during the birth hospitalization when limited colostrum volumes make it a challenge to adequately assess the effectiveness of breast milk transfer.[25] Therefore, late preterm infants who are breastfed merit timely post-birth hospitalization discharge follow-up and lactation support.[17,23] Lactation support coupled with regular neonatal weight checks is helpful in averting lactation difficulties and in the early identification of mother-infant pairs prone to lactation failure. Parental education (written and verbal) about neonatal jaundice and when to call the pediatrician is also important.[15] A shortened hospital stay (<48 hours after delivery), although permitted for selected healthy term neonates, is not recommended for late preterm neonates.[26]

EXCLUSIVE BREAST MILK FEEDING

It is likely no coincidence that almost every reported case of kernicterus over the past 2.5 decades has been in breastfed infants.[4] As such, exclusive breast milk feeding, particularly if nursing is not going well and weight loss is excessive, is listed as a major hyperbilirubinemia risk factor in the 2004 AAP practice guideline.[15] What does the association between exclusive breast milk feeding and kernicterus imply with respect to the etiopathogenesis of marked neonatal jaundice? Numerous studies have reported an association between breastfeeding and an increased incidence and severity of hyperbilirubinemia, both during the first few days of life and in the genesis of prolonged neonatal jaundice.[27–31] A pooled analysis of 12 studies that included over 8000 neonates showed a threefold greater incidence in TSB levels of 12.0 mg/dL (205 μmol) or higher, and a sixfold greater incidence in TSB levels of 15 mg/dL (257 μmol) or higher in breastfed infants compared with formula-fed counterparts.[30] Other investigators, however, report that when adequate breastfeeding is established and sufficient lactation support is in place, breastfed infants should be at no greater risk for hyperbilirubinemia than their formula-fed counterparts.[32–35] The later studies suggest that many breastfed infants who develop marked neonatal jaundice do so in the context of a delay in lactation or varying degrees of lactation failure. Indeed, an appreciable percentage of the breastfed infants who develop kernicterus have been noted to have inadequate intake and variable but substantial degrees of dehydration and weight loss.[3,36]

Inadequate breast milk intake, in addition to contributing to dehydration, can further enhance hyperbilirubinemia by increasing the enterohepatic circulation of bilirubin and resultant hepatic bilirubin load. The enterohepatic circulation of bilirubin is already exaggerated in the neonatal period, in part because the newborn intestinal tract is not yet colonized with bacteria that convert conjugated bilirubin to urobilinogen, and because intestinal beta-glucuronidase activity is high.[37,38] Earlier studies in newborn humans and primates suggest that the enterohepatic circulation of bilirubin may account for up to 50% of the hepatic bilirubin load in neonates.[39,40] Moreover, fasting hyperbilirubinemia is largely due to intestinal reabsorption of unconjugated bilirubin,[41,42] an additional mechanism by which inadequate lactation and poor enteral intake may contribute to marked hyperbilirubinemia in some newborns. In the context of limited hepatic conjugation capacity in the immediate postnatal period, any further increase in hepatic bilirubin load likely results in more hyperbilirubinemia. Recent study confirms that early breastfeeding-associated jaundice is associated with a state of relative caloric deprivation[43] and resultant enhanced enterohepatic circulation of bilirubin.[43,44] Breastfeeding-associated jaundice, however, is not associated with increased bilirubin production.[45,46]

Lactation failure, however, is not uniformly present in affected infants, suggesting that other mechanisms may be operative in breastfeeding-associated jaundice, a finding that merits further clinical study. Breast milk feeding may act as an environmental modifier for selected genotypes and thereby potentially predispose to the development of marked neonatal jaundice.[47,48] A recent report lends credence to this possibility, demonstrating that the risk of developing a TSB level of 20 mg/dL (342 μmol/L) or higher associated with breast milk feeding was enhanced 22-fold when combined with expression of a coding sequence gene polymorphism of the (1) bilirubin conjugating enzyme *UGT1A1* (the G211A missense mutation *UGT1A1*6*) or (2) solute carrier organic anion transporter 1B1 (*SLCO1B1*, also known as organic anion transporter polypeptide 2 [*OATP-2*]; the A388G missense variant *SLCO1B1*1b*).[12] SLCO1B1 is a sinusoidal membrane protein putatively involved in facilitating the hepatic uptake of unconjugated bilirubin.[49] This hyperbilirubinemia risk increased to 88-fold when breast milk feedings were combined with the *UGT1A1* and *SLCO1B1* variants.[12] Other investigators have previously reported an association between prolonged (>14 days) breast milk jaundice and expression of a *UGT1A1* gene promoter variant, namely a TA insertion in the TATAA box region, resulting in the variant allele A(TA)$_7$TAA (*UGT1A1*28*) instead of the wild-type allele A(TA)$_6$TAA.[50,51] In recognizing the relationship between breast milk feeding and jaundice, the benefits of breast milk feeds far outweigh the related risk of hyperbilirubinemia. Cases of severe neonatal hyperbilirubinemia with suboptimal breast milk feedings underscore the need for effective lactation support and timely follow-up examinations.

GLUCOSE-6-PHOSPHATE DEHYDROGENASE DEFICIENCY

G6PD deficiency is an X-linked enzymopathy affecting hemizygous males, homozygous females, and a subset of heterozygous females (by way of nonrandom X chromosome inactivation) and is an important cause of severe neonatal hyperbilirubinemia and kernicterus worldwide.[52–55] Although most prevalent in Africa, the Middle East, East Asia, and the Mediterranean, G6PD deficiency has evolved into a global problem as a result of centuries of immigration and intermarriage.[52–55] It is a noteworthy contributor to endemic rates of bilirubin encephalopathy in several developing countries (eg, Nigeria, where approximately 3% of neonatal hospital admissions evidence bilirubin encephalopathy)[56] and accounts for a substantial and disproportionate number of neonates who have kernicterus in the US Pilot Kernicterus registry (20.8% of all reported cases).[4] Although most of the latter cases are African American male infants,[4] other population subgroups in the United States at risk for G6PD deficiency include African American female infants and newborns of East Asian, Greek, Italian (especially Sardinia and Sicily), and Middle Eastern descent.[55]

Current G6PD deficiency prevalence rates in the United States are 12.2% for African American male infants, 4.1% for African American female infants, and 4.3% for Asian male infants (**Table 1**).[57] Even the ethnicity subset characterized as "unknown/other" in this large United States–based cohort showed a G6PD deficiency prevalence of 3.0% in male infants and 1.8% in female infants.[57] In this regard, *G6PD* is remarkable for its genetic diversity (more than 370 variants have been described),[58] and those mutations seen in the United States include, among numerous others, the: (1) *African A–* variants, a group of double-site mutations—all of which share the A376G variant (also known as G6PD A+ when expressed alone; a nondeficient variant)—coupled most commonly with the G202A mutation (G202A;A376G)[52,59] but, on occasion, with the T968C variant (T968C;A376G, also known as G6PD Betica)[52] or the G680T mutation (G680T;A376G);[52] (2) the *Mediterranean* (C563T)[52,59] mutation; (3) the *Canton* (G1376T)[52,59] mutation, and (4) the *Kaiping* (G1388A)[52,59] variant.

Two modes of hyperbilirubinemia presentation have classically been reported in *G6PD*-deficient neonates (with overlap between the two on occasion). The first is an acute, often sudden, unpredictable rise in TSB to potentially hazardous levels precipitated by an environmental trigger (eg, naphthalene in moth balls or infection);[52–55] this mode is difficult to foretell and therefore difficult to anticipate or prevent, and it is often a challenge to ascertain the trigger. The second mode of presentation is low-grade

Table 1
Presence of glucose-6-phosphate dehydrogenase deficiency in United States military personnel by sex and self-reported ethnicity

Ethnicity	Deficiency n (%)		
	Female	Male	Total
American Indian/Alaskan	112 (0.9)	492 (0.8)	604 (0.8)
Asian	465 (0.9)	1658 (4.30)	2123 (3.6)
African American	2763 (4.1)	8513 (12.2)	11,276 (10.2)
Hispanic	842 (1.2)	4462 (2.0)	5304 (1.9)
Caucasian	4018 (0.0)	38,108 (0.3)	42,126 (1.3)
Unknown/other	228 (1.8)	1641 (3.0)	1869 (2.9)

From Chinevere TD, Murray CK, Grant E, et al. Prevalence of glucose-6-phosphate dehydrogenase deficiency in U.S. Army personnel. Military Medicine: International Journal of AMSUS 2006;171(9):906; with permission.

hemolysis coupled with genetic polymorphisms of the *UGT1A1* gene that reduce *UGT1A1* expression and thereby limit hepatic bilirubin conjugation. These polymorphisms include the $(TA)_7$ dinucleotide repeat TATAA box promoter element (*UGT1A1*28*)[53–55,60] and the G211A coding sequence (UGT1A1*6)[61] variants; the former underlies the Gilbert syndrome phenotype in Caucasians,[62] whereas the latter underlies the Gilbert syndrome phenotype in East Asians.[61,63] Gilbert syndrome is a condition characterized by mild indirect hyperbilirubinemia in the absence of liver disease and clinically overt hemolysis.[62] Kaplan and colleagues[60] were the first to demonstrate dose-dependent genetic interactions between the *UGT1A1*28* promoter variant and G6PD deficiency that enhance neonatal hyperbilirubinemia risk. Other investigators have subsequently confirmed that coupling of G6PD deficiency and other genetically determined hemolytic conditions (eg, hereditary spherocytosis) with hepatic gene variants that adversely impact bilirubin clearance (ie, hepatic bilirubin uptake [*SLCO1B1*] and conjugation [*UGT1A1*]) increases the risk of significant neonatal hyperbilirubinemia.[61,63–65] Coexistent nongenetic factors may also impact hyperbilirubinemia risk in G6PD-deficient African American male neonates, as has been shown in those who are also late preterm and breastfed.[66] Sixty percent of this subgroup demonstrate bilirubin levels greater than 95% (high risk zone) on the bilirubin nomogram of Bhutani and colleagues[21] (odds ratio: 10.2; 95% confidence interval [CI]: 1.35–76.93).[66]

Because African Americans as a group have a lower incidence of neonatal hyperbilirubinemia (**Fig. 3**)[67] than the rest of the population[14,20,67] (odds ratio: 0.43 for bilirubin level that exceeded or was within 1 mg/dL [17 μmol/L] of 2004 AAP hour-specific phototherapy treatment threshold;[14] odds ratio: 0.56 for TSB ≥20 mg/dL [342 μmol/L][20]), numeric instruments designed to predict hyperbilirubinemia risk in newborns deduct points for black race.[11,13] This lower overall hyperbilirubinemia incidence, however, may belie the hyperbilirubinemia risk for G6PD-deficient African American newborns, leading some to caution that African American neonates who have overt jaundice (male or female) merit special attention and follow-up because such infants represent exceptions to this general pattern, a subset of which might be G6PD deficient. It may be that when an African American infant develops notable jaundice, he or she is at equal or perhaps even greater risk (if G6PD deficient) for hazardous hyperbilirubinemia. Consistent with this assertion, Kaplan and colleagues[68] reported that 48.4% of G6PD-deficient African American neonates developed a TSB level of 75% or higher and 21.9%

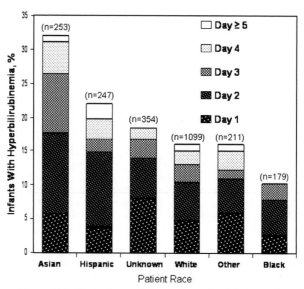

Fig. 3. Incidence of hyperbilirubinemia on different days after birth as a function of mother's race. Hyperbilirubinemia was defined as a TSB level of 5 mg/dL (86 μmol/L) or higher at 24 hours of age or less, 10 mg/dL (171 μmol/L) or higher at 24 to 48 hours of age, or 13 mg/dL (223 μmol/L) or higher thereafter. (*From* Newman TB, Easterling J, Goldman ES, et al. Laboratory evaluation of jaundice in newborns. Frequency, cost and yield. Am J Dis Child 144(3):355. Copyright © 1990, American Medical Association. All rights reserved; with permission.)

developed a TSB level of 95% or higher. In contrast, Keren and colleagues[14] reported that the presence of clinical jaundice or a G6PD mutation was not associated with the development of significant hyperbilirubinemia in black infants or black male infant cohorts. This matter merits further clinical study and clarification.

Although there has been discussion on the potential utility of screening for G6PD deficiency in the United States,[69] no consensus has emerged on whether or how best to screen for this condition in the United States and point-of-care testing during the birth hospitalization in not routinely practiced. Other countries (eg, Israel, Taiwan [Singapore])[70,71] have adopted various point-of-care G6PD screening strategies, some that target specific at-risk population subgroups, and others that screen population-wide, with reported success in reducing the prevalence of severe hyperbilirubinemia and kernicterus.

ABO HEMOLYTIC DISEASE

Hemolytic disease related to ABO incompatibility is a major risk factor for severe hyperbilirubinemia in the 2004 AAP practice guideline[15] and, for all intents and purposes, is limited to infants of blood group A or B born to mothers who are blood group O.[72,73] Although this association exists in approximately 15% of pregnancies, only a small fraction of such infants develop significant hyperbilirubinemia.[72,73] More specifically, of type A or B infants born to mothers who are blood group O, only approximately one third have a positive direct Coombs' test, and of those who have a positive direct Coombs' test, only approximately 15% will evidence a peak serum bilirubin level of 12.8 mg/dL (219 μmol/L) or higher.[73] Infants born of ABO-incompatible mother-infant pairs who have a negative direct Coombs' test appear, as a group, to be at no greater risk for developing significant hyperbilirubinemia than their ABO-compatible counterparts, regardless of the infant's indirect Coombs' test status.[73] Thus, evidence of symptomatic ABO hemolytic disease is found in only about 5% of ABO-incompatible mother-infant pairs and, in most circumstances, a positive direct Coombs' test appears to be necessary but not sufficient.[73–75] The diagnosis of symptomatic ABO hemolytic disease should be considered in infants who develop marked jaundice in the context of ABO incompatibility with a positive direct Coombs' test, often accompanied by microspherocytosis on red cell smear.[72–74] Underscoring the importance of a positive direct Coombs' test in support of the diagnosis of ABO hemolytic disease, Herschel and colleagues[74] recently concluded that in newborns of ABO-incompatible mother-infant pairs who have a negative direct Coombs' test and significant hyperbilirubinemia, a cause other than isoimmunization should be sought.

Despite the difficulty in predicting its development, symptomatic ABO hemolytic disease does occur, often with clinical jaundice detected within the first 12 to 24 hours of life; hence, the term "icterus praecox" was ascribed to this condition in its seminal description by Halbrecht[76] in 1944. The early rapid rise in TSB levels during the first 24 hours of life to the 10 to 15 mg/dL range or slightly higher is typically followed by a plateau at 15 to 20 mg/dL on the second day of life.[72,77] Hyperbilirubinemia secondary to ABO hemolytic disease was recognized decades ago to be controllable with phototherapy in most cases,[72,77] and even more so using current intensive photo-therapy strategies with special blue fluorescent lamps.[78] The addition of intravenous immune globulin to the therapeutic armamentarium against immune-mediated (posi-tive direct Coombs' test) hyperbilirubinemia has proved effective in reducing hemo-lysis[79] and the need for exchange transfusion in ABO hemolytic disease (number needed to treat: 2.7).[80] Few affected infants who have ABO hemolytic disease ever develop hyperbilirubinemia to levels requiring exchange transfusion,[72,81] although preparations for possible double-volume exchange should be made when exchange thresholds are approached.[15] Routine screening of all ABO-incompatible cord blood has been recommended in the past[82] and remains common practice in some nurs-eries.[83] The current literature,[73,83,84] however, suggests that such routine screening is probably not warranted given the low yield and cost, consistent with the tenor of recommendations of the American Association of Blood Banks.[85] A blood type and Coombs' test is indicated, however, in the evaluation of any newborn who has early or clinically significant jaundice.

EAST ASIAN ETHNICITY

Neonates of East Asian ethnicity encompassing the populations of mainland China, Hong Kong, Japan, Macau, Korea, and Taiwan evidence a higher incidence of hyper-bilirubinemia than other ethnicities (see **Fig. 3**)[67] and an overall increased risk for a TSB level of 20 mg/dL (342 μmol/L) or greater (odds ratio: 3.1; 95% CI: 1.5–6.3).[11] As such, East Asian ancestry is listed as a major risk factor for severe hyperbilirubinemia in the 2004 AAP clinical practice guideline.[15] Investigators have speculated as to the nature of this phenomenon, invoking potential population differences in the incidence of ABO hemolytic disease and G6PD deficiency and in environmental exposures to Chinese materia medica, among others.[86] There is little doubt that G6PD deficiency is an important contributor to hyperbilirubinemia risk in East Asian newborns. Innate ethnic variation in hepatic bilirubin clearance[86] also contributes to the biologic basis of hyper-bilirubinemia risk in Asian newborns as revealed by genetic analysis of enzymatic vari-ants that modulate bilirubin metabolism. Four different *UGT1A1* coding sequence variants: G211A (*UGT1A1*6*); C686A (*UGT1A1*27*); C1091T (*UGT1A1*73*); and

T1456G (*UGT1A1*7*) have been described in East Asian populations, each associated with a Gilbert syndrome phenotype.[12,87] Of these, the *UGT1A1*6* variant is predominant, with an allele frequency of 11% to 13% in East Asians[87] (as high as 30% in neonates who have TSB levels of 15 mg/dL [257 μmol/L])[88] or higher and an associated significant decrease in UGT1A1 enzyme activity.[89] Hepatic *SLCO1B1* gene variants are also prevalent in East Asian populations,[12,90] and the *SLCO1B1*1b* variant is demonstrated to enhance neonatal hyperbilirubinemia risk.[12] As noted in the section on breast milk feeding earlier, coupling the *UGT1A1* and *SLCO1B1* variants enhances hyperbilirubinemia risk, a risk that is further increased when that infant is also exclusively breastfed.[12] The high incidence of neonatal hyperbilirubinemia in East Asian populations appears to be at least partly attributable to the prevalence of these hepatic gene polymorphisms.

JAUNDICE OBSERVED IN THE FIRST 24 HOURS OF LIFE

Jaundice appearing in the first 24 hours of life has long been regarded as an abnormal clinical finding and an indication for a bilirubin measurement.[15] Approximately 2.8% of newborns evidence jaundice within 18 hours of life and 6.7% within 24 hours (**Fig. 4**).[91] As contrasted with nonjaundiced newborns on the first day of life, newborns who have overt jaundice in the first 24 hours of life are more likely to receive phototherapy (18.9% versus 1.7%; relative risk: 10.1; 95% CI: 4.2–24.4)[91] and to develop a TSB level of 25 mg/dL (428 μmol/L) or higher (odds ratio: 2.9; 95% CI: 1.6–5.2).[91]

CEPHALOHEMATOMA OR SIGNIFICANT BRUISING

Internal hemorrhage, ecchymoses, and other extravascular blood collections enhance the bilirubin load on the liver. Extravascular red cells have a markedly shortened life span, and their heme fraction is quickly catabolized to bilirubin by tissue macrophages that contain heme oxygenase and biliverdin reductase.[92] Thus, cephalohematoma, subdural hemorrhage, massive adrenal hemorrhage, and marked bruising can be associated with increased serum bilirubin levels and typically manifest 48 to 72 hours

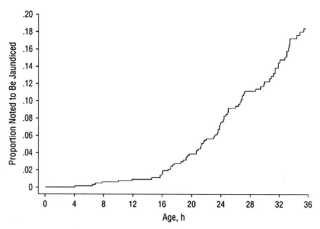

Fig. 4. Cumulative proportion of newborns noted to be jaundiced as a function of postnatal age in hours (h). (*From* Newman TB, Liljestrand P, Escobar GJ. Jaundice noted in the first 24 hours after birth in a managed care organization. Arch Pediatr Adolesc Med 156(12):1246, copyright © 2002, American Medical Association. All rights reserved; with permission.)

following the extravasation of blood.[92] This temporal pattern is consistent with the evolution of ecchymoses and bilirubin formation in situ and also accounts for why extravascular blood can cause prolonged indirect hyperbilirubinemia.[92] An unusual but dramatic example of how extravascular blood can contribute to the genesis of hyperbilirubinemia is found in reports of marked jaundice associated with the delayed absorption of intraperitoneal blood in infants who received fetal intraperitoneal red cell transfusions.[93,94] In one such case, 13 exchange transfusions were necessary to control the hyperbilirubinemia that resolved only when approximately 87 mL of packed red cells were evacuated from the intraperitoneal cavity.[93] In this instance, the intraperitoneal blood hematocrit of 60% had the potential to contribute up to approximately 600 mg of bilirubin to the infant's bilirubin load over time. Although other causes of extravasation are generally not associated with such large amounts of sequestered blood and resultant bilirubin load, they can nevertheless contribute to the development of jaundice.

PREVIOUS SIBLING TREATED WITH PHOTOTHERAPY

A history of a previous sibling treated with phototherapy is an identified risk factor for hyperbilirubinemia,[11,95] most notable at higher TSB levels (>15 mg/dL [257 μmol/L]).[96] This relationship may reflect recurrent ABO or Rh hemolytic disease[97] or exposure to a common environmental factor in addition to a shared genetic background.[95] It is known that the recurrence rate of ABO hemolytic disease is high; 88% in infants of the same blood type as their index sibling, with almost two thirds of the affected infants requiring treatment.[98] An excess risk in sibs independent of other hyperbilirubinemia risk factors expected to recur in sibships (including breastfeeding, lower gestational age, and hemolytic disease), however, suggests that genetic rather than environmental effects are responsible.[95,96] Consistent with this hypothesis, there is a higher concordance level in TSB between monozygotic (identical) as opposed to dizygotic (fraternal) twins when controlled for confounders known to modulate neonatal bilirubinemia.[99] Regardless of the etiopathogenesis, a previous sibling treated with phototherapy is a risk factor for hyperbilirubinemia.[11,15]

COMBINING CLINICAL RISK FACTOR ASSESSMENT WITH PREDISCHARGE BILIRUBIN MEASUREMENT

Three recent clinical studies suggest that combining clinical risk factor analysis with a birth hospitalization predischarge measurement of TSB or TcB will improve the prediction of subsequent hyperbilirubinemia risk.[13,14,16] An hour-specific predischarge TSB or TcB level in the high risk zone (>95%) using the percentile-based bilirubin nomogram described by Bhutani and colleagues[21] is itself a major risk factor (see **Box 1**) for severe hyperbilirubinemia.[21,100] Not surprisingly, the clinical factors most predictive of hyperbilirubinemia risk when combined with the risk-zone characterization are lower gestational age and exclusive breastfeeding.[11,13,14,16] On the basis of these recent reports, the authors of a commentary that provides clarifications on the 2004 AAP clinical practice guidelines on the management of hyperbilirubinemia in the newborn infant 35 or more weeks of gestation recommend universal predischarge bilirubin screening to help assess the risk of subsequent severe hyperbilirubinemmia.[101] Recently published data further suggest that predischarge bilirubin screening is associated with a reduction in the incidence of TSB levels of 25 mg/dL (428 μmol/L) or higher,[102,103] possibly by increasing the use of phototherapy.[103] The efficacy and cost-effectiveness of a combined percentile-based risk-zone clinical risk factor analysis in preventing bilirubin encephalopathy is unknown.[101]

SUMMARY

A myriad of demographic, environmental, and genetic factors have been identified as risks for developing severe hyperbilirubinemia. Late preterm gestational age, exclusive breastfeeding, G6PD deficiency, ABO hemolytic disease, East Asian ethnicity, jaundice observed in the first 24 hours of life, cephalohematoma or significant bruising, and a previous sibling treated with phototherapy are highlighted as major risk factors in the 2004 AAP guideline[15] and reviewed herein. It increasingly appears that combining a predischarge TSB or TcB measurement with other clinical risk factors will better predict which neonates are at greatest risk and will help caretakers formulate birth hospitalization management plans and postdischarge outpatient follow-up and evaluation.[101]

REFERENCES

1. Perlstein MA. The late clinical syndrome of posticteric encephalopathy. Pediatr Clin North Am 1960;7(3):665–87.
2. Watchko JF. Kernicterus and the molecular mechanisms of bilirubin-induced CNS injury in newborns. Neuromolecular Med 2006;8(4):513–29.
3. Maisels MJ, Newman TB. Kernicterus in otherwise healthy, breast-fed term newborns. Pediatrics 1995;96(4):730–3.
4. Bhutani VK, Johnson LH, Maisels MJ, et al. Kernicterus: epidemiological strategies for its prevention through systems-based approaches. J Perinatol 2004; 24(10):650–62.
5. Ip S, Chung M, Kulig J, et al. An evidence-based review of important issues concerning neonatal hyperbilirubinemia. Pediatrics 2004;114(1):e130–53.
6. Ebbesen F. Recurrence of kernicterus in term and near-term infants in Denmark. Acta Paediatr 2000;89(10):1213–7.
7. Hansen TWR. Kernicterus: an international perspective. Semin Neonatol 2002; 7(2):103–9.
8. Kaplan M, Hammerman C. Understanding and preventing severe hyperbilirubinemia: is bilirubin neurotoxicity really a problem in the developed world? Clin Perinatol 2004;31(3):555–75.
9. Ryan AS, Wenjun Z, Acosta A. Breastfeeding continues to increase into the new millennium. Pediatrics 2002;110(6):1103–9.
10. Curtin SC, Kozak LJ. Decline in US cesarean delivery rate appears to stall. Birth 1998;25(4):259–62.
11. Newman TB, Xiong B, Gonzales VM, et al. Prediction and prevention of extreme neonatal hyperbilirubinemia in a mature health maintenance organization. Arch Pediatr Adolesc Med 2000;154(11):1140–7.
12. Huang MJ, Kua KE, Teng HC, et al. Risk factors for severe hyperbilirubinemia in neonates. Pediatr Res 2004;56(5):682–9.
13. Newman TB, Liljestrand P, Escobar GJ. Combining clinical risk factors with serum bilirubin levels to predict hyperbilirubinemia in newborns. Arch Pediatr Adolesc Med 2005;159(2):113–9.
14. Keren R, Luan X, Friedman S, et al. A comparison of alternative risk-assessment strategies for predicting significant neonatal hyperbilirubinemia in term and near-term infants. Pediatrics 2008;121(1):e170–9.
15. American Academy of Pediatrics. Management of hyperbilirubinemia in the newborn infant 35 or more weeks of gestation. Pediatrics 2004;114(1):297–316.

16. Maisels MJ, DeRidder JM, Kring EA, et al. Routine transcutaneous bilirubin measurements combined with clinical risk factors improves the prediction of subsequent hyperbilirubinemia. J Perinatol 2009, in press.

17. Watchko JF. Hyperbilirubinemia and bilirubin toxicity in the late preterm infant. Clin Perinatol 2006;33(4):839–52.

18. Kaplan M, Muraca M, Vreman HJ, et al. Neonatal bilirubin production–conjugation imbalance: effect of glucose-6-phosphate dehydrogenase deficiency and borderline prematurity. Arch Dis Child Fetal Neonatal Ed 2005;90(2):F123–7.

19. Kawade N, Onish S. The prenatal and postnatal development of UDP-glucuronyltransferase activity towards bilirubin and the effect of premature birth on this activity in the human liver. Biochem J 1981;196(1):257–60.

20. Newman TB, Escobar GJ, Gonzales VM, et al. Frequency of neonatal bilirubin testing and hyperbilirubinemia in a large health maintenance organization. Pediatrics 1999;104(5):1198–203.

21. Bhutani VK, Johnson L, Sivieri EM, et al. Predictive ability of a predischarge hour-specific serum bilirubin for subsequent significant hyperbilirubinemia in healthy term and near-term newborns. Pediatrics 1999;103(1):6–14.

22. Keren R, Luan X, Tremont K, et al. Visual assessment of jaundice in term and late preterm infants. Arch Dis Child Fetal Neonatal Ed 2009, in press.

23. Bhutani VK, Johnson L. Kernicterus in late preterm infants cared for as term healthy infants. Semin Perinatol 2006;30(2):89–97.

24. Wang ML, Dorer DJ, Fleming MP, et al. Clinical outcomes of near-term infants. Pediatrics 2004;114(2):372–6.

25. Neifert MR. Prevention of breastfeeding tragedies. Pediatr Clin North Am 2001; 48(2):273–97.

26. American Academy of Pediatrics. Care of the neonate. In: Lockwood CJ, Lemons JA, editors. Guideline for perinatal care. 6th edition. Elk Grove Village (IL): American Academy of Pediatrics, American College of Obstetrics and Gynecology; 2007. p. 227–30.

27. Kivlahan C, James EJP. The natural history of neonatal jaundice. Pediatrics 1984;74(3):364–70.

28. Linn S, Schoenbaum SC, Monson RR, et al. Epidemiology of neonatal hyperbilirubinemia. Pediatrics 1985;75(4):770–4.

29. Maisels MJ, Gifford K, Antle CE, et al. Normal serum bilirubin levels in the newborn and the effect of breast feeding. Pediatrics 1986;78(5):837–43.

30. Schneider AP. Breast milk jaundice in the newborn. A real entity. JAMA 1986; 255(23):3270–4.

31. Hansen TWR. Bilirubin production, breast-feeding and neonatal jaundice. Acta Paediatr 2001;90(7):716–23.

32. Nielsen HE, Haase P, Blaabjerg J, et al. Risk factors and sib correlation in physiological neonatal jaundice. Acta Paediatr 1987;76(3):504–11.

33. Rubaltelli FF. Unconjugated and conjugated bilirubin pigments during perinatal development IV: the influence of breast-feeding on neonatal hyperbilirubinemia. Biol Neonate 1993;64(2–3):104–9.

34. De Carvalho M, Klaus MH, Merkatz RB. Frequency of breastfeeding and serum bilirubin concentration. Am J Dis Child 1982;136(8):737–8.

35. Yamauchi Y, Yamanouchi I. Breast-feeding frequency during the first 24 hours after birth in full term neonates. Pediatrics 1990;86(2):171–5.

36. Johnson LH, Bhutani VK, Brown AK. System-based approach to management of neonatal jaundice and prevention of kernicterus. J Pediatr 2002;140(4):396–403.

37. Takimoto M, Matsuda I. β-glucuronidase activity in the stool of newborn infant. Biol Neonate 1971;18(1):66–70.
38. Gourley GR. Perinatal bilirubin metabolism. In: Gluckman PD, Heymann MA, editors. Perinatal and pediatric pathophysiology. A clinical perspective. Boston: Hodder and Stoughton; 1993. p. 437–9.
39. Poland RD, Odell GB. Physiologic jaundice: the enterohepatic circulation of bilirubin. N Engl J Med 1971;284(1):1–6.
40. Gartner LM, Lee K-S, Vaisman S, et al. Development of bilirubin transport and metabolism in the newborn rhesus monkey. J Pediatr 1977;90(4):513–31.
41. Gartner U, Goeser T, Wolkoff AW. Effect of fasting on the uptake of bilirubin and sulfobromopthalein by the isolated perfused rat liver. Gastroenterology 1997; 113(5):1707–13.
42. Fevery J. Fasting hyperbilirubinemia: unraveling the mechanism involved. Gastroenterology 1997;113(5):1798–800.
43. Bertini G, Carlo C, Tronchin M, et al. Is breastfeeding really favoring early neonatal jaundice. Pediatrics 2001;107(3):e41. Available at: http://www.pediatrics.org/cgi/content/full/107/3/e41.
44. Maisels MJ. Epidemiology of neonatal jaundice. In: Maisels MJ, Watchko JF, editors. Neonatal jaundice. Amsterdam: Harwood Academic Publishers; 2000. p. 37–49.
45. Stevenson DK, Bortoletti AL, Ostrander CR, et al. Pulmonary excretion of carbon monoxide in the human infant as an index of bilirubin production. IV: effects of breast-feeding and caloric intake in the first postnatal week. Pediatrics 1980; 65(6):1170–2.
46. Hintz SR, Gaylord TD, Oh W, et al. Serum bilirubin levels at 72 hours by selected characteristics in breastfed and formula-fed term infants delivered by cesarean section. Acta Paediatr 2001;90(7):776–81.
47. Watchko JF. Vigintiphobia revisited. Pediatrics 2005;115(6):1747–53.
48. Watchko JF. Genetics and the risk of neonatal hyperbilirubinemia. Pediatr Res 2004;56(5):677–8.
49. Cui Y, Konig J, Leier I, et al. Hepatic uptake of bilirubin and its conjugates by the human organic anion transporter SLC21A6. J Biol Chem 2001;276(13): 9626–30.
50. Monaghan G, McLellan A, McGeehan A, et al. Gilbert's syndrome is a contributory factor in prolonged unconjugated hyperbilirubinemia of the newborn. J Pediatr 1999;134(4):441–6.
51. Maruo Y, Nishizawa K, Sato H, et al. Association of neonatal hyperbilirubinemia with bilirubin UDP-glucuronosyltransferase polymorphism. Pediatrics 1999; 103(6):1224–7.
52. Beutler E. G6PD deficiency. Blood 1994;84(11):3613–36.
53. Valaes T. Neonatal jaundice in glucose-6-phosphate dehydrogenase deficiency. In: Maisels MJ, Watchko JF, editors. Neonatal jaundice. Amsterdam: Harwood Academic Publishers; 2000. p. 67–72.
54. Valaes T. Severe neonatal jaundice associated with glucose-6-phosphate dehydrogenase deficiency: pathogenesis and global epidemiology. Acta Paediatr Suppl 1994;394:58–76.
55. Kaplan M, Hammerman C. Glucose-6-phosphate dehydrogenase deficiency: a hidden risk for kernicterus. Semin Perinatol 2004;28(5):356–64.
56. Oguniesi TA, Dedeke IOF, Adekanmbi AF, et al. The incidence and outcome of bilirubin encephalopathy in Nigeria: a bi-centre study. Niger J Med 2007;16(4): 354–9.

57. Chinevere TD, Murray CK, Grant E, et al. Prevalence of glucose-6-phosphate dehydrogenase deficiency in U.S. Army personnel. Mil Med 2006;171(9): 905–7.
58. Beutler E. Glucose-6-phosphate dehydrogenase deficiency: a historical perspective. Blood 2008;111(1):16–24.
59. Lin Z, Fontaine JM, Freer DE, et al. Alternative DNA-based newborn screening for glucose-6-phosphate dehydrogenase deficiency. Mol Genet Metab 2005; 86(1–2):212–9.
60. Kaplan M, Renbaum P, Levy-Lahad E, et al. Gilbert syndrome and glucose-6-phosphate dehydrogenase deficiency: a dose-dependent genetic interaction crucial to neonatal hyperbilirubinemia. Proc Natl Acad Sci U S A 1997;94(22): 12128–32.
61. Huang CS, Chang PF, Huang MJ, et al. Glucose-6-phosphate dehydrogenase deficiency, the UDP-glucuronsyltransferase 1A1 gene, and neonatal hyperbilirubinemia. Gastroenterology 2002;123(1):127–33.
62. Bosma PJ, Roy Chowdhury J, Bakker C, et al. The genetic basis of the reduced expression of bilirubin UDP-glucuronosyltransferase 1 in Gilbert's syndrome. N Engl J Med 1995;333(18):1171–5.
63. Huang CS. Molecular genetics of unconjugated hyperbilirubinemia in Taiwanese. J Biomed Sci 2005;12(3):445–50.
64. Iolascon A, Faienza MF, Moretti A. UGT1 promoter polymorphism accounts for increased neonatal appearance of hereditary spherocytosis. Blood 1998; 91(3):1093–4.
65. Watchko JF, Lin Z, Clark RH, et al. The complex multifactorial nature of significant hyperbilirubinemia in neonates. EPAS 2009;5500.2
66. Kaplan M, Herschel M, Hammerman C, et al. Neonatal hyperbilirubinemia in African American males: the importance of glucose-6-phosphate dehydrogenase deficiency. J Pediatr 2006;149(1):83–8.
67. Newman TB, Easterling J, Goldman ES, et al. Laboratory evaluation of jaundice in newborns. Frequency, cost and yield. Am J Dis Child 1990;144(3):364–8.
68. Kaplan M, Herschel M, Hammerman C, et al. Hyperbilirubinemia among African American glucose-6-phosphate dehydrogenase-efficient neonates. Pediatrics 2004;114(2):e213–9.
69. A Planning Conference: Utility of Screening for G6PD Deficiency to Prevent Severe Neonatal Hyperbilirubinemia. Bethesda, MD, May 11–12, 2007.
70. Kaplan M, Merob P, Regev R. Israel guidelines for the management of neonatal hyperbilirubinemia and prevention of kernicterus. J Perinatol 2008;28(6): 389–97.
71. Padilla CD, Therrell BL. Newborn screening in the Asia Pacific region. J Inherit Metab Dis 2007;30(4):490–506.
72. Naiman JL. Erythroblastosis fetalis. In: Oski FA, Naiman JL, editors. Hematologic problems in the newborn. Philadelphia: W.B. Saunders; 1982. p. 326–32.
73. Ozolek JA, Watchko JF, Mimouni F. Prevalence and lack of clinical significance of blood group incompatibility in mothers with blood type A or B. J Pediatr 1994; 125(1):87–91.
74. Herschel M, Karrison T, Wen M, et al. Isoimmunization is unlikely to be the cause of hemolysis in ABO-incompatible but direct antiglobin test-negative neonates. Pediatrics 2002;110(1):127–30.
75. Kaplan M, Na'amad M, Kenan A, et al. Failure to predict hemolysis and hyperbilirubinemia by IgG subclass in blood group A or B infants born to group O mothers. Pediatrics 2009;123(1):e132–7.

76. Halbrecht I. Role of hemagglutinins anti-A and anti-B in pathogenesis of jaundice of the newborn (icterus neonatorum precox). Am J Dis Child 1944;68(4):248–9.
77. Cashore WJ. Neonatal hyperbilirubinemia. In: Oski FA, DeAngelis CD, Feigin RD, et al, editors. Principles and practice of pediatrics. Philadelphia: J.B. Lippincott; 1990. p. 399–408.
78. Maisels MJ, McDonagh AF. Phototherapy for neonatal jaundice. N Engl J Med 2008;358(9):920–8.
79. Hammerman C, Vreman HJ, Kaplan M, et al. Intravenous immune globulin in neonatal immune hemolytic disease: does it reduce hemolysis. Acta Paediatr 1996;85(11):1351–3.
80. Gottstein R, Cooke RW. Systematic review of intravenous immunoglobulin in haemolytic disease of the newborn. Arch Dis Child Fetal Neonatal Ed 2003; 88(1):F6–10.
81. Watchko JF. Indirect hyperbilirubinemia in the neonate. In: Maisels MJ, Watchko JF, editors. Neonatal jaundice. Amsterdam: Harwood Academic Publishers; 2000. p. 51–66.
82. Hubinont PO, Bricoult A, Ghysdael P. ABO mother-infant incompatibilities. Am J Obstet Gynecol 1960;79(3):593–600.
83. Leistikow EA, Collin MF, Savastano GD, et al. Wasted health care dollars. Routine cord blood type and Coombs' testing. Arch Pediatr Adolesc Med 1995;149(10):1147–51.
84. Quinn MW, Weindling AM, Davidson DC. Does ABO incompatibility matter? Arch Dis Child 1988;63(10):1258–60.
85. Judd WJ, Luban NLC, Ness PM, et al. Prenatal and perinatal immunohematology: recommendations for serologic management of the fetus, newborn infant, and obstetric patient. Transfusion 1990;30(2):175–83.
86. Ho NK. Neonatal jaundice in Asia. Baillieres Clin Haematol 1992;5(1):131–42.
87. Huang CS, Luo GA, Huang MJ, et al. Variations of the bilirubin uridine-glucuronosyl transferase 1A1 gene in healthy Taiwanese. Pharmacogenetics 2000; 10(6):539–44.
88. Huang CS, Chang PF, Huang MJ, et al. Relationship between bilirubin UDP-glucuronosyl transferase 1A1 gene and neonatal hyperbilirubinemia. Pediatr Res 2002;52(4):601–5.
89. Yamamoto K, Sato H, Fujiyama Y, et al. Contribution of two missense mutations (G71R and Y486D) of the bilirubin UDP glycosyltransferase (UGT1A1) gene to phenotypes of Gilbert's syndrome and Crigler-Najjar syndrome type II. Biochim Biophys Acta 1998;1406(3):267–73.
90. Kim EY, Cho DY, Shin HJ, et al. Duplex pyrosequencing assay of the 388A>G and 521T>C SLCO1B1 polymorphisms in three Asian populations. Clin Chim Acta 2008;388(1–2):68–72.
91. Newman TB, Liljestrand P, Escobar GJ. Jaundice noted in the first 24 hours after birth in a managed care organization. Arch Pediatr Adolesc Med 2002;156(12): 1244–50.
92. Odell GB. Neonatal hyperbilirubinemia. New York: Grune and Stratton; 1980. p. 56–7.
93. Wright K, Tarr PI, Hickman RO, et al. Hyperbilirubinemia secondary to delayed absorption of intraperitoneal blood following intrauterine transfusion. J Pediatr 1982;100(2):302–4.
94. Rajagopalan I, Katz BZ. Hyperbilirubinemia secondary to hemolysis of intrauterine intraperitoneal blood transfusion. Clin Pediatr 1984;23(9):511–2.

95. Gale R, Seidman DS, Dollberg S, et al. Epidemiology of neonatal jaundice in the Jerusalem population. J Pediatr Gastroenterol Nutr 1990;10(1):82–6.
96. Khoury MJ, Calle EE, Joesoef RM. Recurrence risk of neonatal hyperbilirubinemia in siblings. Am J Dis Child 1988;142(10):1065–9.
97. Maisels MJ. Jaundice in the newborn. Pediatr Rev 1982;3(X):305–19.
98. Katz MA, Kanto WP, Korotkin JH. Recurrence rate of ABO hemolytic disease of the newborn. Obstet Gynecol 1982;59(5):611–4.
99. Ebbesen F, Mortensen BB. Difference in plasma bilirubin concentration between monozygotic and dizygotic newborn twins. Acta Paediatr 2003;92(5):569–73.
100. Bhutani V, Gourley GR, Adler S, et al. Non-invasive measurement of total serum bilirubin in a multiracial predischarge newborn population to assess the risk of severe hyperbilirubinemia. Pediatrics 2000;106(2):e17.
101. Maisels MJ, Bhutani VK, Bogen D, et al. Management of hyperbilirubinemia in the newborn infant 35 or more weeks of gestation—an update with clarifications. Pediatrics 2009, in press.
102. Eggert LD, Wiedmeier SE, Wilson J, et al. The effect of instituting a prehospital-discharge newborn bilirubin screening program in an 18-hospital health system. Pediatrics 2006;117(5):e855–62.
103. Kuzniewicz MW, Escobar GJ, Newman TB. The impact of universal bilirubin screening on severe hyperbilirubinemia and phototherapy use in a managed care organization. Pediatrics 2009, in press.

Group B Streptococcus and Early-Onset Sepsis in the Era of Maternal Prophylaxis

Joyce M. Koenig, MD*, William J. Keenan, MD

KEYWORDS

- Group B *Streptococcus* • Sepsis • Pneumonia • Meningitis
- Neonate • Newborn • Review

HISTORICAL ASPECTS OF MATERNAL PUERPERAL SEPSIS AND GROUP B *STREPTOCOCCUS* AS A CAUSATIVE AGENT

Puerperal sepsis (or "childbed fever") has been associated with maternal morbidity and mortality for centuries.[1] The controversial figure, Ignác Semmelweiss, a Hungarian obstetrician who practiced in Vienna in the early to mid-1800s, was the first to identify an infectious mode of transmission of puerperal sepsis.[2,3] Semmelweiss, in a key observation, linked the septic death of a colleague after an autopsy of a woman with puerperal sepsis to an infectious agent in "decaying matter," a contentious idea at a time when puerperal sepsis was thought to occur solely in women. His observations led to his strong espousal of hand washing before the examination of patients. These speculations of an organic causative agent in puerperal sepsis helped to lay the groundwork for the germ theory of infection several decades later.[4,5]

Group B *Streptococcus* (*Streptococcus agalactiae*; GBS) was first identified as a cause of puerperal sepsis in 1935 when Lancefield and Hare[6] observed differences in the hemolytic culture characteristics of two types of streptococci obtained from autopsies of women who had puerperal sepsis. Fry[7] subsequently reported several cases of fatal puerperal sepsis related to group B streptococcal disease. The use of antibiotics, initially sulfa drugs, followed by penicillin, dramatically decreased mortality attributable to puerperal sepsis. It was not until the early 1960s, however, that an association was observed between GBS infection in mothers and their newborn infants.[8,9] Subsequent studies showed that although all known GBS serotypes could cause maternal infection, type III was associated with most invasive neonatal disease (meningitis).[10]

This work was supported in part by grant HD047401 from the National Institutes of Health and the Pediatric Research Institute, Cardinal Glennon Children's Medical Center Foundation.
Division of Neonatal-Perinatal Medicine, Department of Pediatrics, E. Doisy Research Building, Saint Louis University, 1100 South Grand Boulevard, Saint Louis, MO 63104, USA
* Corresponding author.
E-mail address: koenijm@slu.edu (J.M. Koenig).

GBS can cause significant maternal morbidity, particularly endometritis, chorioamnionitis, and bacteremia.[11] In a multiregional surveillance study that followed the initial recommendations (1992) of the American Academy of Pediatrics (AAP) for GBS prophylaxis (but before the 1996 Centers for Disease Control and Prevention [CDC] consensus guidelines), Zaleznik and colleagues[12] determined a maternal GBS attack rate of 0.3 per 1000 deliveries. The incidence of maternal GBS infection showed wide variation among sites, ranging from 0.1 per 1000 deliveries in Seattle to 0.8 per 1000 deliveries in Houston, a difference thought to reflect regional obstetric practices. Most (96%) women presented with bacteremia, and there was no associated mortality. Maternal disease had an adverse effect on fetal or neonatal outcome, however; 28% of affected mothers had pregnancy loss attributable to miscarriage or stillbirth or delivered an infant who developed GBS early-onset sepsis (EOS).

Historically, GBS began to be described in the 1960s as a significant causative organism for life-threatening infections in infants less than 3 months of age.[11] GBS was the most commonly identified organism in infected neonates in the first week of life before the establishment of universal screening of pregnant women for GBS colonization and prophylactic measures. In a 2000 multisite surveillance study conducted in eight states, the incidence of invasive GBS disease was lowest in children aged 3 months to 14 years, representing 2% of total cases compared with 20% occurring in the first week after birth. The risk for dying from GBS disease was twice as high in the older infants compared with the neonates, however.[13] In addition, GBS disease was responsible for 33% of infections in subjects 65 years of age or older, who had the highest case fatality rate (15%) compared with all other age groups. Although universal screening measures and aggressive maternal GBS prophylaxis have accounted for both a significant decrease in the incidence of invasive EOS GBS disease in neonates and of invasive disease in pregnant women, GBS remains a prominent cause of infection-related morbidity and mortality in the elderly with underlying chronic disease and in immunocompromised hosts.[14–17]

GBS infection acquired from the colonized birth canal during labor or after membrane rupture can lead to miscarriage, stillbirth, prematurity, or invasive neonatal disease.[11] Early-onset GBS infections are strongly linked to maternal colonization, although only a fraction of cases of late-onset disease in infants have a similar association.[11,18] Vaginal colonization with GBS is acquired from the gastrointestinal tract, and a large proportion of healthy adults are reportedly colonized.[19] Colonized women are typically asymptomatic, and urinary tract infections with GBS may also have few associated clinical symptoms.[20–22] In the absence of intrapartum antibiotic prophylaxis (IAP), exposure of the term newborn to the colonized mother infrequently causes infection and leads to asymptomatic neonatal colonization without infection in approximately 75% of exposed infants.[18] The neonatal attack rate of GBS infection through this vertical transmission ranges from 1 to 2 per 1000 live births. In the 1980s, Boyer and Gotoff[23] determined that women colonized with GBS in the presence of other risk factors (birth weight [BW] <2.5 kg, ruptured membranes for >18 hours, intrapartum fever) versus women who were GBS culture-negative before delivery were 24 times more likely to have neonates with EOS attributable to GBS. Maternal GBS bacteriuria has been associated with a high risk for neonatal EOS.[20]

NEONATAL RISK FOR INVASIVE GROUP B *STREPTOCOCCUS* DISEASE: HOST IMMUNOLOGIC FACTORS

As a group, neonates are at risk for infections, and this is particularly so in preterm neonates.[24–26] When compared with older children and adults, neonates have an intrinsic limitation in their capacity to produce neutrophils and a subsequent susceptibility to exhaustion of marrow reserves during times of increased use, such as sepsis.[27,28] In addition, those neutrophils that are produced have impairments of numerous functions important to the clearance of microbes, including marrow egress, adhesion to the microvascular endothelium, chemotaxis, and bactericidal function.[24,28–36] Perhaps as a compensatory mechanism, neonatal neutrophils have a prolonged functional life span, which can potentially delay their clearance and prolong inflammatory and cytotoxic processes.[37–39] Relative deficiencies in circulating levels of GBS-specific antibody and complement in the context of neutrophil dysfunction heighten the neonatal susceptibility to GBS infection.[24,40–51] Furthermore, studies have also shown that vernix caseosa, which is sparse in the preterm infant, contains proteins important to host defense functions, including antimicrobial peptides and factors that promote opsonization and inhibit protease activity.[52]

NEONATAL RISK FOR INVASIVE GROUP B *STREPTOCOCCUS* DISEASE: BACTERIAL VIRULENCE FACTORS

Capsular polysaccharides (CPSs) expressed by GBS and identified by serotyping assist in bacterial evasion of host defense by interfering with their ingestion by phagocytes. More virulent strains of encapsulated GBS can produce increased amounts of polysaccharides. Lancefield and Hare[6] was the first to serotype GBS, and she identified the prominence of serotype III in neonatal meningitis, subsequently confirmed by others. GBS expresses 9 (and possibly 10) unique serotypes, and most invasive neonatal GBS disease in the United States has been associated with types Ia, II, and III in addition to a more recent prevalence of type V.[53]

   Another important virulence factor of GBS is related to its ability to attach to the vascular endothelium and epithelium, particularly of the vaginal tissue and chorionic membranes in addition to the neonatal lungs, which is a prerequisite for invasiveness and disease.[54] The more virulent invasive strains of GBS have been found to have a greater capacity for adherence, and this has been particularly evident in studies of serotype III GBS.[53–55] Environmental factors, including ambient oxygen concentration, may contribute to bacterial adherence as well.[56] Additional virulence factors have been reviewed.[57]

NEONATAL EARLY-ONSET INFECTION AND GROUP B *STREPTOCOCCUS*

Neonatal EOS is an infection occurring in the first week of life in term newborns and in the first 72 hours of life in very low birth weight (VLBW) neonates.[58] This gestational age-adjusted difference in the definition of EOS accounts for the higher acquisition of nosocomial organisms as causative agents of sepsis in VLBW neonates after 3 days of hospitalization. Gram-positive bacteria were the most commonly identified causative organisms of neonatal sepsis in the early part of the twentieth century.[11] Lancefield and Hare[6] identified GBS as a contributing factor in often-fatal puerperal and neonatal sepsis in the 1930s. In the 1970s, GBS became the most common causative agent of EOS, whereas gram-negative organisms had been the most common cause of EOS in the early antibiotic era. Before the era of maternal prophylaxis, GBS had a reported national incidence of approximately 2 per 1000 live births and was associated with 50% mortality in affected neonates.[18,59] Over the past decade, the approaches to maternal prophylaxis have resulted in a remarkable decrease the incidence of GBS to its current rate of 0.3 per 1000 live births.[60]

   Early-onset invasive disease attributable to GBS most commonly presents in neonates during the first day after birth (60%–70% of cases reported in multicenter trials).[12,13] One third (32%) of cases were identified between 24 and 48 hours of life, whereas only 8% of cases occurred in infants greater than 2 days of age.[12] Early-onset GBS infections may be invasive and cause nonfocal bacteremia (the most common presentation), pneumonia (**Fig. 1**), or meningitis and, less commonly, joint and bone involvement.[11] In contrast, infants with GBS infections after the first week of life ("late-onset sepsis") commonly present with bacteremia but more frequently (nearly one quarter of cases) develop meningitis (**Fig. 2**) than infants who have EOS caused by GBS.

EARLY-ONSET SEPSIS AND RISK FOR NEONATAL DEATH

Death attributable to EOS is inversely related to gestational age and birth weight. Surveillance data obtained before the release of the initial 1996 CDC consensus statement showed an overall case fatality rate of 16% for infants who had GBS EOS.[12] Approximately 65% of these deaths occurred in neonates weighing less than 2500 g. The CDC assessed the effects of IAP on EOS and late-onset sepsis occurring in two periods (1985–1991 and 1995–1999) using a national data set.[61] Mortality attributable to EOS decreased from 24.9 per 100,000 live births to 15.6 per 100,000 live births, potentially reflecting adherence to GBS prophylactic regimens.

GROUP B *STREPTOCOCCUS*, EARLY-ONSET SEPSIS, AND THE ROLE OF INTRAPARTUM PROPHYLAXIS

In the 1970s, Larsen and Sever[62] used a rhesus monkey model to investigate the biology of peripartum GBS infection. Cerebral inoculation of GBS types 1c and III was uniformly fatal, whereas intravenous or intra-amniotic inoculation with GBS just before delivery resulted in neonatal pneumonia and meningitis but variable mortality.[63] Studies designed to assess the utility of antibiotics under these conditions showed a significant protective effect, even in the presence of intracerebral infection. In 1979, Yow and colleagues[64] showed the effectiveness of single-dose ampicillin in averting the peripartum transmission of GBS by colonized mothers to their neonates. In that study of women colonized with GBS, none of the 34 women who received

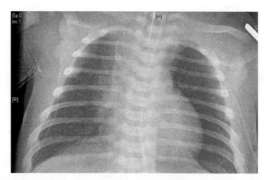

Fig. 1. Typical chest radiograph of a newborn with GBS pneumonia. CXR of a term infant with GBS and a small left-sided pneumothorax. Infant was delivered to a mother with unknown GBS and ruptured membranes for 7 hours. Infant required mild resuscitation, then developed progressive respiratory distress and required intubation. A sepsis work-up was performed and antibiotics were started; culture of a tracheal aspirate was positive for GBS. Infant was discharged home in good health on DOL 11. (*Courtesy of* A. Ali, MD, St. Louis, MO.)

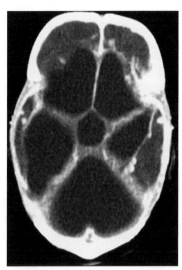

Fig. 2. Head CT scan of a 3-week-old male newborn after late-onset GBS meningitis. The CT scan performed 27 days later showed virtually no normal cortex. He was able to breathe without a respirator but was unable to suck. (*Courtesy of* Carol J. Baker, MD, Houston, TX.)

intrapartum ampicillin during labor delivered colonized infants. In contrast, 58% of infants born to the untreated cohort were colonized. Subsequent clinical trials confirmed the utility of intrapartum antibiotics in significantly preventing neonatal EOS attributable to GBS.[65–68] In these trials, the treatment of colonized women with intrapartum ampicillin or penicillin dramatically reduced the incidence of EOS attributable to GBS, with reported ranges of effectiveness from 25% to 100%. In one study, Boyer and Gotoff[65] observed that colonized women identified at 26 to 28 weeks of gestation who received intrapartum parenteral antibiotics during labor (and who exhibited other risk factors, including preterm labor, prolonged membrane rupture, or fever) had a reduction in the rate of vertically transmitted colonization from 51% to 9% and a decrease in EOS from 6% to 0%.

In 1992, the American Academy of Pediatrics made recommendations for a prophylactic treatment approach to maternal GBS colonization to diminish the incidence of neonatal infection.[69] In an early multiregional surveillance study after these initial recommendations, Zaleznik and colleagues[12] reviewed data in pregnant women and neonates from indigent care and private facilities in Seattle, Minneapolis/St. Paul, Pittsburgh, and Houston during a period from 1993 to 1996. The combined attack rate for GBS EOS in all study sites was lower (0.8 per 1000 live births) than the expected rate of 2 per 1000 live births, based on earlier surveillance data. Attack rates depended on the region, however, ranging from the highest rate of 1.3 per 1000 live births in Houston to a rate of 0.6 per 1000 live births in Minneapolis/St. Paul. Attack rates were highest for African-American and Hispanic women. Low birth weight (<2500 g) was a significant risk factor for GBS EOS (2.1 versus 0.7 per 1000 live births for infants weighing ≥2500 g); however, 75% of the cases occurred in near-term or term infants.

The 1992 AAP recommendations received uneven acceptance. In 1996, the CDC[70–72] released a consensus statement developed with the ACOG and AAP. In that policy statement, strategies that involved universal screening of pregnant women for GBS colonization at 35 to 37 weeks of gestation or a risk-based approach (fever ≥38°C

[104.5°F], premature membrane rupture ≥18 hours, <37 weeks of gestation, or established GBS colonization) were equally acceptable alternatives. Subsequent surveillance studies revealed that almost 50% of neonatal EOS GBS infections were not identified using the risk-based approach.[73,74] A multicenter analysis of surveillance data (1993–1998) showed a striking (65%) decline in the incidence of GBS EOS, confirming the efficacy of screening-triggered treatment of colonized mothers (**Fig. 3**).[13] The general protective effect of GBS prophylaxis was also confirmed by the CDC in its report of national surveillance data for GBS disease in 12.5 million persons during a similar time period.

A large (n = 600,000) retrospective cohort study conducted by the Active Bacterial Core Surveillance Team at the CDC suggested the greater efficacy of universal screening over the risk-based approach. Based on the results of these and other studies, the CDC reissued its most current guidelines in 2002, endorsed by the AAP and ACOG, specifically to promote universal screening for GBS at 35 to 37 weeks of gestation and the treatment of colonized women with IAP.[75,76] To help narrow the use of intrapartum antibiotics, the guidelines did not recommend that women with GBS-negative cultures within 5 weeks of delivery receive GBS prophylaxis in the presence of intrapartum risk factors. In an attempt to enhance the sensitivity of rectovaginal cultures, the revised guidelines outlined a detailed approach to the collection and processing of cultures. In addition, new algorithms were included regarding GBS prophylaxis for threatened preterm delivery and the management of neonates exposed to intrapartum prophylaxis. This refocused approach led to an additional decline in GBS-related EOS to a reported incidence of 0.3 per 1000 live births in term neonates, which has surpassed the established goals of Healthy People 2010 of achieving an incidence of 0.5 per 1000 live births for EOS (**Fig. 4**).[13,77] Concurrently, mortality associated with GBS EOS in term infants also dropped dramatically. Although the initial dramatic decrease in the incidence of GBS EOS was reflective of declines among African-American neonates, analysis of more recent data continues to reveal a several-fold higher incidence of GBS EOS in African-American versus white infants.[13,60,78,79]

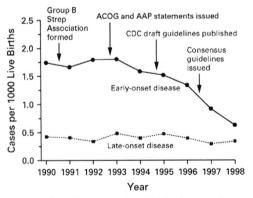

Fig. 3. Incidence of early- and late-onset invasive GBS in three active surveillance areas (California, Georgia, and Tennessee), 1990 through 1998, and activities for the prevention of GBS. Live births for 1998 were approximated on the basis of 1997 data. *Arrows* designate the dates when prevention activities occurred. (*From* Schrag SJ, Zywicki S, Farley MM, et al. Group B streptococcal disease in the era of intrapartum antibiotic prophylaxis. N Engl J Med 2000;342:16; with permission.)

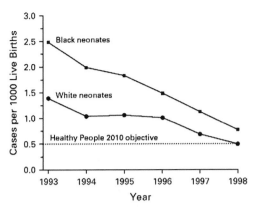

Fig. 4. Incidence of early-onset invasive GBS in black neonates and white neonates in four active surveillance areas (California, Georgia, Tennessee, and Maryland), 1993 through 1998. The Healthy People 2010 objectives, released by the US Department of Health and Human Services, constitute a national prevention strategy for substantially improving the health of people in the United States. Live births for 1998 were approximated on the basis of 1997 data. (*From* Schrag SJ, Zywicki S, Farley MM, et al. Group B streptococcal disease in the era of intrapartum antibiotic prophylaxis. N Engl J Med 2000;342:17; with permission.)

PERSISTENCE OF GROUP B *STREPTOCOCCUS* DISEASE DESPITE UNIVERSAL SCREENING

Despite the significant decrease in the incidence of GBS EOS after the inception of the 1996 CDC guidelines for prophylaxis, a sizable number of infants develop GBS disease annually, particularly in the VLBW infant population.[58,80] Of concern are reports that many of these infants developed GBS EOS in the absence of evidence for maternal colonization. Potential explanations for these occurrences may be related to the acquisition of colonization after a negative screen result (in one study, 8.5% of women with initially negative cultures were colonized at delivery), discordance between antenatal screening and colonization (studies have determined that some women who are negative at their initial screening may be colonized at delivery), effects of undocumented outpatient antibiotics, and uneven techniques in the acquisition or processing of specimens for culture.[81] False-negative rates ranging from 4% to 8% have been reported.[82]

Puopolo and colleagues[82] prospectively reviewed single-center data from three periods encompassing the years 1997 to 2003, which reflected changes in obstetric approaches to GBS prophylaxis, using a screening-based protocol. In this study, the attack rate for GBS EOS was 0.37 per 1000 live births, a decrease in incidence that mirrored rates reported for other institutions. In affected neonates, nearly two thirds of mothers (82% of term gestations) had a negative GBS culture screen. Nineteen of 25 GBS-negative mothers of infected neonates presented with at least one intrapartum risk factor, but only a small fraction (<20%) received intrapartum prophylaxis and in only one case was prophylaxis initiated more than 4 hours before delivery. Twelve of 17 infected term infants had no or mild symptoms. Those treated empirically based on risk factors with subsequent positive blood cultures remained clinically stable. In contrast, 7 of 8 preterm infants with GBS EOS presented with clinical evidence of sepsis. These data indicated a protective effect of early empiric antibiotic therapy in neonates at risk for EOS and underscored the importance of evaluating even well-appearing infants for possible sepsis in the presence of any maternal risk factors, despite a negative GBS status in the mother. These researchers concluded that the relatively high false-negative maternal screening incidence indicates the need for rapid identification of at-risk deliveries.

EFFECT OF UNIVERSAL SCREENING FOR GROUP B *STREPTOCOCCUS* IN VERY LOW BIRTH WEIGHT NEONATES

Despite the dramatic impact of universal screening at 36 weeks of gestation on the incidence of and mortality associated with GBS EOS in term infants, its effect in VLBW neonates has been less apparent. Data from several multicenter surveillance studies associated with the National Institutes of Child Health and Human Development (NICHD) Neonatal Research Network VLBW registry from three study periods have been compared: 1991 to 1993, 1998 to 2000, and 2002 to 2003. Stoll and colleagues[80,83] reported that the attack rate of EOS attributable to GBS declined significantly between the first two periods (from 5.9 to 1.7 per 1000 live births) but did not change between the last two study periods (1.8 per 1000 live births). The case fatality rate markedly dropped during the first periods (the most recent data report a rate of 2.6%), although GBS EOS remains a significant cause of neonatal death in the preterm population (19.9%), with the highest mortality observed in VLBW neonates (35% in a 2003 study).

Therapeutic approaches to GBS-colonized women identified early in gestation and who present with premature membrane rupture or are in labor have lacked consistency and have been hampered by a lack of data. Although prophylactic antibiotics reduce transmission of GBS from a colonized mother to her infant, this approach may not completely prevent neonatal disease.[84] The cause(s) of the disparate prophylactic effectiveness of maternal GBS screening between term and VLBW neonates remain(s) enigmatic. One potential explanation involves the pronounced immunoincompetence of fetuses and extremely premature neonates.[24,26] In addition, screening early in gestation and prophylaxis may be ineffective. Boyer and colleagues[81] reported that 8.5% of women with negative cultures at 26 to 28 weeks of gestation were GBS-positive at the time of delivery.

GROUP B *STREPTOCOCCUS* PROPHYLAXIS AND ALTERATIONS IN THE PROFILE OF CAUSATIVE ORGANISMS IN EARLY-ONSET SEPSIS

Mounting evidence shows that the increasing use of intrapartum antibiotics as part of GBS prophylaxis has altered the profile of microorganisms causing EOS. Universal screening measures and IAP have resulted in a dramatic decrease in GBS as a causative organism, but there has been a dramatic shift toward gram-negative organisms as a cause of EOS in VLBW infants.

Surveillance data were prospectively collected from 16 centers belonging to the NICHD Neonatal Research Network VLBW registry during a 13-year period. Stoll and colleagues[80,83] reviewed these data during three time periods to assess the pathogens associated with EOS in VLBW neonates. In VLBW neonates, EOS was described as infection occurring in the first 72 hours of life in the presence of clinical symptoms and a positive blood culture. In the latter two periods, there were no changes in birth weight, gender, or gestational age among cohorts. The rate of EOS in neonates weighing 401 to 1500 g remained relatively stable during this period (15–19 of 1000 live births); however, the pattern of distribution for associated pathogens underwent a significant change.

Gram-positive organisms predominated during the first period, causing 56% of EOS; this was primarily attributable to GBS. After the 1996 institution of CDC guidelines, there was a precipitous decline in the attack rate of GBS, from 5.9 per 1000 live births in 1991 to 1993 to 1.7 per 1000 live births in 1998 to 2000; this did not change further in the last period evaluated (1.8 per 1000 live births) (**Table 1**).[81] The incidence of EOS attributable to *Escherichia coli* more than doubled between these two periods, from 3.2 to 6.8 per 1000 live births, and did not change in the last period evaluated (7.0 per 1000 live births). In 1998 to 2000, EOS was primarily associated with gram-negative bacteria (61%), and nearly three-quarters of these cases were attributable to *E. coli*, followed by *Hemophilus influenzae* (8%), Citrobacter (2%), and others (**Table 2**). Less than half (37%) of EOS infections were attributable to gram-positive infections, with 11% of the total attributable to GBS. One disturbing trend over the periods studied was the gradual increase in the incidence of EOS attributable to coagulase-negative *Staphylococcus*, which accounted for nearly 15% of gram-positive EOS in the period from 2002 to 2003.

GROUP B *STREPTOCOCCUS* PROPHYLAXIS AND THE EMERGENCE OF BACTERIAL RESISTANCE

Increasing evidence has linked the administration of maternal intrapartum antibiotics with the emergence of resistant bacterial strains. GBS remains sensitive to penicillin. Cases of resistance to erythromycin and clindamycin, antibiotics frequently given to women with documented penicillin allergy, have been reported, however.[85] In 2002, recommendations were made in partial response to the emerging frequency of GBS resistance to erythromycin and clindamycin to measure antibiotic sensitivities of GBS in high-risk penicillin-sensitive woman.[75]

A major concern is the increasing incidence of antibiotic resistance in gram-negative organisms, particularly *E. coli*. In the NICHD VLBW registry, analysis of 39 isolates in the cohort from 2002 to 2003 showed an 85% resistance to ampicillin.[80] Analysis of maternal intrapartum antibiotic exposure showed a marked increase in antibiotic use from the earliest cohort studied compared with 69% of mothers who received antibiotics in 2002 to 2003. A significantly higher proportion of neonates with *E. coli* sepsis were born to mothers who had received ampicillin within 72 hours of delivery (1.1% versus 0.4%). Although the CDC guidelines for IAP outline the preferential use of penicillin in the absence of known allergy, surveillance data indicated that ampicillin was used for IAP in 49% of cases.

The results of the VLBW registry analysis have reflected similar trends in other institutions. In a single-institution retrospective review of three periods encompassing 1979 to 2006, Bizzarro and colleagues[86] observed an increase in antibiotic use (from 16% to 85%) paralleling the adoption of the CDC guidelines for GBS prophylaxis. In VLBW neonates, the incidence of ampicillin-resistant *E. coli* increased dramatically, from 0% in the first period (1979–1992) to 64% in the latest period (1997–2006). Colonization with resistant organisms was associated with lower birth weights, lower gestational ages, and exposure to antenatal antibiotics. In an analysis of data (1998–2000) from San Francisco and Atlanta for the CDC Active Bacterial Core surveillance, the rates of ampicillin-resistance in EOS attributable to *E. coli* in preterm infants increased from 29% (2 of 7 infants) in 1998 to 84% (16 of 18 infants) in 2000.[87] *E. coli*-associated mortality tended to be more common in ampicillin-resistant cases (26%) compared with those that were sensitive to ampicillin (5%). Ampicillin-resistant *E. coli* infections increased during the study period in preterm but not term infants, a possible reflection of prolonged exposure of the preterm group to antibiotics. Eighty-two percent of mothers who delivered preterm infants with EOS with an ampicillin-resistant organism had received antenatal antibiotics compared with 40% of mothers of term infants with resistant disease.

Table 1
Rates of early-onset sepsis and associated pathogens in 1991 to 1993 and 1998 to 2000

Early-Onset Sepsis	1991–1993		1998–2000	
	No. Infected/Total No.	Rate Per 1000 Live-Born VLBW Infants	No. Infected/Total No.	Rate Per 1000 Live-Born VLBW Infants
Any	147/7606	19.3	84/5447	15.4
Gram-positive	83/7606	10.9	31/5447	5.7[a]
Group B streptococci	45/7606	5.9	9/5447	1.7[b]
Gram-negative	63/7606	8.3	51/5447	9.4
Escherichia coli	24/7606	3.2	37/5447	6.8[c]
Fungus	1/7606	0.1	2/5447	0.4

Data from the period from 1991 to 1993 are from Stoll and colleagues. *P* = .007 for the change in the distribution of pathogens between the two periods; there was no significant change in the overall rate of sepsis. VLBW infants are defined as infants weighing between 401 and 1500 g. When the three centers that were not included in the earlier birth cohort are excluded from the analysis, the rates of group B streptococci and *E. coli* in the more recent birth cohort are 2.1 per 1000 live-born VLBW infants and 7.3 per 1000 live-born VLBW infants, respectively, and the changes remain significant (*P* = .003).

[a] *P* = .002 for the comparison with the earlier period.
[b] *P*<.001 for the comparison with the earlier period.
[c] *P* = .004 for the comparison with the earlier period.

From Stoll BJ, Hansen N, Fanaroff AA, et al. Changes in pathogens causing early-onset sepsis in very-low-birth-weight infants. N Engl J Med 2002;347:243; with permission.

Table 2
Distribution of pathogens among 84 cases of early-onset sepsis occurring in 5447 infants born between September 1, 1998, and August 31, 2000

Organism	No. With Sepsis (%)
Gram-negative organisms	51 (60.7)
Escherichia coli	37 (44.0)
Haemophilus influenzae	7 (8.3)
Citrobacter	2 (2.4)
Other[a]	5 (6.0)
Gram-positive organisms	31 (36.9)
Group B Streptococcus	9 (10.7)
Viridans Streptococcus	3 (3.6)
Other streptococci[b]	4 (4.8)
Listeria monocytogenes	2 (2.4)
Coagulase-negative Staphylococcus[c]	9 (10.7)
Other[d]	4 (4.8)
Fungi	2 (2.4)
Candida albicans	2 (2.4)
Total	84 (100)

Seven of the 84 infants had two positive blood cultures for the same organism.
[a] Other gram-negative organisms included Klebsiella (in 1 infant), Bacteroides (in 2 infants), Eikenella corrodens (in 1 infant), and Stenotrophomonas maltophilia (in 1 infant).
[b] Other streptococci included group A Streptococcus (in 1 infant) and three cases in which the species was unknown.
[c] Of 18 positive blood cultures for coagulase-negative staphylococci, 1 met the criteria for definite infection and 8 met the criteria for possible infection; in the other 9 cultures, the organism was considered to be a contaminant (see the Methods section).
[d] Other gram-positive organisms included Staphylococcus aureus (in 1 infant), Bacillus (in 2 infants), and Peptostreptococcus (in 1 infant).
From Stoll BJ, Hansen N, Fanaroff AA, et al. Changes in pathogens causing early-onset sepsis in very-low-birth-weight infants. N Engl J Med 2002;347:242; with permission.

Conversely, Schrag and colleagues[88] reported a lack of an association between IAP and EOS attributable to ampicillin-resistant E. coli. Although more than half of infected subjects had been exposed to intrapartum antibiotics, those with ampicillin-resistant E. coli did not have a greater exposure to intrapartum antibiotics in general, although they were exposed to more doses of penicillin or ampicillin, possibly a reflection of factors linked to prematurity or maternal infection. The strongest identified risk factors for E. coli sepsis were prematurity, particularly 33 weeks or less of gestation, followed by maternal fever and prolonged membrane rupture. Univariate analysis controlling for intrapartum fever revealed an association between IAP and E. coli infection in general (ampicillin-resistant and ampicillin-sensitive). When separating the analysis based on gestational age, exposure to IAP for 4 or more hours actually reduced the odds for E. coli infection in term infants, indicative of a protective effect.

Increased emergence of ampicillin-resistant E. coli EOS has also been reported in other countries. Analysis of single-institution data from Madrid showed a preferential increase of resistant E. coli EOS among preterm but not term neonates, a finding that was not paralleled by a significantly greater use of intrapartum antibiotics.[89] Retrospective analysis in one hospital in New Zealand confirmed the preponderance of

E. coli infection in premature infants, with more than half being resistant to amoxicillin.[90]

ECONOMIC COSTS OF PERIPARTUM GROUP B *STREPTOCOCCUS* DISEASE AND ITS PREVENTION

Peripartum GBS infection is associated with significant morbidity and mortality and causes maternal septicemia, septic abortion, stillbirth, and premature delivery. In addition, neonatal GBS infection significantly prolongs hospitalization and has been associated with developmental delay, blindness, deafness, and other neurologic impairments. Although the emotional toll of these complications cannot be numerically assessed, the economic costs are significant. A study of one California health maintenance organization correlated an incidence of EOS GBS of 0.1% from 1989 to 1983 with a calculated cost of $2.8 million.[91] The initiation of a risk-based approach (1994–1995) resulted in a decreased incidence of EOS paralleling those reported in multicenter surveys (0.04%). The investigators estimated that nearly two thirds of EOS GBS cases had been prevented by this strategy, representing 65.5 life-years saved attributable to averted cases and a net cost savings of $1.1 million.

Studies of the economic impact of strategies to prevent GBS EOS have determined a marked increase in the use of maternal intravenous antibiotics (in one study, from 27% in 1998 to 41% in 2002) and have cataloged the contribution of this practice to the emergence of resistant organisms.[92,93] Maternal prophylaxis has also been associated with increased early antibiotic use in term neonates and a longer hospital stay.[92,94] A recent single-institution study from Switzerland assessed GBS early-onset disease in the context of risk factors and cost-effectiveness of different preventative strategies.[95] From March 2005 to 2006, the maternal colonization rate was 21% and risk factors were present in 37% of women at the time of delivery. Although the risk-based approach was associated with a lower direct cost compared with a screening approach, these researchers suggested universal screening as the more effective regimen in the presence of a high maternal colonization rate.

ALTERNATIVE STRATEGIES TO PREVENTION OF GROUP B *STREPTOCOCCUS* EARLY-ONSET SEPSIS

Although universal screening measures have had a significant and positive impact on EOS attributable to GBS, this approach is not fail-safe and early-onset GBS disease remains a major public health issue. In addition, evidence has linked the emergence of resistant organisms to IAP administration. An increasing number of investigators have become proponents of alternative approaches to minimize the need for antenatal prophylaxis and its attendant risks.

Combination approaches to the screening or prophylaxis of mothers and their newborns have been explored with some success. In one trial from Italy, neonates delivered to screened mothers were themselves cultured and treated with a course of prophylactic amoxicillin, resulting in a decrease in EOS and late-onset GBS disease (from an incidence of 0.74 to 0.048 per 1000 live births at the end of the study). Further studies are required to assess the cost-benefits of targeted approaches, in addition to unintended consequences, however, particularly with respect to microbial resistance patterns. For example, prophylactic oral administration of amoxicillin-clavulanate for prematurely ruptured membranes or preterm labor was associated with an increased risk for necrotizing enterocolitis.[96]

The administration of prophylactic vaccines is the most promising approach to the prevention of neonatal GBS disease.[97] A major rationale for the vaccination of women against GBS is the fact that most (85%–90%) pregnant women lack protective anti-bodies at the time of delivery.[98] In a decision analytic model, effective maternal vacci-nation in combination with a screening approach was predicted to prevent 66% of peripartum GBS infections and 1 of 25 preterm births.[99] Vaccines based on CPS expression and conjugated to tetanus toxoid have shown particular therapeutic potential.[98,100–105] In early trials, maternal immune responses to polysaccharide vaccines were variable, although in a study directed by Baker and colleagues,[102] 75% of infants born to women who responded to a type III polysaccharide vaccine had protective antibody levels 2 months after delivery. Conjugation of CPS vaccines to tetanus toxoid has improved antigenic responses in recipients. A high proportion (93%–100%) of immunized women exhibited a fourfold increase in type-specific anti-body responses after immunization, although this number was lower (80%) for those receiving the type 1b conjugated vaccine.[106] Importantly, antibody levels were detect-able 2 years after immunization. Nevertheless, although substantial evidence has shown these vaccines to be promising deterrents to GBS disease in the United States, the participation by pharmaceutical companies has been hesitant.[97] The goal of a universally effective vaccine and a successful immunization strategy remains elusive. The development of efficacious vaccines with global relevance has been hindered by changes in the prominence of various GBS serotypes and antigenicity patterns over time, in addition to regional variations in human populations.[107–109]

Conventional approaches to the development of numerous vaccines have been augmented by novel DNA, genomic, and protein technologies and are rapidly being superseded by such techniques as reverse vaccinology, in which pathogen-specific genomic sequences are used to screen for potential protein candidates for vaccine development.[109–111] A thorough discussion of GBS vaccine development and novel approaches, which is beyond the scope of this article, has been elegantly reviewed elsewhere.[106,109]

Alternative approaches to the eradication of GBS colonization have been consid-ered, including the development of topical agents that can target GBS. One approach involving the use of chlorhexidine as a vaginal disinfectant has been favored by some because of low cost, lack of impact on the development of antibiotic resistance, and its potential use in undeveloped areas. Although a systematic review of the literature was consistent with a decrease in neonatal GBS colonization of neonates, this was not associated with a reduction in early-onset neonatal disease.[112] One novel agent, aqueous allicin, a substance derived from garlic, has been shown to have potent bactericidal activity against GBS isolates in culture.[113] Another consideration involves bacteriophage lysins, which are cell wall hydrolases that render bacteria vulnerable to lysis.[114] In vivo studies in neonatal mice have shown the potent and wide-spectrum bactericidal activity of a bacteriophage lysin, PlyGBS, against GBS colonization. Inter-esting possibilities of this approach include potential utility in cases of antibiotic resis-tance, its rapid action, and the apparent lack of toxicity.

An approach involving the use of rapid diagnostic tests could help to guide manage-ment shortly before delivery, particularly in cases in which GBS status is unknown or when cultures are negative in the presence of risk factors. One such test involves a rapid polymerase chain reaction (PCR) assay, which has been shown to match or exceed the sensitivity of culture-based approaches,[115] the commercial version of which has been approved by the US Food and Drug Administration (FDA) for this purpose.[116] In a Stanford University cost analysis of a hypothetical cohort, a PCR-based strategy resulted in a net cost benefit, less maternal antibiotic use, fewer neonatal GBS infections, and a lower incidence of GBS-related infant death and disability compared with the current universal screening approach.[117]

SUMMARY

The changing face of EOS has been associated with the wide adoption of consensus guidelines to detect and treat women with GBS colonization. The utility of these guidelines, promulgated by the CDC and endorsed by the AAP and ACOG, has stood the test of time and experience. Faithful adherence to a universal screening approach across institutions has dramatically decreased maternal and early-onset neonatal GBS disease and has lowered the incidence of GBS EOS to a level that achieves the goal outlined in Healthy People 2010. Unintended consequences of increased intrapartum antibiotic exposure, particularly to ampicillin, include an increasing prevalence of gram-negative bacteria causing EOS, particularly of resistant strains, however. Morbidity and mortality attributable to EOS related to GBS and other organisms remain significant, especially in VLBW neonates.

Despite an era of marked success with universal screening, GBS continues to be an important cause of EOS, and thus remains a significant public health issue. Measures that augment its diagnosis and prevention are imperative. Improved eradication of GBS colonization and disease may involve universal screening in conjunction with rapid diagnostic technologies or other novel approaches. Given the complications and potential limitations associated with maternal intrapartum prophylaxis, however, vaccines may be the most effective means of preventing neonatal GBS disease. Although efficacious against most serotypes associated with GBS disease in the United States, the global utility of conjugated GBS vaccines may be hampered by the variability of serotypes in diverse populations and geographic locations. Modern technologies, such as those involving proteomics and genomic sequencing, are likely to hasten the development of a universal vaccine against GBS.

REFERENCES

1. Loudon I. Deaths in childbed from the eighteenth century to 1935. Med Hist 1986;30:1–41.
2. Raju TN. Ignac Semmelweis and the etiology of fetal and neonatal sepsis. J Perinatol 1999;19:307–10.
3. Noakes TD, Borresen J, Hew-Butler T, et al. Semmelweis and the aetiology of puerperal sepsis 160 years on: an historical review. Epidemiol Infect 2008;136: 1–9.
4. Pasteur. On the germ theory. Science 1881;2:420–2.
5. Baxter AG. Louis Pasteur's beer of revenge. Nat Rev Immunol. 2001;1:229–32.
6. Lancefield RC, Hare R. The serological differentiation of pathogenic and non-pathogenic strains of hemolytici streptococci. J Exp Med 1935;61:335–49.
7. Fry RM. Fatal infections by hemolytic Streptococcus group B. Lancet 1938;1: 199–201.
8. Hood M, Janney A, Dameron G. Beta hemolytic streptococcus group B associated with problems of the perinatal period. Am J Obstet Gynecol 1961;82: 809–18.
9. Eickhoff TC, Klein JO, Daly AK, et al. Neonatal sepsis and other infections due to group B beta-hemolytic streptococci. N Engl J Med 1964;271:1221–8.
10. Baker CJ, Barrett FF. Group B streptococcal infections in infants. The importance of the various serotypes. JAMA 1974;230:1158–60.
11. Edwards MS, Baker CJ. Group B streptococcal infections. In: Remington JS, Klein JO, editors. Infectious diseases of the fetus and newborn infant. 5th edition. Philadelphia: Saunders; 2001. p. 1091–156.

12. Zaleznik DF, Rench MA, Hillier S, et al. Invasive disease due to group B Strep-tococcus in pregnant women and neonates from diverse population groups. Clin Infect Dis 2000;30:276–81.

13. Schrag SJ, Zywicki S, Farley MM, et al. Group B streptococcal disease in the era of intrapartum antibiotic prophylaxis. N Engl J Med 2000;342:15–20.

14. Edwards MS, Baker CJ. Group B streptococcal infections in elderly adults. Clin Infect Dis. 2005;41:839–47.

15. Edwards MS, Rench MA, Palazzi DL, et al. Group B streptococcal colonization and serotype-specific immunity in healthy elderly persons. Clin Infect Dis 2005; 40:352–7.

16. Amaya RA, Baker CJ, Keitel WA, et al. Healthy elderly people lack neutrophil-mediated functional activity to type V group B Streptococcus. J Am Geriatr Soc 2004;52:46–50.

17. Huang PY, Lee MH, Yang CC, et al. Group B streptococcal bacteremia in non-pregnant adults. J Microbiol Immunol Infect 2006;39:237–41.

18. Baker CJ, Barrett FF. Transmission of group B streptococci among parturient women and their neonates. J Pediatr 1973;83:919–25.

19. Schuchat A. Epidemiology of group B streptococcal disease in the United States: shifting paradigms. Clin Microbiol Rev 1998;11:497–513.

20. Wood EG, Dillon HC Jr. A prospective study of group B streptococcal bacteriuria in pregnancy. Am J Obstet Gynecol 1981;140:515–20.

21. Persson K, Christensen KK, Christensen P, et al. Asymptomatic bacteriuria during pregnancy with special reference to group B streptococci. Scand J Infect Dis 1985;17:195–9.

22. Persson K, Bjerre B, Elfstrom L, et al. Group B streptococci at delivery: high count in urine increases risk for neonatal colonization. Scand J Infect Dis 1986;18:525–31.

23. Boyer KM, Gadzala CA, Burd LI, et al. Selective intrapartum chemoprophylaxis of neonatal group B streptococcal early-onset disease. I. Epidemiologic ratio-nale. J Infect Dis 1983;148:795–801.

24. Wilson CB. Immunologic basis for increased susceptibility of the neonate to infection. J Pediatr 1986;108:1–12.

25. Koenig JM, Yoder MC. White cell disorders in the neonate. In: Spitzer AR, editor. Intensive care of the fetus and neonate. 2nd edition. Philadelphia: Elsevier Mosby; 2005.

26. Koenig JM, Yoder MC. Neonatal neutrophils: the good, the bad, and the ugly. Clin Perinatol 2004;31:39–51.

27. Christensen RD, Rothstein G, Hill HR, et al. Fatal early onset group B strepto-coccal sepsis with normal leukocyte counts. Pediatr Infect Dis 1985;4:242–5.

28. Christensen RD, Rothstein G. Exhaustion of mature marrow neutrophils in neonates with sepsis. J Pediatr 1980;96:316–8.

29. Shigeoka AO, Santos JI, Hill HR. Functional analysis of neutrophil granulocytes from healthy, infected, and stressed neonates. J Pediatr 1979;95:454–60.

30. Shigeoka AO, Charette RP, Wyman ML, et al. Defective oxidative metabolic responses of neutrophils from stressed neonates. J Pediatr 1981;98:392–8.

31. Anderson DC. Neonatal neutrophil dysfunction. Am J Pediatr Hematol Oncol 1989;11:224–6.

32. Quie PG. Antimicrobial defenses in the neonate. Semin Perinatol 1990;14:2–9.

33. Ohman L, Tullus K, Katouli M, et al. Correlation between susceptibility of infants to infections and interaction with neutrophils of Escherichia coli strains causing neonatal and infantile septicemia. J Infect Dis 1995;171:128–33.

34. Kallman J, Schollin J, Schalen C, et al. Impaired phagocytosis and opsonisation towards group B streptococci in preterm neonates. Arch Dis Child Fetal Neonatal Ed 1998;78:F46–50.
35. Yost CC, Cody MJ, Harris ES, et al. Impaired neutrophil extracellular trap (NET) formation: a novel innate immune deficiency of human neonates. Blood 2009; [epub ahead of print].
36. Stroobant J, Harris MC, Cody CS, et al. Diminished bactericidal capacity for group B Streptococcus in neutrophils from "stressed" and healthy neonates. Pediatr Res 1984;18:634–7.
37. Allgaier B, Shi M, Luo D, et al. Spontaneous and Fas-mediated apoptosis are diminished in umbilical cord blood neutrophils compared with adult neutrophils. J Leukoc Biol. 1998;64:331–6.
38. Hanna N, Vasquez P, Pham P, et al. Mechanisms underlying reduced apoptosis in neonatal neutrophils. Pediatr Res 2005;57:56–62.
39. Koenig JM, Stegner JJ, Schmeck AC, et al. Neonatal neutrophils with prolonged survival exhibit enhanced inflammatory and cytotoxic responsiveness. Pediatr Res 2005;57:424–9.
40. Baker CJ, Edwards MS, Kasper DL. Role of antibody to native type III polysaccharide of group B Streptococcus in infant infection. Pediatrics 1981;68: 544–9.
41. Edwards MS, Kasper DL, Jennings HJ, et al. Capsular sialic acid prevents activation of the alternative complement pathway by type III, group B streptococci. J Immunol 1982;128:1278–83.
42. Anderson DC, Hughes BJ, Edwards MS, et al. Impaired chemotaxigenesis by type III group B streptococci in neonatal sera: relationship to diminished concentration of specific anticapsular antibody and abnormalities of serum complement. Pediatr Res 1983;17:496–502.
43. Edwards MS, Kasper DL, Nicholson-Weller A, et al. The role of complement in opsonization of GBS. Antibiot Chemother 1985;35:170–89.
44. Givner LB, Baker CJ, Edwards MS. Type III group B Streptococcus: functional interaction with IgG subclass antibodies. J Infect Dis 1987;155:532–9.
45. Patterson LE, Baker CJ, Rench MA, et al. Fibronectin and age-limited susceptibility to type III, group B Streptococcus. J Infect Dis 1988;158:471–4.
46. Smith CL, Baker CJ, Anderson DC, et al. Role of complement receptors in opsonophagocytosis of group B streptococci by adult and neonatal neutrophils. J Infect Dis 1990;162:489–95.
47. Campbell JR, Baker CJ, Edwards MS. Deposition and degradation of C3 on type III group B streptococci. Infect Immun 1991;59:1978–83.
48. Noya FJ, Baker CJ, Edwards MS. Neutrophil Fc receptor participation in phagocytosis of type III group B streptococci. Infect Immun 1993;61:1415–20.
49. Edwards MS, Rench MA, Hall MA, et al. Fibronectin levels in premature infants with late-onset sepsis. J Perinatol 1993;13:8–13.
50. Berger M. Complement deficiency and neutrophil dysfunction as risk factors for bacterial infection in newborns and the role of granulocyte transfusion in therapy. Rev Infect Dis 1990;12(Suppl 4):S401–9.
51. Christensen RD, Brown MS, Hall DC, et al. Effect on neutrophil kinetics and serum opsonic capacity of intravenous administration of immune globulin to neonates with clinical signs of early-onset sepsis. J Pediatr 1991;118:606–14.
52. Tollin M, Bergsson G, Kai-Larsen Y, et al. Vernix caseosa as a multi-component defence system based on polypeptides, lipids and their interactions. Cell Mol Life Sci 2005;62:2390–9.

53. Rowen JL, Baker CJ. Group B streptococcal infections. In: Feigin RD, Cherry JD, editors. Textbook of pediatric infectious diseases. 4th edition. Philadelphia: W.B. Saunders Company; 1998. p. 1089–106.
54. Gibson RL, Soderland C, Henderson WR Jr, et al. Group B streptococci (GBS) injure lung endothelium in vitro: GBS invasion and GBS-induced eicosanoid production is greater with microvascular than with pulmonary artery cells. Infect Immun 1995;63:271–9.
55. Tamura GS, Kuypers JM, Smith S, et al. Adherence of group B streptococci to cultured epithelial cells: roles of environmental factors and bacterial surface components. Infect Immun 1994;62:2450–8.
56. Johri AK, Padilla J, Malin G, et al. Oxygen regulates invasiveness and virulence of group B streptococcus. Infect Immun 2003;71:6707–11.
57. Liu GY, Nizet V. Extracellular virulence factors of group B streptococci. Front Biosci 2004;9:1794–802.
58. Stoll BJ, Gordon T, Korones SB, et al. Early-onset sepsis in very low birth weight neonates: a report from the National Institute of Child Health and Human Development Neonatal Research Network. J Pediatr 1996;129:72–80.
59. Barton LL, Feigin RD, Lins R. Group B beta hemolytic streptococcal meningitis in infants. J Pediatr 1973;82:719–23.
60. Centers for Disease Control and Prevention. Perinatal group B streptococcal disease after universal screening recommendations—United States, 2003–2005. MMWR Morb Mortal Wkly Rep 2007;56:701–5.
61. Lukacs SL, Schoendorf KC, Schuchat A. Trends in sepsis-related neonatal mortality in the United States, 1985–1998. Pediatr Infect Dis J 2004;23:599–603.
62. Larsen JW, Sever JL. Group B Streptococcus and pregnancy: a review. Am J Obstet Gynecol 2008;198:440–8.
63. Larsen JW Jr, London WT, Palmer AE, et al. Experimental group B streptococcal infection in the rhesus monkey. I. Disease production in the neonate. Am J Obstet Gynecol 1978;132:686–90.
64. Yow MD, Mason EO, Leeds LJ, et al. Ampicillin prevents intrapartum transmission of group B streptococcus. JAMA 1979;241:1245–7.
65. Boyer KM, Gotoff SP. Prevention of early-onset neonatal group B streptococcal disease with selective intrapartum chemoprophylaxis. N Engl J Med 1986;314:1665–9.
66. Garland SM, Fliegner JR. Group B Streptococcus (GBS) and neonatal infections: the case for intrapartum chemoprophylaxis. Aust N Z J Obstet Gynaecol 1991;31:119–22.
67. Matorras R, Garcia-Perea A, Madero R, et al. Maternal colonization by group B streptococci and puerperal infection; analysis of intrapartum chemoprophylaxis. Eur J Obstet Gynecol Reprod Biol 1991;38:203–7.
68. Tuppurainen N, Hallman M. Prevention of neonatal group B streptococcal disease: intrapartum detection and chemoprophylaxis of heavily colonized parturients. Obstet Gynecol 1989;73:583–7.
69. Committee on Infectious Disease; Committee on Fetus and Newborn. Guidelines for prevention of group B streptococcal (GBS) infection by chemoprophylaxis. Pediatrics 1992;90:775–8.
70. Centers for Disease Control and Prevention. Prevention of perinatal group B streptococcal disease: a public health perspective. MMWR Recomm Rep 1996;45(RR-7):1–24.

71. American College of Obstetricians and Gynecologists, Committee on Obstetric Practice. Prevention of early-onset group B streptococcal disease in newborns. Washington, DC: American College of Obstetricians and Gynecologists; 1996. [Opinion 173].

72. American Academy of Pediatrics Committee on ID Committee on Fetus and Newborn. Revised guidelines for prevention of early-onset group B streptococcal (GBS) disease. Pediatrics 1997;99:489–96.

73. Centers for Disease Control and Prevention. Early-onset group B streptococcal disease—United States, 1998–1999. JAMA 2000;284:1508–10.

74. Centers for Disease Control and Prevention. Group B strep prevention (GBS, baby strep, group B streptococcal bacteria). Available at: http://www.cdc.gov/groupbstrep/hospitals/hospitals_guidelines.htm.

75. Centers for Disease Control and Prevention. Prevention of perinatal group B streptococcal disease: revised guidelines from the CDC. MMWR Recomm Rep 2002;51(RR-11):1–24.

76. Baker CJ. CDC revises group B strep prevention guidelines. AAP News 2002; 21(3):118.

77. Phares CR, Lynfield R, Farley MM, et al. Epidemiology of invasive group B streptococcal disease in the United States, 1999–2005. JAMA 2008;299: 2056–65.

78. Lijoi D, Di CE, Ferrero S, et al. The efficacy of 2002 CDC guidelines in preventing perinatal group B streptococcal vertical transmission: a prospective study. Arch Gynecol Obstet 2007;275:373–9.

79. Centers for Disease Control and Prevention. Trends in perinatal group B streptococcal disease—United States, 2000–2006. MMWR Morb Mortal Wkly Rep 2009;58:109–12.

80. Stoll BJ, Hansen NI, Higgins RD, et al. Very low birth weight preterm infants with early onset neonatal sepsis: the predominance of gram-negative infections continues in the National Institute of Child Health and Human Development Neonatal Research Network, 2002–2003. Pediatr Infect Dis J 2005;24: 635–9.

81. Boyer KM, Gadzala CA, Kelly PD, et al. Selective intrapartum chemoprophylaxis of neonatal group B streptococcal early-onset disease. II. Predictive value of prenatal cultures. J Infect Dis 1983;148:802–9.

82. Puopolo KM, Madoff LC, Eichenwald EC. Early-onset group B streptococcal disease in the era of maternal screening. Pediatrics 2005;115:1240–6.

83. Stoll BJ, Hansen N, Fanaroff AA, et al. Changes in pathogens causing early-onset sepsis in very-low-birth-weight infants. N Engl J Med 2002;347:240–7.

84. Alvarez JR, Williams SF, Ganesh VL, et al. Duration of antimicrobial prophylaxis for group B streptococcus in patients with preterm premature rupture of membranes who are not in labor. Am J Obstet Gynecol 2007;197:390–4.

85. Chen KT, Puopolo KM, Eichenwald EC, et al. No increase in rates of early-onset neonatal sepsis by antibiotic-resistant group B Streptococcus in the era of intrapartum antibiotic prophylaxis. Am J Obstet Gynecol 2005;192:1167–71.

86. Bizzarro MJ, Dembry LM, Baltimore RS, et al. Changing patterns in neonatal Escherichia coli sepsis and ampicillin resistance in the era of intrapartum antibiotic prophylaxis. Pediatrics 2008;121:689–96.

87. Hyde TB, Hilger TM, Reingold A, et al. Trends in incidence and antimicrobial resistance of early-onset sepsis: population-based surveillance in San Francisco and Atlanta. Pediatrics 2002;110:690–5.

88. Schrag SJ, Hadler JL, Arnold KE, et al. Risk factors for invasive, early-onset *Escherichia coli* infections in the era of widespread intrapartum antibiotic use. Pediatrics 2006;118:570–6.

89. Alarcon A, Pena P, Salas S, et al. Neonatal early onset *Escherichia coli* sepsis: trends in incidence and antimicrobial resistance in the era of intrapartum antimicrobial prophylaxis. Pediatr Infect Dis J 2004;23:295–9.

90. Jones B, Peake K, Morris AJ, et al. *Escherichia coli*: a growing problem in early onset neonatal sepsis. Aust N Z J Obstet Gynaecol 2004;44:558–61.

91. Mohle-Boetani JC, Lieu TA, Ray GT, et al. Preventing neonatal group B streptococcal disease: cost-effectiveness in a health maintenance organization and the impact of delayed hospital discharge for newborns who received intrapartum antibiotics. Pediatrics 1999;103:703–10.

92. Glasgow TS, Speakman M, Firth S, et al. Clinical and economic outcomes for term infants associated with increasing administration of antibiotics to their mothers. Paediatr Perinat Epidemiol 2007;21:338–46.

93. Schuchat A. Group B Streptococcus. Lancet 1999;353:51–6.

94. Platt R, son-Mitty J, Weissman L, et al. Resource utilization associated with initial hospital stays complicated by early onset group B streptococcal disease. Pediatr Infect Dis J 1999;18:529–33.

95. Rausch AV, Gross A, Droz S, et al. Group B Streptococcus colonization in pregnancy: prevalence and prevention strategies of neonatal sepsis. J Perinat Med 2009;37:124–9.

96. Kenyon SL, Taylor DJ, Tarnow-Mordi W. Broad-spectrum antibiotics for preterm, prelabour rupture of fetal membranes: the ORACLE I randomised trial. ORACLE Collaborative Group. Lancet 2001;357:979–88.

97. Edwards MS. Group B streptococcal conjugate vaccine: a timely concept for which the time has come. Hum Vaccin 2008;4:444–8.

98. Baker CJ, Kasper DL. Group B streptococcal vaccines. Rev Infect Dis 1985;7: 458–67.

99. Sinha A, Lieu TA, Paoletti LC, et al. The projected health benefits of maternal group B streptococcal vaccination in the era of chemoprophylaxis. Vaccine 2005;23:3187–95.

100. Baker CJ, Paoletti LC, Wessels MR, et al. Safety and immunogenicity of capsular polysaccharide-tetanus toxoid conjugate vaccines for group B streptococcal types Ia and Ib. J Infect Dis 1999;179:142–50.

101. Baker CJ, Paoletti LC, Rench MA, et al. Use of capsular polysaccharide-tetanus toxoid conjugate vaccine for type II group B Streptococcus in healthy women. J Infect Dis 2000;182:1129–38.

102. Baker CJ, Rench MA, McInnes P. Immunization of pregnant women with group B streptococcal type III capsular polysaccharide-tetanus toxoid conjugate vaccine. Vaccine 2003;21:3468–72.

103. Baker CJ, Paoletti LC, Rench MA, et al. Immune response of healthy women to 2 different group B streptococcal type V capsular polysaccharide-protein conjugate vaccines. J Infect Dis 2004;189:1103–12.

104. Margarit I, Rinaudo CD, Galeotti CL, et al. Preventing bacterial infections with pilus-based vaccines: the group B Streptococcus paradigm. J Infect Dis 2009; 199:108–15.

105. Healy CM, Baker CJ. Prospects for prevention of childhood infections by maternal immunization. Curr Opin Infect Dis. 2006;19:271–6.

106. Edwards MS. Vaccines against group B Streptococcus. In: Levine MM, Kaper JB, Rappuoli R, et al, editors. New generation vaccines. 3rd edition. New York, Basel: Marcel Dekker, Inc.; 2004. p. 711–21.

107. Lachenauer CS, Kasper DL, Shimada J, et al. Serotypes VI and VIII predominate among group B streptococci isolated from pregnant Japanese women. J Infect Dis 1999;179:1030–3.

108. Hickman ME, Rench MA, Ferrieri P, et al. Changing epidemiology of group B streptococcal colonization. Pediatrics 1999;104:203–9.

109. Johri AK, Paoletti LC, Glaser P, et al. Group B Streptococcus: global incidence and vaccine development. Nat Rev Microbiol 2006;4:932–42.

110. Mora M, Donati C, Medini D, et al. Microbial genomes and vaccine design: refinements to the classical reverse vaccinology approach. Curr Opin Microbiol 2006;9:532–6.

111. Rappuoli R. Reverse vaccinology. Curr Opin Microbiol 2000;3:445–50.

112. Stade B, Shah V, Ohlsson A. Vaginal chlorhexidine during labour to prevent early-onset neonatal group B streptococcal infection. Cochrane Database Syst Rev 2004;3:CD003520.

113. Cutler RR, Odent M, Hajj-Ahmad H, et al. In vitro activity of an aqueous allicin extract and a novel allicin topical gel formulation against Lancefield group B streptococci. J Antimicrob Chemother 2009;63:151–4.

114. Cheng Q, Nelson D, Zhu S, et al. Removal of group B streptococci colonizing the vagina and oropharynx of mice with a bacteriophage lytic enzyme. Antimicrobial Agents Chemother 2005;49:111–7.

115. Natarajan G, Johnson YR, Zhang F, et al. Real-time polymerase chain reaction for the rapid detection of group B streptococcal colonization in neonates. Pediatrics 2006;118:14–22.

116. Picard FJ, Bergeron MG. Laboratory detection of group B Streptococcus for prevention of perinatal disease. Eur J Clin Microbiol Infect Dis 2004;23:665–71.

117. Haberland CA, Benitz WE, Sanders GD, et al. Perinatal screening for group B streptococci: cost-benefit analysis of rapid polymerase chain reaction. Pediatrics 2002;110:471–80.

Prenatal Diagnosis of Congenital Heart Disease

Pei-Ni Jone, MD[a], Kenneth O. Schowengerdt, Jr., MD[b],*

KEYWORDS

- Fetal echocardiography • Prenatal diagnosis
- Neonatal heart disease

Fetal echocardiography, an accurate and safe method to diagnose congenital heart disease, has become widely used in pediatric cardiology and perinatology. It allows detailed prenatal diagnosis of suspected or known congenital heart disease and serves as a general screening tool for possible congenital heart disease. With the advent of better technology, fetal echocardiography can delineate the details of fetal cardiac anatomy, thus broadening our understanding of the development of the fetal heart and fetal cardiac defects. Outcomes of infants with severe cardiac malformations may improve with prenatal diagnosis of congenital heart disease.[1–3] Fetal echocardiography allows for improved counseling of families after a prenatal diagnosis of congenital heart disease; it allows them to better anticipate the expected course of the pregnancy, and leads to a better understanding of the postnatal prognosis. It also allows for referral of mothers with affected fetuses to tertiary cardiac care centers for timely neonatal management. The early diagnosis of congenital heart disease allows prompt evaluation of genetic syndromes and analysis of the fetal karyotype. Prenatal detection of arrhythmias by fetal echocardiography allows for in utero treatment in many instances. Fetal echocardiography can also serve to identify patients for in utero cardiac interventions that may be performed at certain select centers.

GOALS OF FETAL ECHOCARDIOGRAPHY

The goals of fetal echocardiography are to exclude congenital heart disease and, when present, to diagnose the specific malformations of the heart. It serves as a diagnostic tool for determining fetal cardiac anatomy and fetal arrhythmias. Fetal echocardiography provides a better understanding of fetal cardiac anatomy and developmental malformations of the heart, such as development of hypoplastic

---

[a] Division of Pediatric Cardiology, University of Colorado, Denver, CO, USA
[b] Pediatric Cardiology, Cardinal Glennon Children's Medical Center, Saint Louis University School of Medicine, 1465 S. Grand Boulevard, Saint Louis, MO 63104, USA
* Corresponding author.
E-mail address: schowko@slu.edu (K.O. Schowengerdt).

Pediatr Clin N Am 56 (2009) 709–715
doi:10.1016/j.pcl.2009.04.002   pediatric.theclinics.com
0031-3955/09/$ – see front matter © 2009 Elsevier Inc. All rights reserved.

ventricles related to obstruction of the respective outflow tracts. Fetal echocardiography may also serve as a navigator for fetal cardiac interventions in selected instances.

SCREENING WITH FETAL ECHOCARDIOGRAPHY

The optimal transabdominal fetal echocardiogram can be performed at 16 weeks of pregnancy and onwards. However, typical general obstetric ultrasounds for low risk pregnancies are performed at 18 to 22 weeks gestation. By this time, details of the fetal cardiac anatomy can be well visualized and evaluated, such as the atrioventricular and ventriculoarterial connections. Fetal echocardiographic images actually may be difficult to obtain beyond 28 to 30 weeks gestation because of fetal rib shadowing, fetal position, or maternal body habitus.

INDICATIONS OF FETAL ECHOCARDIOGRAPHY

Pregnancies at high risk for structural, functional, or rhythm-related fetal heart disease constitute indications for fetal echocardiographic assessment. Indications for fetal echocardiography can be stratified into three categories: fetal, maternal, and familial.[4–7] These are outlined in **Box 1**. Increased nuchal thickening in the first trimester has been associated with an increased incidence of congenital heart disease.[8–14] This increase in nuchal thickening may be associated with left-sided

---

Box 1
Indications for fetal echocardiography

Fetal

    Abnormal screening obstetric ultrasound

    Extracardiac anomalies (omphalocele, duodenal atresia, VACTERL, spina bifida)

    Chromosomal abnormalities (trisomies, microdeletions)

    Increased first-trimester nuchal translucency measurement

    Nonimmune hydrops

    Tachyarrhythmias

    Bradyarrhythmias

Maternal

    Diabetes

    Phenylketonuria

    Teratogen exposure

    Maternal congenital heart defect

Familial

    Previous child with congenital heart defect

    Paternal congenital heart defect

    Tuberous sclerosis

    Noonan syndrome

    Velocardiofacial syndrome

obstructive lesions or chromosomal abnormalities with possible associated cardiac defects such as trisomy 21 and Turner syndrome.[10,13]

ADVANTAGES OF FETAL ECHOCARDIOGRAPHY

Fetal echocardiography provides potential benefits for both the neonate and the family. Prenatal diagnosis of congenital heart disease allows for more specific family counseling to be rendered, and allows parents to ask questions related to the pregnancy and postnatal prognosis. A detailed explanation of the potential cardiac surgical procedures that the infant will require and their timing can be provided, with the opportunity for parents to prepare emotionally before birth. Arrangements for delivery at a tertiary care center providing neonatal cardiac care can and should be made. Neonatal hypoxemia and acidosis can be prevented by early institution of prostaglandin E infusion for ductal dependent lesions immediately after delivery. It should also be mentioned that a negative fetal echocardiogram could provide needed reassurance to the family who had had a previous child with a congenital heart defect.

Studies show improved postnatal outcome when a prenatal diagnosis of congenital heart disease is made.[3,15,16] Prenatal diagnosis is associated with decreased preoperative morbidity, decreased incidence of acidosis, reduced risk of hemodynamic compromise, and better end-organ perfusion.[17] Thus, fetal echocardiography can play an important role in identifying fetuses with types of congenital heart disease requiring specific early postnatal therapy, especially those with ductal dependent lesions such as critical left heart obstructive lesions, transposition of great arteries, and pulmonary atresia. Franklin and colleagues[1] demonstrated that infants with a prenatal diagnosis of severe coarctation had improved survival compared with those with a postnatal diagnosis, with cardiovascular collapse and death being more common in the latter group.

Fetal echocardiography is also useful in diagnosing and managing fetal arrhythmias. M-mode tracings of the atria and ventricles can delineate the fetal rhythm. Isolated premature atrial and ventricular contractions in the fetus are benign and do not require treatment. Tachyarrhythmias in the fetus, most commonly fetal supraventricular tachycardia, can be controlled by treatment of the mother with antiarrhythmic agents.[18] In utero treatment of fetal arrhythmias has been useful in preventing hydrops and fetal demise. Jaeggi and colleagues[19] have demonstrated that a prenatal diagnosis of complete atrioventricular block was associated with high fetal and neonatal mortality, and was often associated with anti-Rho or anti-La antibodies. In this case, maternal treatment with steroids or sympathomimetics may be beneficial to the fetus whose bradycardia has resulted in decompensated heart failure.[20] Identifying congenital complete heart block prenatally can prepare families and health care providers for the need for delivery at a tertiary center should the fetus require temporary or permanent pacing after delivery.

SPECTRUM OF CONGENITAL HEART DISEASE DIAGNOSED BY FETAL ECHOCARDIOGRAPHY

Using current state-of-the-art echocardiographic equipment and methods, fetal echocardiography can diagnose major cardiac malformations in detail. The spectrum of ventricular hypoplasia syndromes such as hypoplastic left heart syndrome, unbalanced atrioventricular canal defect, severe tricuspid stenosis, or tricuspid atresia can be readily seen in the four-chamber view (**Fig. 1**). As the fetus relies on the ductus arteriosus for survival, ductal flow patterns are routinely assessed. A prenatal diagnosis of hypoplastic left heart syndrome is particularly important, as normal somatic growth of the fetus can occur in this setting and these infants may appear normal

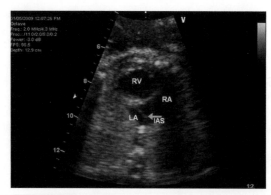

Fig. 1. Fetal echocardiogram demonstrating finding of hypoplastic left heart syndrome. Note the enlarged right atrium (RA) and right ventricle (RV). The left atrium (LA) is small, and there is no appreciable left ventricular cavity. The interatrial septum (IAS) is identified by the arrow.

for varying periods after delivery. Only after the ductus arteriosus begins to close do these infants become hemodynamically compromised. Often, severe acidosis is present when the diagnosis is suspected. Right-sided lesions encompassing the spectrum of tetralogy of Fallot include varying degrees of obstruction or atresia of the right ventricular outflow tract (**Fig. 2**). These lesions can best be visualized by examining the outflow tracts anterior to the four- chamber view. The branch pulmonary arteries can also be visualized using the outflow tract views and their relative size assessed. Retrograde filling of the branch pulmonary arteries from the aorta by way of the ductus arteriosus may be seen, indicative of severe pulmonary stenosis or pulmonary atresia. The ductus arteriosus may be small or tortuous depending on the severity of the obstruction of the right ventricular outflow tract.

Transposition of the great arteries, double-outlet right ventricle, and subaortic ventricular septal defects can also be diagnosed prenatally by fetal echocardiography. Fetuses with these lesions will grow and be tolerant of these defects because of the unique features of the fetal circulation.[5]

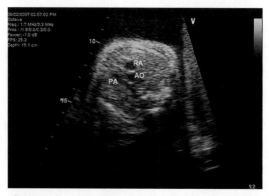

Fig. 2. Fetal echocardiogram demonstrating findings consistent with tetralogy of Fallot. The right ventricular outflow tract is not well visualized, and the pulmonary arteries (PA) are hypoplastic. The size discrepancy with the aorta (AO) is apparent.

Major cardiac malformations should be followed serially by fetal echocardiography as progressive alterations in flow may affect growth of cardiac structures over time; for example, the development of ventricular hypoplasia in the setting of significant outflow obstruction. In addition, assessment of left atrial size, restriction of flow across the foramen ovale, and pulmonary venous flow patterns can be useful in identifying those infants with hypoplastic left heart syndrome at high risk of morbidity and mortality after birth.[21]

Mild defects such as mild coarctation of the aorta and mild valvar stenoses can be observed in utero; but, because of the unique fetal circulation, fetal development is not affected. The large ductus arteriosus allows equalization of systolic blood pressure in the great arteries, thus a pressure gradient does not develop in utero.[5] A subtle clue suggesting mild coarctation is a dilated right ventricle resulting from increased systemic vascular resistance.[22]

Tricuspid regurgitation and mitral regurgitation can be seen readily in the four-chamber view by fetal echocardiography. Severe tricuspid regurgitation can result in severe heart failure and hydrops fetalis (**Fig. 3**).[23] The causes of tricuspid regurgitation are right ventricular volume overload (severe pulmonic stenosis or constriction of the ductus arteriosus), ventricular dysfunction or dilation (cardiomyopathy), or structural abnormalities of the tricuspid valve (Ebstein anomaly, dysplastic tricuspid valve, and common atrioventricular canal). Mitral regurgitation is less common. Severe mitral regurgitation can cause similar effects of volume overload of the left heart.

LIMITATIONS OF FETAL ECHOCARDIOGRAPHY

Fetal echocardiography, like other ultrasound tests, is operator dependent and relies on the expertise of the pediatric cardiologist and screening perinatologist. Technical limitations include poor fetal positioning in which the fetal lie does not allow for adequate image acquisition and difficult imaging due to maternal body habitus. In obese gravid patients, image acquisition is poor and scanning the fetus becomes difficult. Multiple fetuses also create a shadowing phenomenon that may not allow adequate cardiac visualization. Small ventricular septal defects are difficult to visualize and identification of a secundum atrial septal defect versus flow through the foramen ovale can be difficult. Importantly, total anomalous pulmonary venous return may be difficult to diagnose in utero because the pulmonary veins carry little blood flow prenatally.[24]

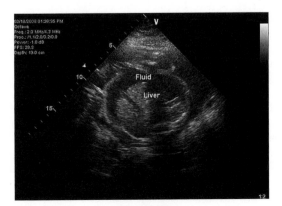

Fig. 3. Prominent ascites seen in a case of fetal hydrops.

FETAL CARDIAC INTERVENTIONS

Fetal echocardiography serves as a guide for fetal cardiac catheter-based interventions. Several specialized centers offer catheter-based interventions in utero to dilate stenosis of the pulmonary or aortic valves.[25] Evidence suggests that early relief of severe outflow tract obstruction can reverse the progression of ventricular hypoplasia in some instances by improving flow and thereby creating a stimulus for growth of the ventricle.[26] Prenatal diagnosis of congenital heart defects is crucial in identifying patients who are suitable candidates for fetal cardiac intervention. A severely restrictive atrial septal defect in hypoplastic left heart syndrome can be dilated in utero to prevent fetal demise or minimize morbidity and mortality after birth. Fetal cardiac intervention is an evolving field and warrants further research to provide in utero treatment for the fetus who would otherwise not survive.

SUMMARY

Advancements in the field of fetal echocardiography have had a significant impact within the fields of pediatric cardiology, perinatology, and neonatology. A detailed and accurate prenatal diagnosis of congenital heart disease allows for improved counseling of the parents, not only regarding the prognosis for their affected child, but also the potential risks in future pregnancies. Prenatal diagnosis may guide the timing and optimal location of delivery. Infants with significant congenital heart disease should be delivered at a tertiary care center with pediatric cardiology and congenital heart surgery support. A prenatal diagnosis allows appropriate planning and consultation between the cardiologist and neonatologist before the delivery to optimize the care of the newborn and prevent postnatal hemodynamic compromise that can occur with severe cardiac malformations. If immediate interventions are anticipated, these can be planned so that they may occur in a timely way.

In addition to identifying structural heart disease, fetal echocardiography has been shown to be accurate in diagnosing and managing fetal arrhythmias. Appropriate treatment of these rhythm disturbances can prevent fetal demise and the morbidity and mortality associated with severe hydrops.

Finally, fetal echocardiography is able to identify potential candidates for in utero cardiac intervention and serves as the imaging guidance technique for these procedures. Future advancement may lead to additional techniques that alter the natural history of abnormal cardiac development and improve survival.

REFERENCES

1. Franklin O, Burch M, Manning N, et al. Prenatal diagnosis of coarctation of the aorta improves survival and reduces morbidity. Heart 2002;87:67–9.
2. Maeno YV, Kamenir SA, Sinclair B, et al. Prenatal features of ductus arteriosus constriction and restrictive foramen ovale in d-transposition of the great arteries. Circulation 1999;99:1209–14.
3. Tworetzky W, McElhinney DB, Reddy VM, et al. Improved surgical outcome after fetal diagnosis of hypoplastic left heart syndrome. Circulation 2001;103:1269–73.
4. Boughman JA, Berg KA, Astemborski JA, et al. Familial risks of congenital heart defect assessed in a population-based epidemiologic study. Am J Med Genet 1987;26:839–49.
5. Cohen MS. Fetal diagnosis and management of congenital heart disease. Clin Perinatol 2001;28:11–29, v–vi.
6. Snider AR. Two-dimensional and Doppler echocardiographic evaluation of heart disease in the neonate and fetus. Clin Perinatol 1988;15:523–65.

7. Shipp TD, Bromley B, Hornberger LK, et al. Levorotation of the fetal cardiac axis: a clue for the presence of congenital heart disease. Obstet Gynecol 1995;85:97–102.
8. Devine PC, Simpson LL. Nuchal translucency and its relationship to congenital heart disease. Semin Perinatol 2000;24:343–51.
9. Hafner E, Schuller T, Metzenbauer M, et al. Increased nuchal translucency and congenital heart defects in a low-risk population. Prenat Diagn 2003;23:985–9.
10. Hyett J, Perdu M, Sharland G, et al. Using fetal nuchal translucency to screen for major congenital cardiac defects at 10–14 weeks of gestation: population based cohort study. BMJ 1999;318:81–5.
11. Hyett JA, Perdu M, Sharland GK, et al. Increased nuchal translucency at 10–14 weeks of gestation as a marker for major cardiac defects. Ultrasound Obstet Gynecol 1997;10:242–6.
12. Makrydimas G, Sotiriadis A, Ioannidis JP. Screening performance of first-trimester nuchal translucency for major cardiac defects: a meta-analysis. Am J Obstet Gynecol 2003;189:1330–5.
13. Nicolaides KH. Nuchal translucency and other first-trimester sonographic markers of chromosomal abnormalities. Am J Obstet Gynecol 2004;191:45–67.
14. Zosmer N, Souter VL, Chan CS, et al. Early diagnosis of major cardiac defects in chromosomally normal fetuses with increased nuchal translucency. Br J Obstet Gynaecol 1999;106:829–33.
15. Chang AC, Huhta JC, Yoon GY, et al. Diagnosis, transport, and outcome in fetuses with left ventricular outflow tract obstruction. J Thorac Cardiovasc Surg 1991;102:841–8.
16. Verheijen PM, Lisowski LA, Stoutenbeek P, et al. Prenatal diagnosis of congenital heart disease affects preoperative acidosis in the newborn patient. J Thorac Cardiovasc Surg 2001;121:798–803.
17. Bonnet D, Coltri A, Butera G, et al. Detection of transposition of the great arteries in fetuses reduces neonatal morbidity and mortality. Circulation 1999;99:916–8.
18. Simpson LL. Fetal supraventricular tachycardias: diagnosis and management. Semin Perinatol 2000;24:360–72.
19. Jaeggi ET, Hamilton RM, Silverman ED, et al. Outcome of children with fetal, neonatal or childhood diagnosis of isolated congenital atrioventricular block. A single institution's experience of 30 years. J Am Coll Cardiol 2002;39:130–7.
20. Groves AM, Allan LD, Rosenthal E. Therapeutic trial of sympathomimetics in three cases of complete heart block in the fetus. Circulation 1995;92:3394–6.
21. Taketazu M, Barrea C, Smallhorn JF, et al. Intrauterine pulmonary venous flow and restrictive foramen ovale in fetal hypoplastic left heart syndrome. J Am Coll Cardiol 2004;43:1902–7.
22. Hornberger LK, Sahn DJ, Kleinman CS, et al. Antenatal diagnosis of coarctation of the aorta: a multicenter experience. J Am Coll Cardiol 1994;23:417–23.
23. Hornberger LK, Sahn DJ, Kleinman CS, et al. Tricuspid valve disease with significant tricuspid insufficiency in the fetus: diagnosis and outcome. J Am Coll Cardiol 1991;17:167–73.
24. Yeager SB, Parness IA, Spevak PJ, et al. Prenatal echocardiographic diagnosis of pulmonary and systemic venous anomalies. Am Heart J 1994;128:397–405.
25. Kohl T, Sharland G, Allan LD, et al. World experience of percutaneous ultrasound-guided balloon valvuloplasty in human fetuses with severe aortic valve obstruction. Am J Cardiol 2000;85:1230–3.
26. Hornberger LK, Sanders SP, Rein AJ, et al. Left heart obstructive lesions and left ventricular growth in the midtrimester fetus. A longitudinal study. Circulation 1995;92:1531–8.

Index

Note: Page numbers of article titles are in **boldface** type.

Pediatr Clin N Am 56 (2009) 717–730
doi:10.1016/S0031-3955(09)00050-9
0031-3955/09/$ – see front matter © 2009 Elsevier Inc. All rights reserved.

pediatric.theclinics.com

Moving?

Make sure your subscription moves with you!

To notify us of your new address, find your **Clinics Account Number** (located on your mailing label above your name), and contact customer service at:

E-mail: elspcs@elsevier.com

800-654-2452 (subscribers in the U.S. & Canada)
314-453-7041 (subscribers outside of the U.S. & Canada)

Fax number: 314-523-5170

Elsevier Periodicals Customer Service
11830 Westline Industrial Drive
St. Louis, MO 63146

*To ensure uninterrupted delivery of your subscription, please notify us at least 4 weeks in advance of move.